The Anatomy & Physiology

SECOND EDITION

Survival Manual

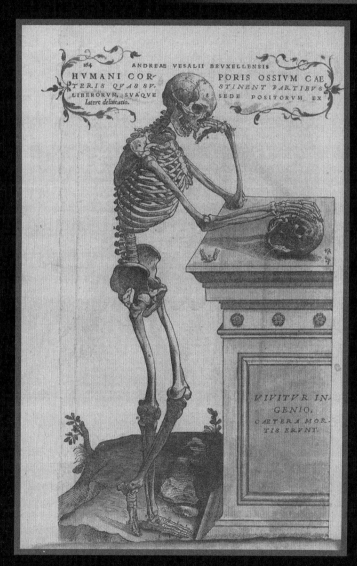

Michael Robert WEINTRAUB

Kendall Hunt
publishing company

Dedication

For all my students,
teachers
and most of all
my wife Jenny
whose love, patience and confidence made this project a reality.

Cover images and Unit opener images from Vesalius, Andreas. *De corporis humani fabrica libri septem.* (Basel: Johannes Oporinus, 1543).

Kendall Hunt
publishing company

www.kendallhunt.com
Send all inquiries to:
4050 Westmark Drive
Dubuque, IA 52004-1840

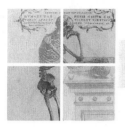

Contents

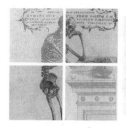

Surviving Anatomy and Physiology

Greetings Future Health Care Professionals!

Okay, let's just skip the warm and fuzzy intro and go for the tough love: these are without a doubt going to be the two hardest prerequisite courses in your pre-professional career, period. They will not only form the foundation of your knowledge of the workings of the human body, but serve as the proving ground for paraprofessional programs such as Nursing, Radiology and Respiratory Technology, Occupational Therapy, Paramedic, and Physician Assistant. As a pre-professional college student in the '70s (MD, DC, DO, DPM, DDS), it was Organic Chemistry, but for today's aspiring RN, RT, PA, and OT, it's A&P 1 and 2. And it's not gettin' any easier out there. Over the past two decades of teaching I've watched Nursing and Radiology programs "up the ante" from a minimum grade of C to as high as B. Even Respiratory Tech and LPN programs have dropped the one semester basic A&P course and now require a C in the "full metal jacket" version that this book addresses.

Although many "survivors" who are out there in the field working at their chosen profession will tell you how much "stuff" that we instructors tried to cram between their auricles is never used, these two semesters are more about developing personal work and study habits that prepare you for the learning experience that's ahead in clinical training. Remember, you're going to be caring for sick people; they'll be anxious, frightened, vulnerable, fragile—*and depending on you to help them.* More so, a recent Gallop Poll has listed the Registered Nurse as the most trusted professional in the country. (College professors only ranked five, which was still way above lawyers and used car dealers).

So how do we get there from here? There's surviving, and then there's THRIVING. The adage *"Failing to plan is planning to fail"* can never be made more true than with a course like this. So let's make a plan for success:

1. **Have a comfortable course load for the semester.**

    Your classroom hours only make up 20% of the time you'll need on a weekly basis to study and learn your course material. I recommend at least 9–10 hours of home study time for lecture and 3–4 hours for lab—over and above the 6 hours you'll be spending in the class/lab. And that doesn't include "over-time" in preparing for major unit exams and lab practicals. So to the fulltime student, do not treat this semester as an all-you-eat buffet and cram as many classes in under the flat rate credits-per-semester umbrella to get the most of your tuition dollar. Likewise to the part-time student, forget your personal deadlines and treat this like the NYC marathon. Anyone who finishes IS a winner regardless of how long it takes to get there *so pace yourself with the number of classes you take per semester.*

2. **Attend all your class meetings.**

    Many schools have mandatory attendance requirements; others allow students to come and go as they please. But in any case, I have never met an A student who only shows up for the exams. Without question, A&P is like life: you get back what you put into it. And the more you're immersed in the process, the better you'll absorb the coursework. *Be there, aloha.*

3. **Be an active classroom participant.**

That starts with paying attention, which is something you can't do if you're half asleep wearing dark sunglasses, using ear buds or Bluetooth, texting your friends, or whatever else you're doing on your cell phone. (Oh, how I hate watching students texting during class.). You know that if you did any of that nonsense at your job, you won't have that job very much longer. And *this* is part of your future job—*Learning*.

Learning begins with taking notes. Sure, there's the class textbook—and of course this book!—but taking notes integrates both the left and right sides of the brain, and the more forms of stimuli that you use, the better your memory becomes. Writing while listening and watching is the trifecta in this race. So write and draw whatever your instructor puts on the board, whether they do it the good old-fashioned way by hand (my preference) or on the screen. And if you can't keep up with your instructor's pace, then record the lectures. This is where iPods and smartphones come in handy as a learning tool besides listening to music or playing Angry Birds.

And, most important: Not sure of what you just heard? Got questions? Then ask them!

And don't ask your friend sitting next to you either—they're probably as clueless as you. It's the person at the front of the classroom who's being paid to be there for just that reason. Here's another old adage: "He who is afraid to ask is ashamed to learn." I've always thought that was a bit accusatory, so, how 'bout this one instead: "You're paying for this!" Professors may "profess" but we're here to teach. And if you're still not getting the answer then get to him/her at the end of class--don't go home without it.

4. And if you walk out of lecture and still feel completely lost, don't panic. Inscribed over the Temples to Aesculapius, the God of Healing is: "*Know Thyself.*" This means as soon as you know you're having trouble with the course then go for tutoring. NOW! All colleges offer free science tutorials. In many cases the tutors are former A&P students who have excelled at the class and just want to help others find their way through this jungle of Greek and Latin terms. And the sooner you admit you need some hand-holding, the sooner you'll be able to take off the training wheels and work successfully on your own. Remember what I said about "being afraid to ask"? There's certainly no reason to be embarrassed by going for tutoring; on the contrary, it's commendable.

5. **The Three "R's".**

That's "review, review, review."

Once lecture is over the real work begins. First, rewrite your notes, legibly, while listening to the recorded lecture to fill in any missing gaps. Write as if you were preparing a report. Then, review the assigned pages in the lecture text; "hearing" the material in another "voice" can give you a better understanding of the material.

And then:

6. **Use this book!**

I created the "Survival Manual" as a learning tool to assist my students in their after class learning experience. It is designed as a "fill-in-the-blank" exam that self-tests you to see where your strengths and weaknesses are. Use a pencil so that you can erase and re-test yourself, over and over and over. Yes, it's easy enough to get the answers from the key at the end of the unit, but they're there only for you to check to see how well you're really doing. In fact, it's better to refer to your notes for the answers because if you find that the information is missing then now you know you need to record the lectures. Keep in mind that most instructors want you to know what we've covered in class. We embellish the topic with our own input (especially healthcare professionals like myself) rather than simply reciting the textbook for you. In fact, that's why we're here: to bring the topic alive!

Once you've filled in the correct answers you will have a "review book" on the subject to study from. One aspect you'll note is that often enough the answers to one question are found in the wording of the question following it, thus making for repetition of facts during review. This assists in memory building.

Another way to use this book is to fill in the answers and highlight text as you follow along during lecture. Many students have found that it allows them to keep up with their instructors while they add notes in between the lines and in the margins. And when it comes to pre-exam reviews, the workbook acts as a checklist for topics of concentration.

Just remember, this is a tool, and we need to use tools correctly to get the most from them. And of course, the more you put into this class, the more you will get out of it.

Go For It!

Yours in Success,

Dr. Michael R. Weintraub

P.S.:   Got questions?
Contact Dr. W: drmrweintraub@gmail.com

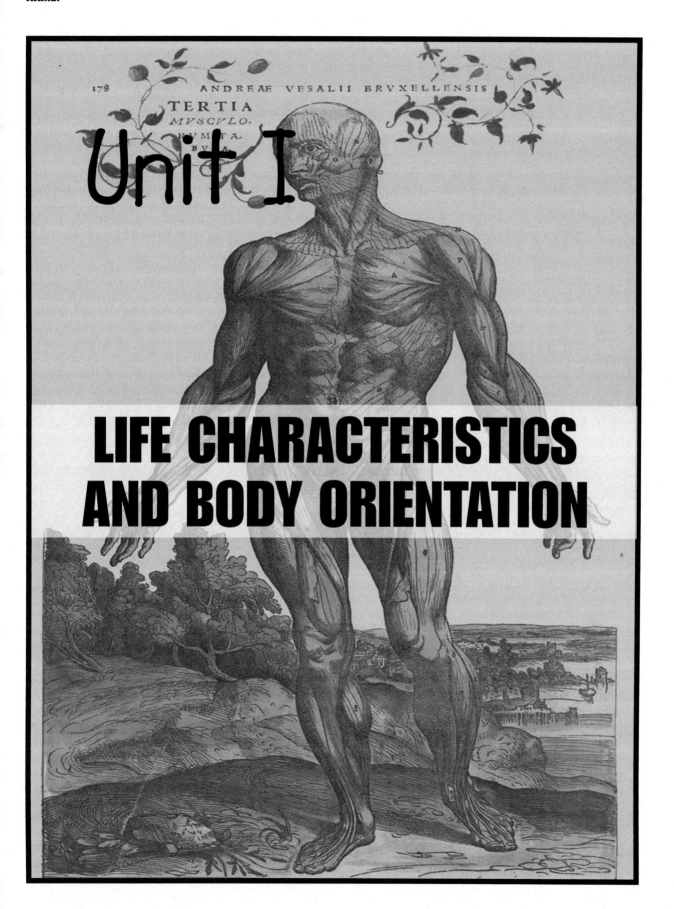

Unit I

LIFE CHARACTERISTICS
AND BODY ORIENTATION

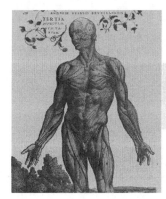

Part 1: Life Characteristics

1. Define Biology: _____
    _____ .

2. If biology is the study of life or living things, then "anatomy" is the study of _____
    _____ .

3. "Physiology" is the study of how living things _____ .

4. Define Irritability: _____
    _____ .

5. Define Adaptation: _____
    _____ .

6. Define Metabolism: _____
    _____ .

7. Metabolism includes the chemical processes of _____, the breakdown of large
    compounds, and _____, the release of energy from glucose.

8. Define Growth and Repair: _____
    _____ .

9. Growth and Repair involves the chemical process of _____ and cellular replication
    or _____ .

10. Define Reproduction: _____
    _____ .

    Reproduction in bacteria is identical to mitosis whereas reproduction in humans involves the
    cellular process of _____, which produces sperm and ova, collectively known as
    _____ .

11. Define Homeostasis: _____
    _____ .

12. Maintaining the internal environment within acceptable limitations implies that homeostasis is not a static but _____ _____.

13. In order to maintain a dynamic equilibrium, homeostatic mechanisms involve three components: a _____, _____ _____, and an _____.

14. Receptors detect internal changes and signal the control center; this is _____.

15. The control center responds by stimulating the effector; this is _____.

16. Effectors are _____, _____ or _____ _____.

17. When an effector does the opposite or counters the stimulus, it is called a _____ _____ System.

18. When an effector enhances the stimulus, it is called a _____ _____ System.

19. How is a cell defined? _____

20. If the cell is the basic unit of structure and function, what is a tissue? _____ _____

21. What is an organ? _____

22. What is an organ system? _____

Which organ system:

23. Transports nutrients and respiratory gases to the tissues? _____

24. Rids the body of nitrogen-based metabolic wastes by filtering the blood? _____

25. Regulates homeostasis by use of hormones? _____

26. Houses immune cells and collects interstial fluid? _____

27. Exchanges gases between the external environment and blood? _____

28. Performs catabolism? _____

29. Regulates and coordinates all other organ systems? _____

30. Creates a protective boundary between the internal and external environments? _____

31. Which two systems combine to perform movement and locomotion? _____ and _____

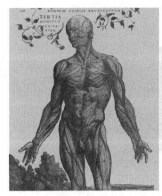

Part 2: Body Planes and Sections

32. What is the anatomical neutral position for the human body? _____
_____, _____ _____, and palms _____
_____.

33. Which plane divides the body into front and back halves? _____

34. What term also means frontal? _____

35. Which plane divides the body into left and right halves? _____.

36. Which term implies a sagittal section to the right or left of the midline? _____

37. Which plane divides the body into top and bottom halves? _____

38. A section cut at an angle is called an _____ section.

39. Transverse sections are also referred to as _____ and as a _____
_____.

40. A coronal section to the front of the body midline is described as being _____.

41. What other term implies anterior for the human body? _____

42. A coronal section towards the back of the body midline is described as _____.

43. What other term implies posterior? _____

44. One would describe the location of the sternum as _____ / _____ to the
heart, and the spine as _____ / _____ to the heart.

45. A parasagittal section that moves away from the body midline to the right or left is also described as
_____.

46. A transverse section that is towards the head is described as being _____.

47. What other term implies "head ward"? _____

48. If superior and cephalad describe the location of head relative to the waist, what terms would be
appropriate to describe the location of the feet relative to the waist? _____ and
_____.

49. What term would be used to describe a structure that is on the opposite side of the body? _____

50. If contralateral is the opposite side, what term implies "on the same side"? _____

51. The arms and legs are properly called the _____ and _____ _____, respectively.

52. What term implies that a structure of the upper or lower extremity is closer to the body (approximates)? _____ What term implies it is further away (at a distance)? _____

53. One would describe the location of the elbow as being _____ to the shoulder, but _____ to the wrist.

54. If a structure is closer to the surface than another, it is described as being _____.

55. One would describe the skin as being superficial to the muscles, but the muscles are _____ to the skin.

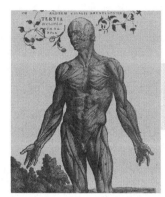

Part 3: **Surface Anatomy**

56. Which term is used to describe the head? _____

Which term is used to describe the following cephalic areas?

57. forehead: _____

58. nose: _____

59. eyes: _____

60. ears: _____

61. mouth: _____

62. cheeks: _____

63. chin: _____

64. base of the skull: _____

65. What term is used to indicate the neck? _____

66. What is the proper name for the breast-bone? _____ And for the collar-bone?
_____

67. Which muscle originates on the sternum and clavicle, and inserts on the mastoid process behind the ear?
_____ (_____)

68. Which muscle creates the outline of the shoulder? _____

69. What are the three borders of the "Posterior triangle"? _____, _____, and
_____

70. The posterior region of the shoulder is named for the "shoulder blade"; this is properly called the
_____ region.

71. The lateral aspect of the shoulder is named for the _____ process of the scapula. What is
the proper name of the armpit? _____

72. Which muscle creates the anterior border of the axilla? _____ _____
    Which muscle creates the posterior border? _____ _____

73. The trunk is subdivided into upper and lower areas commonly called the _____ and
    _____, respectively.

74. The chest is properly called the _____; the abdomen can be subdivided into three areas:
    the upper _____, _____, and lower _____.

75. The area of the thorax overlying the pectoralis muscle is referred to as the _____ region,
    but the area of the nipple is properly called the _____ area.

76. The most inferior point of the pelvic region is called the _____.

77. Below the pubis is the _____ area.

78. The posterior surface of the thorax and abdomen is called the _____.

79. The central region of the dorsum is named for the underlying spinal column, the _____
    area.

80. The regions flanking the lower vertebral area are the _____ areas; the inferior-most point
    of the vertebral area is the _____ area.

81. The inferior-most area of the body, posterior to the genital area and anterior to the anus, is called the
    _____ area.

82. The term for the upper arm is _____ and for the forearm is _____.

83. The brachial and antebrachial areas are separated by the anterior surface of the elbow; this is called the
    _____ area.

84. The posterior surface of the antecubital/elbow is called the _____ area.

85. The hand is subdivided into three areas: _____, _____, and
    _____.

86. The wrist is named for the bones which comprise it and is called the _____ area. The
    hand is called the _____ area and the fingers _____.

87. The manual area is noted for its anterior or _____ surface and its _____
    or posterior surface.

88. Unlike the other four digits, the thumb is properly called the _____.

89. The lateral surface of the hip joint is called the _____ area.

90. The buttock is properly called the _____ area.

91. The groin is referred to as the _____ area.

92. The thigh is called the _____ area.

93. The anterior surface of the knee is known as the _____, and its posterior surface as the _____ area.

94. The leg is noted for three surfaces; the anterior shin or _____, the lateral _____ or _____, and the posterior calf or _____.

95. Like the hand, the foot is also divided into three areas: the ankle or _____, _____, and toes or _____.

96. The pedal area is noted for its superior surface, the _____, and inferior or _____ surface.

97. The name for the big toe is _____. The heel is named for the largest of the tarsal bones of the ankle, and called the _____ area.

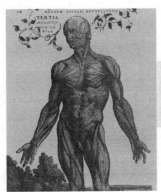

Part 4: Body Cavities

98. The body is divided into two major cavities, the _____ and _____.

99. The Dorsal Cavity consists of the bony vaults that protect the Central Nervous System and is subdivided into _____ and _____ Cavities.

100. The Ventral Body Cavity is subdivided by what structure? _____

101. Superior to the diaphragm is the _____ Cavity, and inferior to it is the _____ Cavity.

102. The Thoracic Cavity is further subdivided into the Left and Right _____ Cavities, the _____ and the _____ Cavity.

103. The Pleural Cavities are created by two serous membranes surrounding each lung; the _____ pleura overlies the lung and the _____ pleura lines the thoracic wall. The cavity is _____ filled.

104. Like the Pleural Cavity, the Pericardial Cavity is fluid-filled with a visceral and parietal layer. The Pericardial Cavity lies within the Mediastinum. What other two structures are located within the Mediastinum? _____ and _____

105. The Abdominopelvic Cavity is further subdivided into the upper _____ and lower _____ Cavities.

106. The lower Pelvic Cavity is within the pelvic bones, but both contain a fluid-filled serous membrane-lined cavity, the _____ Cavity.

107. The Peritoneal Cavity is noted for its _____ _____ lining the abdominal wall, and its _____ _____ covering the surface of the organs.

108. The Visceral Peritoneum is also known as a _____.

109. The Abdominopelvic Cavity can be subdivided into nine regions; the top row from right to left is the Right _____, _____, and Left _____.

110. What organs are noted in the Right Hypochondriac? _____ and _____
_____ Epigastric? _____ and _____
Left Hypochondriac? _____ and _____ Regions.

111. The middle row from right to left includes the Right _____, _____, and
Left _____ Regions.

112. The Right Lumbar is noted for the _____ _____, the Umbilical for
the _____ _____, and the Left Lumbar for the _____
_____.

113. The lower row from right to left includes the Right _____ or _____, the
_____, and the Left _____ or _____ Regions.

114. The Right Iliac/Inguinal is noted for the _____ and _____ in females,
the Hypogastric for the _____, _____ (♀) and _____
(♂), and the Left Iliac/Inguinal for the _____ _____.

115. When dividing into quadrants, at what point is the cavity cut transversely and sagittally?
_____

Unit I: Life Characteristics and Body Orientation

Part 1: Characteristics of Life

1. the study of life and living things
2. the structure of living things
3. function
4. detect a change in the environment
5. respond to a change
6. obtain nutrition and convert it to energy to do work
7. catabolism and oxidation
8. development from a primitive zygote to a mature adult form, and the replacement of cells and tissues within certain limitations
9. anabolism, mitosis
10. production of progeny/offspring. meiosis, gametes
11. maintain one's internal environment within acceptable limitations
12. dynamic equilibrium
13. receptor, control center and effector
14. irritability
15. adaptation
16. glands, muscles or motor nerves
17. negative feedback
18. positive feedback
19. the basic unit of structure and function
20. a group of cells of similar size, ,shape, and function
21. any structure composed of two or more tissues that perform a function
22. a group of organs that perform a general life function
23. cardiovascular
24. urinary
25. endocrine
26. lymphatic
27. respiratory
28. digestive
29. nervous
30. integumentary
31. muscular and skeletal

Part 2: Body Planes and Sections

32. standing upright, facing forward, and palms facing forward
33. frontal
34. coronal
35. midsagittal
36. parasagittal
37. transverse
38. horizontal, cross section
39. oblique
40. anterior
41. ventral
42. posterior
43. dorsal
44. anterior/ventral, posterior/dorsal
45. lateral
46. superior
47. cephalad
48. inferior and caudal
49. contralateral
50. ipsilateral
51. upper and lower extremities
52. proximal; distal
53. distal, proximal
54. superficial
55. deep

Part 3: Surface Anatomy

56. cephalic
57. frontal
58. nasal
59. ocular
60. otic
61. oral
62. buccal
63. mental
64. occipital
65. cervical
66. sternum, clavicle
67. sternocleidomastoideus (SCM)
68. trapezius
69. SCM, trapezius and clavicle
70. scapular
71. acromium; axilla
72. pectoralis major; latissimus dorsi
73. chest and abdomen

74. thorax; abdominal, umbilical and pelvic
75. pectoral, mammary
76. pubis
77. genital
78. dorsum
79. vertebral
80. lumbar; sacral
81. perineal
82. brachial, antebrachial
83. antecubital
84. olecranal
85. wrist, hand, and fingers
86. carpal, manual and digital
87. palmar, dorsum
88. pollux
89. coxal
90. gluteal
91. inguinal
92. femoral
93. patellar, popliteal
94. crural, fibular or peroneal, sural
95. tarsal, pedal and digital
96. dorsum, plantar
97. hallux, calcaneal

Part 4: Body Cavities

98. Dorsal and Ventral
99. Cranial and Vertebral
100. The diaphragm
101. Thoracic, Abdominopelvic
102. Pleural, Mediastinum, Pericardial
103. visceral, parietal. fluid filled
104. trachea and esophagus
105. Abdominal, Pelvic
106. Peritoneal
107. parietal peritoneum, visceral peritoneum
108. serosa
109. hypochondriac, epigastric, hypochondriac
110. liver and gallbladder; stomach and pancreas, stomach and spleen
111. lumbar, umbilical, lumbar
112. ascending colon, small intestine, descending colon
113. iliac/inguinal, hypogastric, iliac inguinal
114. appendix and ovaries; bladder, uterus, and prostate; sigmoid colon
115. umbilical

Unit I: **Take a Test!**

1. "Biology" is defined as the study of:
   - a) things natural
   - b) life and living things
   - c) organic polymers
   - d) all of these

2. An organism's response to a change in its external environment is called:
   - a) adaptation
   - b) metabolism
   - c) growth and repair
   - d) irritability
   - e) homeostasis

3. Which process/processes would be included in metabolism:
   - a) oxidation
   - b) catabolism
   - c) anabolism
   - d) a and b
   - e) a, b and c

4. Anabolism is associated with which characteristic:
   - a) irritability
   - b) adaptation
   - c) metabolism
   - d) homeostasis
   - e) growth and repair

5. An organism's ability to maintain its internal environment:
   - a) homeostasis
   - b) growth and repair
   - c) metabolism
   - d) irritability
   - e) adaptation

6. Which would be considered a negative feedback system:
   - a) platelets secret hormones to attract more platelets making a blood clot
   - b) when calcium is high the thyroid secretes calcitonin to store it as bone
   - c) during childbirth uterine contractions push the child's head into the cervix, stretching it causing another contraction
   - d) a and b
   - e) a, b and c

7. Which of the following would be considered an effector in a feedback system:
   - a) muscle
   - b) gland
   - c) motor nerve
   - d) a and b
   - e) a, b and c

8. Which is the correct order of organization from *smallest to largest*:
   - a) organ, tissue, cell, organelle, organic compound, atom
   - b) atom, organic compound, organelle, cell, tissue, organ
   - c) organic compound, organelle, cell, atom, tissue, organ
   - d) atom, organelle, organic compound, tissue, cell, organ
   - e) cell, organelle, atom, organic compound, organ, tissue

9. Which type of section divides the body into left and right halves:
   a) coronal
   b) midsagittal
   c) transverse
   d) oblique

10. A section cutting through the body on an angle is referred to as being:
    a) coronal
    b) midsagittal
    c) transverse
    d) oblique

11. Which term means "superior":
    a) anterior
    b) caudal
    c) cephalad
    d) ventral
    e) posterior

12. Which term is same as "dorsal":
    a) anterior
    b) caudal
    c) cephalad
    d) ventral
    e) posterior

13. Which term is same as "caudal":
    a) anterior
    b) inferior
    c) cephalad
    d) ventral
    e) posterior

14. Which term means implies that one structure is closer to the body than another:
    a) ipsilateral
    b) contralateral
    c) proximal
    d) distal
    e) deep

15. Which term means implies that one structure is on the opposite side of the body:
    a) ipsilateral
    b) contralateral
    c) proximal
    d) distal
    e) deep

16. Which term is used for the neck:
    a) cervical
    b) thorax
    c) axilla
    d) inguinal
    e) perineal

17. The chin :
    a) frontal
    b) mental
    c) orbit
    d) otic
    e) buccal

18. The eye :
    a) frontal
    b) mental
    c) orbit
    d) otic
    e) buccal

19. Which term is used for the armpit:
    a) cervical
    b) thorax
    c) axilla
    d) inguinal
    e) perineal

20. Which term is used for the groin:
    a) cervical
    b) thorax
    c) axilla
    d) inguinal
    e) perineal

21. Which term is used for the chest:
    a) cervical
    b) thorax
    c) axilla
    d) inguinal
    e) perineal

22. Which term is used for the pelvic floor:
    a) cervical
    b) thorax
    c) axilla
    d) inguinal
    e) perineal

23. Which term is used for the arm:
    a) brachial
    b) carpal
    c) tarsal
    d) popliteal
    e) coxal

24. Which term is used for the back of the knee:
    a) brachial
    b) carpal
    c) tarsal
    d) popliteal
    e) coxal

25. Which term is used for the wrist:
    a) brachial
    b) carpal
    c) tarsal
    d) popliteal
    e) coxal

26. Which term is used for the hip:
    a) brachial
    b) carpal
    c) tarsal
    d) popliteal
    e) coxal

27. Which term is used for the ankle:
    a) brachial
    b) carpal
    c) tarsal
    d) popliteal
    e) coxal

28. The Liver is located in the:
    a) Right Upper Quadrant
    b) Left Upper Quadrant
    c) Right Lower Quadrant
    d) Left Lower Quadrant

29. The Appendix is located in the:
    a) Right Upper Quadrant
    b) Left Upper Quadrant
    c) Right Lower Quadrant
    d) Left Lower Quadrant

30. The Spleen is located in the:
    a) Right Upper Quadrant
    b) Left Upper Quadrant
    c) Right Lower Quadrant
    d) Left Lower Quadrant

31. Which of the following would be found in the Mediastinum:
    a) Liver
    b) Esophagus
    c) Stomach
    d) Urinary Bladder
    e) Kidney

32. The Lungs are located in the:
    a) Mediastinum
    b) Dorsal Body Cavity
    c) Pleural Cavity
    d) Abdominal Cavity
    e) Peritoneal Cavity

33. Which of the following would be found in the Pelvic Cavity:
   a) Liver
   b) Urinary Bladder
   c) Lungs
   d) Esophagus
   e) Heart

34. Which of the following would be found in the Epigastric Region:
   a) Liver
   b) Esophagus
   c) Stomach
   d) Urinary Bladder
   e) Kidney

35. Which of the following would be found in the Hypogastric Region:
   a) Liver
   b) Esophagus
   c) Stomach
   d) Urinary Bladder
   e) Kidney

36. Which lines the wall of the Thoracic Cavity:
   a) Visceral Peritoneum
   b) Parietal Peritoneum
   c) Visceral Pleura
   d) Parietal Pleura

37. Which covers the external surface of organs within the abdominal cavity:
   a) Visceral Peritoneum
   b) Parietal Peritoneum
   c) Visceral Pleura
   d) Parietal Pleura

38. Which form the dorsal body cavity:
   a) cranial cavity
   b) vertebral
   c) thoracic
   d) a and b
   e) a, b and c

39. Which is not part of the ventral body cavity:
   a) thoracic cavity
   b) mediastinum
   c) pericardial cavity
   d) cranial cavity
   e) pelvic cavity

40. Which is found within the thoracic cavity:
   a) pleural cavity
   b) mediastinum
   c) pericardial cavity
   d) a and b
   e) a, b and c

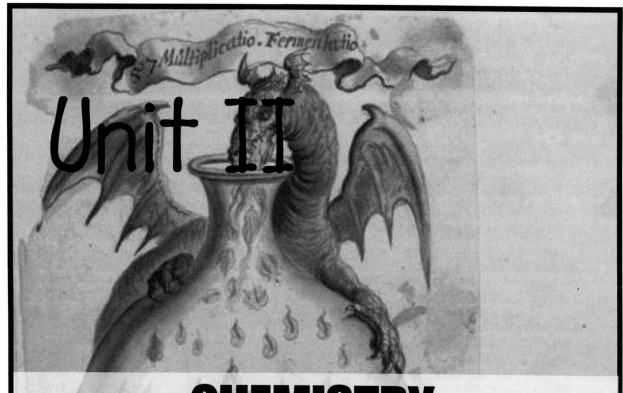

Unit II

CHEMISTRY: THE FOUNDATION OF LIFE

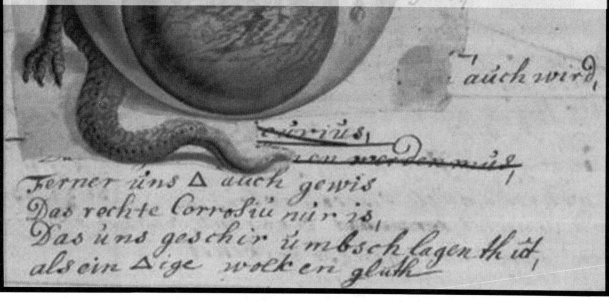

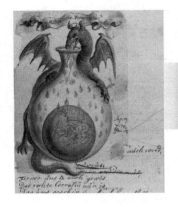

Part I: The Chemistry of Life

1. Define Element: _____
    _____. An _____
    is the smallest portion of an element that still maintains its electrochemical identity.

2. An atom is composed of three particles:
    a) _____ bearing a net _____ charge,
    b) _____ bearing a net _____ charge, and
    c) _____ bearing a net _____ charge.

3. What determines an element's atomic number: _____

4. An element's number of protons is equal to/greater than/lesser than its electrons; therefore, all elements
    therefore bear a net _____ charge.

5. Positively charged protons and neutral neutrons are located within the _____, whereas
    negatively charged electrons _____.

6. The innermost energy level (shell) is filled and becomes stable when it possesses _____ electrons; all
    other shells can become full/stabilize with _____ electrons.

7. What gives an element its electrochemical identity? _____ _____
    _____

8. The outermost energy level of an atom is called the _____ shell; it is the number of free electrons in
    this level that give an element its electrochemical properties.

9. What determines an element's atomic mass: _____.
    What are isotopes: _____.

10. Elements with filled valence shells are classified as _____ and will not combine or interact with other
    atoms whereas those with unfilled shells are considered_____ and will tend to form _____
    with other elements.

11. Combinations of two or more elements in a fixed ratio are called _____.

12. The smallest portion of a compound is called a _____. Compounds are formed by three types of chemical bonds: _____, _____, and _____.

13. In ionic bonds, elements _____ or _____ valence electrons to stabilize their outer shells whereas in covalent bonds, they _____ them.

14. Covalent bonds are extremely _____and will break ionic bonds and are called solvents. What is the most abundant covalent substance? _____. What other group of compounds are covalently bonded: _____.

15. Elements with 1-3 valence electrons will accept/donate their electrons giving them a net _____ charge; elements with 5-7 valence electrons will accept/donate their electrons giving them a net _____charge. Atoms that donate or accept electrons and bear a net charge are called _____.

16. Positively charged ions that have donated 1-3 electrons are called _____; negatively charged elements that have accepted 5-7 electrons are called _____.

17. Cations and anions that are electrically active in living cells are called _____.

18. When a cation is combined with anion it forms a _____.

19. Salts are ionic compounds that will _____ when added to water and form an _____and a _____.

20. An acid releases _____ ions (____) making them _____ donors; bases release _____ ions (_____) and are _____ acceptors.

21. The concentration of H^+/acidity and OH^-/alkalinity is measured on the _____ scale, which ranges from _____-_____, where _____ is most acidic, _____ is most alkaline, and _____ is neutral.

22. When acids (H^+) and bases (OH^-) combine they form a _____ and _____.

23. Water has a pH of _____ and is _____-bonded. Substances that resist changes in pH are known as _____.

24. What do hydrogen bonds do: _____
Is the hydrogen electron exchanged or donated:_____

25. In which compounds are hydrogen bonds found holding molecules together: _____, _____ and _____.

26. The element carbon has _____ valence electrons and forms _____ bonds. In addition to single bonds, carbon can also form: _____, _____, and even _____ between two carbon atoms.

27. What two substances are composed of carbon atoms with quadruple bonds: _____ and _____.

28. What are isomers: _____.

29. When carbon combines with hydrogen the compound is called a _____ .

30. Hydrocarbons are classified as _____ compounds. Compounds without hydrocarbons are called _____.

31. What are the four groups of organic hydrocarbon-based compounds: _____, _____, _____, and _____ _____.

32. These large compounds are also collectively referred to as organic _____.

33. The process by which organic polymers are synthesized is called _____; the process by which compounds disassociate and break down is called _____.

34. When anabolism occurs by the removal of H^+ and OH^- to form water and a new compound, it is referred to as _____ _____; when catabolism occurs by the addition of water to a compound, it is referred to as _____.

35. Carbohydrates have the general chemical formula _____, lipids _____, proteins _____, and nucleic acids _____.

36. Large polymers are composed of smaller subunits called _____. Polymers with identical formulas but different structural distribution are called _____.

37. Carbohydrates, have the formula _____, are subdivided into three categories: _____, _____, and _____.

38. Monosaccharides such as glucose and fructose are also referred to as _____ _____, the building blocks of more complex carbohydrates.

39. Glucose and Fructose are isomers with the same formula _____; how do they differ in structure: ___ _____.

40. Because glucose and fructose have six carbons they are classified as _____. Five-carbon sugars are called _____ and include _____ in DNA and _____ in RNA.

41. Disaccharides are composed of _____ simple sugars and include _____ (cane sugar) and _____ (milk sugar).

42. Sucrose is formed by dehydration synthesis from _____ and _____; an _____ is required in order to break their covalent bond

43. The enzyme _____ is needed to catabolize sucrose; what enzyme is needed for lactose: _____. The inability to produce these enzymes is known as an _____.

44. Polysaccharides include_____, _____, and _____. Monomers are assembled into polysaccharides by _____ _____ which is also known as _____.

45. The covalent bonds linking monosaccharides by dehydration synthesis into di- and polysaccharides are called _____ bonds.

46. Starch and glycogen are polymers of _____. Cellulose, an isomer of _____, is known for forming the _____ _____ of plants and is considered _____ _____ _____.

47. Where is glycogen stored in the human body: the _____ and _____ _____.

48. What term inplies that an atom releases an electron: _____; what term inplies that it accepts an electron: _____.

49. The process by which free energy is released by the oxidation of glucose is called _____ _____.

50. What compound is produced by aerobic respiration: _____

51. Substances that hydrolyze in water are described as being _____.

52. Lipids have the formula _____and are composed of two principal monomers: a backbone molecule called _____ and _____ _____. Lipids do not interact or disassociate in water and are described as being _____.

53. What two functional groups are associated with fatty acids: _____ ($-CH_3$) and _____ ($-COOH$).

54. Which group defines an acid, methyl or carboxyl: _____. What type of group is $-OH$: _____.

55. When glycerol is bound to two fatty acids it forms a _____;

56. Diglycerides form a group of hormones called _____.
When glycerol is bound to three fatty acids it forms a _____.

57. The bonds linking glycerol and fatty acids into triglycerides are called _____ bonds. When glycerol is bound to two fatty acids on one side and a phosphate group on the opposing side it forms a _____. Lipids also include the four-ring compound _____.

58. Triglycerides are also known as _____ _____ _____. Phospholipids form the principal structural element of the _____ _____ and are described as being _____ regarding their interaction with water. Cholesterol is the precursor to the hormone groups called _____ and _____.

59. Triglycerides whose fatty acids possess only single carbon bonds form _____ fats; those that possess two or more double bonds are called _____ fats.

60. Saturated fats are _____ at room temperature, whereas polyunsaturated fats are _____. Where are saturated fats stored in the human body: _____ _____.

61. What term is used for a cooking oil that has been hydrogenated with animal fat/adipose: _____.

62. Proteins have the general formula _____ and are based upon monomers called _____ _____.

63. What two functional groups are associated with amino acids: _____ (−COOH) and _____ (−NH$_2$)

64. Amino acids are linked by _____ bonds, forming the protein's primary structure; a protein's secondary structure gives it a _____ appearance due to _____ bonds.

65. The tertiary structure of proteins is described as _____ and is created by hydrogen and _____ bonds, and _____ forces.

66. Globular proteins can be both structural and functional; what are examples of structural proteins within the cell membrane: _____ proteins and _____ proteins on the external surface.

67. Integral proteins form _____ _____ with pores, _____ receptor sites and _____ for absorption of nutrients. Peripheral proteins form _____ _____ which identify the cell for immunity.

68. Globular proteins also form _____ on the inner surface of the cell membrane and _____ within the cell.

69. Microfilaments are a permanent part of the cell's _____ whereas microtubules are assembled on demand; what do microtubules do: _____.

70. The microfilaments of muscle tissue are _____ and _____; they also known as _____ proteins.

71. Functional proteins include _____, _____ and _____.

72. Enzymes function as _____ _____.

73. How does a catalyst do: _____.

74. What are the two types of energy reactions: _____ and _____.

75. Endergonic Reactions _____ ___ energy whereas Exergonic reactions _____ energy.

76. Anabolism is which type of reaction: _____; Oxidation and Catabolism: _____. Enzymes function in energy releasing exergonic reactions by _____ _____ _____.

77. What is meant by "enzyme specificity": _____.

78. An enzyme's specificity to its substrate or reaction is determined by its _____ _____. Which is used up in an enzyme-substrate reaction?: _____.

79. An enzyme's active site is created by its _____ _____ creating a _____ 'n ____ relationship.

80. Factors affecting enzymes include high _____ and extreme changes in _____; these may result in breaking ____ bonds and alter an enzyme's configuration. This is known as _____.

81. Will lowering an enzyme's temperature break H^+ bonds and cause denaturing? _____. What will happen instead: _____.

82. How is hypothermia related to enzyme activity: _____
_____

83. Nucleic acids have the general formula _____ and are composed of monomers called _____.

84. A typical nucleotide consists of three components: _____ _____,
_____, and _____ _____.

85. The Pentose Deoxyribose is associated with _____ and Ribose with _____. The two Purines are _____ and _____; the three Pyrimidines are _____, _____ and _____.

86. In addition to the nucleotides of DNA and RNA others include _____ and _____.

87. When glucose is oxidized it releases free energy for ADP to bond with _____ to form ATP. When ATP hydrolyzes to power anabolism it always releases lost energy as _____. How does this relate to exercise? _____.

88. The dinucleotides include _____ and _____.

89. During aerobic respiration NAD and FAD combine with _____ released from glucose.

90. The free energy released by H+ electrons is used to couple ADP with P+; the process is referred to as _____ _____.

91. The two DNA purines are _____ and _____; the two DNA pyrimidine bases are _____ and _____.

92. Both DNA and RNA use the Purines Adenine and Guanine, but the two RNA Pyrimidines are _____ and _____.

93. DNA is described as a _____ _____ consisting of two _____ base strands. Nucleotides of an individual base strand (5' or 3') are joined by _____ bonds.

94. Phosphodiester bonds are strong, preventing changes in the DNA sequence. Any change in the DNA sequence is referred to as a _____.

95. The double helix is formed by the joining of complimentary base strands by _____ bonds.

96. The complimentary base pairs joined by hydrogen bonds are limited to: _____ - _____ and _____-_____.

97.   The uncoiled strands of DNA located in the nucleus are referred to as _____.

98.   During Mitosis, chromatin strands will coil into dark staining bodies called _____ which can be moved about by the microtubules of the _____ _____ .

99.   DNA is responsible for gene expression by coding for _____.

100.   DNA codes for enzymes by its base sequence; how many bases are required to code for an amino acid: _____.

101.   What two processes is RNA involved in: _____ _____ and _____ _____

102.   How does RNA assist in DNA replication? _____.

103.   How does RNA assist in Protein synthesis? _____.

104.   When RNA forms the template for replication and the transcript for protein synthesis its nucleotides link into a _____ strand.

105.   In forming a single strand RNA replaces _____ for Thymine during these two processes.

Unit II: The Chemistry of Life

1. Any substance that cannot be synthesized or broken down into smaller particles by a living cell; atom
2. protons, positive; neutrons, neutral; electrons, negative
3. Its number of protons/electrons
4. equal to; neutral
5. nucleus; orbit about the nucleus in energy shells
6. 2; 8
7. the number of free electrons in the outermost shell
8. valence
9. the total number of protons and neutrons in its nucleus
10. inert, unstable, bonds
11. compounds
12. Molecule, ionic, covalent, hydrogen
13. Donate of accept; share
14. Str, negatoveong, water, organic compounds
15. Donate, positive; accept, negative;
16. Cations; anions
17. Electrolytes
18. Salt
19. Disassociate; acid, base
20. hydrogen (H^+), proton; hydroxide (OH^-), proton
21. pH, 1-14, 1, 14, 7
22. salt, water
23. 7, covalently ; buffers
24. they hold complete molecules of other compounds together; No
25. water, proteins, DNA
26. 4, covalent; double, triple, quadruple
27. Graphite, diamonds
28. Compounds with identical chemical formulas but different structural configuration
29. Hydrocarbon
30. Organic; inorganic
31. Carbohydrates, Lipids, Proteins and Nucleic Acids
32. Polymers
33. Anabolism, catabolism
34. Dehydration synthesis; hydrolysis
35. $C_1H_2O_1$, CHO, CHONS, CHONP
36. Monomers; isomers
37. $C_1H_2O_1$, monosaccharides, disaccharides, polysaccharides
38. Simple sugars
39. $C_6H2_2O_6$; glucose is a six-carbon ring, fructose is a five-carbon ring with a side-chain
40. Hexoses; pentoses, Deoxyribose, Ribose
41. Two, sucrose and lactose
42. Glucose and fructose; enzyme
43. Sucrose; lactase; intolerance
44. Starch, glycogen cellulose; dehydration synthesis, anabolism
45. Glycosidic
46. Glucose; glucose, cell wall, non-digestible by humans, forming insoluble dietary fiber
47. Liver, muscle tissue
48. Oxidation; reduction
49. Aerobic respiration
50. ATP
51. Hydrophilic
52. CHO, glycerol, fatty acids; hydrophobic
53. Methyl, carboxyl
54. Carboxyl; hydroxyl
55. Diglyceride
56. Eicosanoids; triglyceride
57. Ester; phospholipid; cholesterol
58. Neutral fats; cell membrane, amphipathic' steroids, androgens
59. Saturated fats; polyunsaturated
60. Solids, liquid/oils; adipose tissue
61. Trans-fats
62. CHONS, amino acids
63. Carboxyl, amine
64. Peptide, coiled, hydrogen
65. Globular, sulfur, ionic
66. Integral, peripheral
67. Transport channels, ligand, cotransporters; antigen markers
68. Microfilaments, microtubules
69. Cytoskeleton; move organelles and chromosomes during mitosis
70. Actin, myosin; contractile

71. Neurotransmitters, hormones, enzymes
72. Organic catalysts
73. Mediate/regulate or speed up a reaction
74. Endergonic, exergonic
75. Use up, release; endergonic, exergonic
76. Reducing activation energy
77. Enzymes work on only one substrate or in one reaction
78. Active site; the substrate
79. Structural configuration, Lock 'n key
80. Temperatures, pH; H^+; denaturing
81. No; reaction speed will slow down and even halt
82. Lowered body temperature slows enzymes for oxidizing glucose, halting ATP production
83. CHONP; nucleotides
84. Pentose sugar, phosphorus, nitrogen base
85. DNA, RNA; adenine and guanine, thymine, cytosine and uracil
86. ADP and ATP
87. Phosphorus, heat; body temperature rises as ATP hydrolyzes to power muscle activity

88. NAD and FAD
89. H^+
90. Oxidative phosphorylation
91. Adenine and guanine; thymine and cytosine
92. Cytosine and uracil
93. Double helix, complimentary; phosphodiester
94. Mutation
95. H^+
96. Adenine-Thymine, Guanine-Cytosine
97. Chromatin
98. Chromosomes, spindle apparatus
99. Enzymes
100. 3
101. DNA replication and protein synthesis
102. It forms a template for the new daughter strand
103. It takes transcription for the polypeptide
104. Single
105. Uracil

Unit II: Take a Test!

1. An element's Atomic Number indicates:
   a) the number of protons   b) the number of electrons
   c) the number of neutrons   d) a and b   e) a, b and c

2. The electrochemical characteristics of an element are determined by:
   a) its total number of protons and electrons
   b) the number of protons and neutrons in its nucleus
   c) the number of electrons in its valence shell
   d) the number of electrons in the nucleus
   e) the number of neutrons

3. An element with the atomic number 6 has _____ electrons in its outermost shell:
   a) 2   b) 3   c) 4   d) 5   e) 7

4. The Atomic Mass of an element is determined by:
   a) its total number of protons and electrons
   b) the number of protons and neutrons in its nucleus
   c) the number of electrons in its valence shell
   d) the number of electrons in the nucleus
   e) the number of neutrons

5. Isoptopes are:
   a) two elements with the same number of protons and neutrons
   b) two elements with the same atomic number but different atomic weight
   c) two compounds with the same chemical formula
   d) compounds that release H^+
   e) inert

6. Which of the following implies that an atom will share electrons to complete its valence shell:
   a) covalent   b) hydrogen
   c) ionic   d) organic   e) inert

7. Electrons are not shared, donated or accepted in which type of bonding:
   a) covalent   b) hydrogen
   c) ionic   d) organic   e) inert

8. Cations are elements which:
   a) donate electrons   b) accept electrons
   c) donate protons   d) accept protons   e) donate neutrons

9. Which of the following is considered an Anion:
   a) Na^+
   b) Ca^{+2}
   c) Cl^-
   d) a and b
   e) a, b and c

10. Compounds which release OH^- when added to water are known as:
    a) acids
    b) isomers
    c) isotopes
    d) bases
    e) organic

11. A substance that resists changes in pH is termed:
    a) acid
    b) base
    c) buffer
    d) electrolyte
    e) salt

12. Which of the following would be considered the most acidic pH:
    a) 6.8
    b) 6.9
    c) 7.0
    d) 7.1
    e) 7.3

13. Which of the following formulas is classified as organic:
    a) H_2O
    b) $C_6H_{12}O_6$
    c) HCl
    d) CO_2
    e) all are organic

14. Glucose has a six-carbon ring, fructose has a five carbon ring with a side chain, nut they are both $C_6H_{12}O_6$: these compounds are considered:
    a) isomers
    b) isotopes
    c) isometrics
    d) isotonics
    e) inert

15. Substances that are attracted to water are called:
    a) hydrophobic
    b) hydrophilic
    c) amphipathic
    d) hydrostatic
    e) hydrolytic

16. Which of the following compounds would have a general formula of $C_1H_2O_1$:
    a) enzyme
    b) cholesterol
    c) DNA
    d) glycogen

17. Which of the following compounds would have a general formula of CHONS:
    a) enzyme
    b) cholesterol
    c) DNA
    d) glycogen

18. Which of the following are considered the monomers of compounds such as cholesterol:
    a) simple sugars
    b) glycerol and fatty acids
    c) amino acids
    d) nucleotides

19. Which of the following are considered the monomers of compounds such as DNA:
    a) simple sugars
    b) glycerol and fatty acids
    c) amino acids
    d) nucleotides

20. The process by which monomers are assembled into polymers is called:
    a) dehydration synthesis
    b) hydrolysis
    c) oxidation
    d) catabolism
    e) a and b

21. The process by which polymers are broken down into monomers is called:
   a) catabolism
   b) hydrolysis
   c) oxidation
   d) dehydration synthesis
   e) a and b

22. The process by which a compound releases an electron is called:
   a) anabolism
   b) oxidation
   c) reduction
   d) dehydration synthesis

23. Monosaccharides are joined to form polymers by which type of linkage:
   a) peptide
   b) ester
   c) glycosidic
   d) phosphodiester
   e) hydrogen

24. Which of the following is a disaccharide:
   a) glucose
   b) lactose
   a) cellulose
   d) starch

25. Starch is stored in human muscle tissue as:
   a) glycogen
   b) cellulose
   c) adipose
   d) glucose

26. Which of the following is a carboxyl group:
   a) $-COOH$
   b) $-CH_3$
   a) $-NH_2$
   d) $-OH$

27. Saturated fats:
   a) are stored as adipose tissue
   b) have single carbon bonds in their fatty acids
   c) are liquids at room temperature
   d) a and b
   e) a, b and c

28. Which of the following is only associated with proteins:
   a) amine group
   b) methyl group
   c) hydroxyl group
   d) carboxyl group

29. A protein's primary structure is accomplished by _____ linkage/bonds:
   a) ester
   b) peptide
   c) glycosidic
   d) phosphodiester
   e) hydrogen

30. Which describes a protein's tertiary structure:
   a) amino acid sequence
   b) coiled
   c) globular
   d) multi-stranded

31. Enzymes act as catalysts by:
   a) donating electrons
   b) accepting electrons
   c) lowering activation energy
   d) forming permanent complexes with the reactants

32. Which of the following reactions would be classified as Exergonic:
    a) catabolism
    b) oxidation
    c) hydrolysis
    d) a and b
    e) a, b and c

33. Which will not denature an enzyme:
    a) high pH
    b) high temperature
    c) low pH
    d) low temperature
    e) only a and b

34. All are classified as Nucleic Acids except:
    a) ATP
    b) DNA
    c) NAD
    d) a and b
    e) all are nucleic acids

35. How does DNA differ from RNA:
    a) DNA is a double helix and RNA is a single strand
    b) DNA uses Deoxyribose and RNA Ribose
    c) DNA use Thymine and RNA uses Uracil
    d) a and b
    e) a, b and c

36. Which of the following is not considered a pyrimidine:
    a) adenine
    b) cytosine
    c) thymine
    d) uracil
    e) they are all pyrimidines

37. All are part of a typical nucleotide except:
    a) nitrogen base
    b) a pentose
    c) phosphate group
    d) glycerol

38. Nucleotides on the same strand are joined by which of the following linkages:
    a) hydrogen
    b) peptide
    c) phosphodiester
    d) ester
    e) glycosidic

39. Which of the following bonds join complementary base pairs in forming the DNA double helix:
    a) hydrogen
    b) peptide
    c) phosphodiester
    d) ester
    e) glycosidic

40. Which of the following purine-pyrimidine complimentary pairs is correct:
    a) thymine-cytosine
    b) thymine-adenine
    c) thymine-uracil
    d) thymine-guanine

1: d, 2: c, 3: c, 4: b, 5: b, 6: a, 7: b, 8: a, 9: c, 10: b, 11: c, 12: a, 13: b, 14: a, 15: b, 16: d, 17: a, 18: b, 19: d, 20: a, 21: e, 22: b, 23: c, 24: b, 25: a, 26: a, 27: d, 28: a, 29: b, 30: c, 31: c, 32: c, 33: d, 34: d, 35: e, 36: a, 37: d, 38: c, 39: a, 40: b

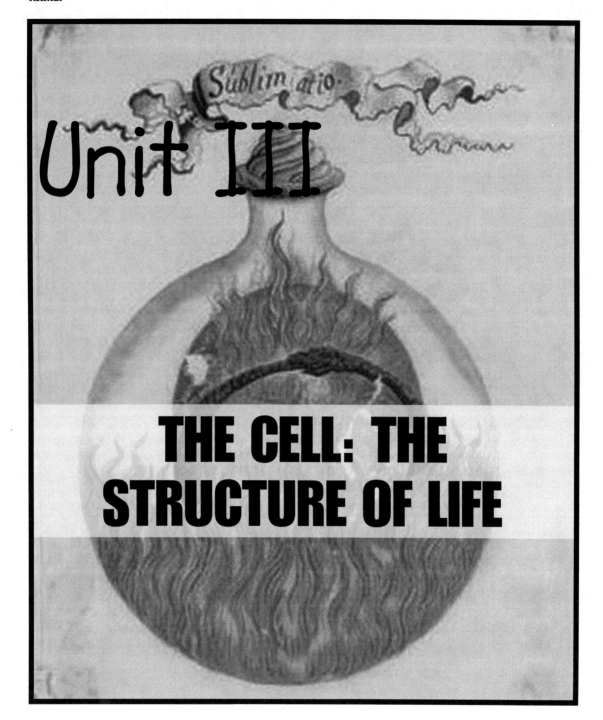

Unit III

THE CELL: THE STRUCTURE OF LIFE

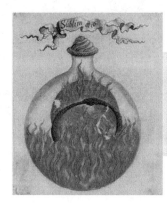

Part 1: Membranes and Transport

1. Cell membranes are principally composed of _____.

2. Phospholipids are composed of a central glycerol molecule bound to two _____ _____ on one side and a _____-bound compound on the other.

3. The fatty acid side of the phospholipid repels/interacts with water and is described as being _____; the phosphate side repels/interacts with water and is described as _____.

4. Because of their opposing hydrophobic _____ and hydrophilic _____ phospholipids are described as being _____.

5. Due to its amphipathic nature the molecule's hydrophobic tails will fold _____ due to the _____ forces exerted by water; this creates a phospholipid _____, also called the _____ membrane.

6. The outer layers of the bilayer plasma membrane are composed of the phospholipid's _____ _____; this forms the basic structural component of the entire _____ System.

7. In addition to the phospholipid bilayer the Cell Membrane is also composed of the lipid _____ and _____ _____.

8. Cholesterol molecules help to _____ the CM. Phospholipids with attached sugar groups are called _____.

9. There are two types of globular proteins: _____ and _____ proteins.

10. Integral proteins are _____ into the plasma membrane; some form _____ which pass from the ECF to the ICF, the openings of which are called _____. Other Integral proteins act as _____ which transport substances across the bilayer.

11. These pores will allow any substance smaller than ____ _____ to pass through. Integral proteins which only face the ECF function as _____ _____ for hormones.

12. Peripheral proteins are not embedded but are _____ to the _____ membrane surface. Some are functional _____; others have sugar chains attached to them and are called _____.

13. Glycoproteins are involved in _____ _____ and, with glycolipids, form the _____ on the cell's surface.

14. Because of the opposing hydrophobic and hydrophilic forces the constituents of the CM are in a constant state of motion or _____; this creates the description of the CM as a _____ _____.

15. Intercellular junctions in which the CMs fuse are called _____ junctions. This forms an _____ barrier between the two cells.

16. Junctions in which cells are held together by scattered linking proteins are called _____.

17. Unlike Tight Junctions and Desmosomes, _____ junctions form _____ which allow the passage of materials between adjacent cells.

18. Because Gap junctions allow the passage of ions they also act as _____ connections between cells.

19. The chemical nature of the CM allows some substances to pass through while blocking others; this is defined as _____ or _____ – _____.

20. The selectively permeable membrane allows substances to pass through by the process of _____.

21. Diffusion is defined as the _____ _____.

22. The four factors affecting the rate of diffusion are: _____, _____, _____ and the _____ of the substance.

23. How does Temperature affect diffusion: _____.

24. How does Pressure affect diffusion: _____.

25. How does Concentration affect diffusion: _____ _____.

26. How does molecular weight affect diffusion: _____ _____.

27. Substances will diffuse across a membrane along an _____ _____ until reaching a _____ _____.

28. The movement of substances along an electrochemical gradient without the expenditure of energy is called _____ _____.

29. Passive Diffusion occurs as either _____ diffusion or _____ diffusion.

30. In Simple diffusion _____-soluble substances move from areas of _____ concentra-tion to _____ concentration.

31. Pore diffusion allows +/− charged _____–_____soluble substances smaller than _____ and to pass through the CM.

32. Non-lipid soluble substances larger than 8 angstroms may enter the cell by _____ diffusion which uses carriers or _____ which bond to the specific substance.

33. The movement of substances against an electrochemical gradient is called _____ _____; these mechanisms are called _____ and require the expenditure of energy in the form of _____.

34. Examples of Active transport using ATP include the _____ pump in nerve potentials, the _____ pump in muscle contraction and the _____ pump in the final stages of oxidation.

35. Pumps work via the use of cotransporter enzymes such as ___/___–____–____ in the Na/K pump and ____–_____–____ in muscle contraction. Substances which "follow" the pumping of Na+ against the gradient do so by what is referred to as _____ active transport.

36. The process by which the cell membrane forms pockets which invaginate to form vesicles containing large substances from the ECF is called _____. The process by which internally formed vesicles migrate to the CM, fuse and expel their contents into the ECF is called _____.

37. Endocytosis and Exocytosis are collectively referred to as _____. Exocytosis is also known as _____.

38. The process by which a cell changes its shape to engulf a particle or microbe is called _____ and is performed by cells called _____.

39. A solution is composed of two components, the _____ which is dissolved in the _____.

40. The movement of solute or dissolved solids through a membrane along an electrochemical gradient is known as _____; the movement of solvent across a membrane from an area of lower solute concentration to higher is called _____.

41. When cells are placed in a solution of identical solute concentration the ECF is described as being _____; solutions of higher solute concentration are _____ and those of lower are _____.

42. Because water movement is limited to a dynamic equilibrium in isotonic solutions there is a 0/net osmosis into/out of the cell. Physiologic saline is also known as _____% _____.

43. Hypertonic solutions result in a 0/net osmosis into/out of the cell; this creates a condition called _____. Hypotonic solutions result in a 0/net osmosis into/out of the cell; this creates a condition called _____.

44. In kidney dialysis the tubing bearing the patient's blood is bathed in a solution which is _____ to toxic metabolites such as _____.

45. The force by which water moves across the membrane from hypo to hypertonic solutions is called _____ _____.

46. The force which resists osmotic pressure is called _____ pressure.

47. Hydrostatic/Osmotic pressure forces water and nutrients from the arterial capillaries into the interstitial spaces whereas Hydrostatic/Osmotic pressure draws water back into the venous capillaries.

48. The process by which hydrostatic pressure forces water and solute across a membrane or through intercellular channels is called _____.

49. Filtration is performed by the _____; the immediate product is called the _____.

50. The process by which filtrate becomes urine is called _____ and involves _____–_____ _____ and _____ _____.

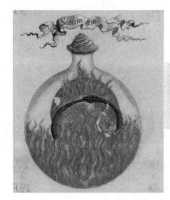

Part 2: The Cell and Cell Cycle

51. The Cell Concept states:
    a) _____,
    b) _____, and
    c) _____.

52. The two principal cell types are _____ and _____.

53. Prokaryotes include single-celled organisms called _____ and differ from eukaryotes in that prokaryotes _____

    _____.

54. The membrane-bound organelles of eukaryotic cells collectively form the _____ System. The intracellular fluid is called _____.

55. Cytosol and the organelles of the Endomembrane System are collectively known as

    _____.

56. How does the Nucleus differ from the Nucleolus:_____

    _____.

57. The Nucleus is noted for strands of DNA called _____; during mitosis and Meiosis these strands condense and coil into _____. The Nucleolus contains the nucleotide _____.

58. What is the function of the Mitochondria _____; the double membrane of the mitochondria is folded into shelves called _____. Mitochondrion supports the theory of endobiosis by possessing its own _____.

59. The Smooth Endoplasmic Reticulum has small cavities called _____ and functions in _____ synthesis and _____.

60. How does the Rough Endoplasmic Reticulum differ from the smooth: _____ _____

    _____.

    Ribosomes synthesize _____.

61. The Golgi Apparatus is responsible for forming the _____ (2°) and _____ (3°) of the polypeptide, refining them into functional proteins such as _____.

62. Vesicles which store digestive enzymes are known as _____ and those storing catalase and oxidase are called _____.

63. Unlike the endomembrane system the cytoskeleton is composed of _____ and _____.

64. Microfilaments include the proteins _____ and _____. Microtubules are composed of proteins called _____ which form building blocks called _____.

65. Actin and Myosin combine for _____ movement whereas tubulin dimers assemble and disassemble to move _____.

66. Microtubules originate at the _____ which is noted for the _____ in mitotic cells.

67. Centrioles form the _____ _____ during mitosis; each centriole is composed of _____ groups of _____ microtubules.

68. Microtubules also form _____ and _____.

69. Flagella, which function by _____; Cilia function by _____ _____. Both are noted for their anchoring _____ _____.

70. The Cell Cycle is divided into two major periods: _____ and _____ also referred to as division.

71. Interphase, the period during which a cell prepares for division, is divided into 3 periods: _____(G1), _____ (S), and _____ (G2).

72. During Growth 1 (G1) the cell synthesizes: _____ _____; During Synthesis (S) _____ is replicated; during Growth 2 (G2) _____ are formed.

73. Mitosis is also referred to as division because: _____
_____.

74. Mitosis can also be defined as the duplication of genetic material maintaining the _____ chromosomal count.

75. The nomenclature indicating Diploid is _____. The Diploid count for human body cells is _____ chromosomes in 23 _____ pairs.

76. The initiation of DNA replication during "Synthesis" of Interphase begins with the unwinding of the double helix by the enzyme _____.

77. After Topoisomerase begins to unwind a section of the DNA polymer, unwinding of the helix is completed by the breaking of _____ bonds between complimentary bases by the enzyme _____.

78. Once bases of the two mother strands are exposed by Helicase, their complimentary bases can be attracted by the formation of a template or _____.

79. The Primer is formed by the enzyme _____ _____. The Primer is a mirror image of the mother strand with one exception: Thymine is replaced by _____.

80. The complimentary bases to the mother strands are delivered to the Primer by the enzyme _____ _____ _____.

81. Each mother strand is identified by its exposed carbon atoms on each end; how is this noted: _____ and _____.

82. The assembling of the new daughter strands progresses in which direction: 3' - 5' or 5'- 3'? _____.

83. Although nucleotides are assembled from 3'-5' they must do so by approaching the replication fork. In what manner is the daughter to the 3'-5' strand assembled: _____ __ _____. In what manner is the 5'-3' strand assembled: ____ _____ _____.

84. What term describes the faster growing 3'-5' strand: _____; what term is describes the slower 5'-3' strand assembled by Okasaki fragments: _____.

85. As DNA Polymerase III delivers nucleotides to form both leading and lagging strands it catalyzes the formation of _____ bonds to the mother strands.

86. Once H+ bonds are formed, nucleotides of both the leading and lagging strands are attached by _____ bonds catalyzed the enzyme _____.

87. Once joined by Ligase, base pairs are "spell-checked" by the enzyme _____ _____ _____. Incorrect pairings (if ever) are removed by the enzyme _____.

88. The ends of chromosomes are noted for non-coding sequences called _____ the gradual loss of which can limit a cell's ability to replicate.

89. Interphase is also noted by the build-up of proteins called _____.

90. Cyclins initiate Mitosis by activating the enzyme _____.

91. Mitosis is subdivided into four phases: _____- _____, _____ and _____.

92. At the start of Mitosis a typical body cell now has _____ chromosomes; duplicated chromosomes are referred as sister _____ and are joined at the _____.

93. Located within the centromere of the joined sister chromatids is the point of attachment for the spindle, the _____.

94. The four principal events of Prophase are:

_____

_____

_____, and

_____.

95. What occurs during Metaphase: _____.

96. What occurs during Anaphase: _____ and _____
_____.

97. During Telophase the new daughter cells are divided by the formation _____ _____;
the separating of the two new cells is called _____.

98. Following cytokinesis the two new cells each begin _____.

99. The Central Dogma implies that ultimately traits are the result of DNA coding for _____.

100. Enzymes are proteins composed of monomers called _____ _____.

101. DNA codes for amino acids by its _____ _____ sequence.

102. Nitrogen bases code for amino acids in groups of _____.

103. Protein Synthesis can be subdivided into _____ and
_____ and involves three types of RNA: mRNA or
_____, tRNA or _____ and rRNA or
_____.

104. Protein transcription uses _____ RNA (_____) and begins by unraveling the portion
of DNA containing the base code with the enzyme _____.

105. After unraveling by Helicase the complimentary strands containing the code are separated by the enzyme
_____ _____. The strand of DNA bearing the code is called the _____
strand.

106. The protein code of the sense strand is preceded by a _____ base sequence; the
protein code is followed by the _____ base code which indicates the protein code has
ended.

107. After exposing the promoter sequence, protein code and terminator base code, the enzyme _____
_____ synthesizes mRNA to form the RNA _____.

108. The RNA transcript formed by RNA Polymerase and mRNA is composed of the complimentary bases to
the DNA code; this is called the _____.

109. In addition to the codon, the mRNA transcript also contains non-coding regions called _____
which will be removed; the remaining coding portions which express traits are called _____.

110. Once introns are removed from the transcript a cap is added to the 5' end and a _____–__–_____ is
added to the 3'; the mature transcript can now leave the nucleus and travel to the _____.

111. Transfer RNA (tRNA) is a _____ strand which is shaped into ____ _____.

112. Each strand of tRNA has a specific _____ _____ attached to it's free end, whereas its
second/central loop carries the 3 base sequence called the _____.

113. The three base sequence anticodon of tRNA is the compliment to the _____ of mRNA and the mirror to the DNA code–with what exception: _____

_____.

114. Ribosomes are subdivided into _____ subunits; the mRNA transcript attaches to the _____ subunit.

115. Amino acids are linked to the free end of tRNA by the enzyme

_____–_____–_____.

116. Protein translation can be divided into three events: _____,
_____ and _____.

117. In order for initiation to begin, initiator tRNA which carries the anticodon for the amino acid _____ must attach to the _____ ribosome subunit.

118. Once tRNA and methionine attach to the smaller subunit, the _____ of the mRNA transcript can attract the _____ of the complimentary tRNA and their respective amino acids and assemble the _____.

119. The process of linking amino acids into a polypeptide is called _____. Amino acid bonds are called _____ bonds.

120. Elongation continues until the _____ codon is reached. After completion the polypeptide travels to the _____ _____ to complete protein synthesis.

121. Any change in the DNA sequence and protein code is termed a _____.

122. Single base substitutions are also called _____ mutations.

123. A point mutation in which the substitution still codes for the same amino acid is called a _____ mutation; one which changes the amino acid for another affecting the polypeptide and its function is called a _____ mutation.

124. An example of a Missense mutation is _____ _____ _____ in which Glutamic HCL is replaced by _____. A point mutation which changes the code to a terminator codon, prematurely ending the polypeptide and its function is called a _____ mutation.

125. Mutations in which bases are added or deleted are called _____ mutations; these generally result is loss of _____ activity.

126. An example of a Frameshift mutation is _____–_____ disease in which there is no _____ enzyme synthesis.

127. The region on a strand of chromatin which codes for a trait is called the _____.

128. Who is credited with outlining the foundations of modern Genetics: _____ _____.

129. What term did Mendel coin for his "invisible agent of heredity": _____; what word is it derived from: _____.

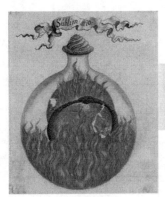

Part 3: Human Genetics

130. Based on his experiments Mendel established three laws of inheritance:
1: _____, 2: _____ and 3: _____ _____.

131. The Law of Dominance states that for a trait to express is requires _____ _____, one from each parent, and that for every trait there exists two variations or _____.

132. What is the principal characteristic of a dominant gene/allele: _____
_____; and of a recessive gene/allele: _____
_____.

133. The genetic composition of an individual trait is called the _____ whereas the physical expression/appearance of the trait is its _____.

134. A genotype composed of two identical alleles is _____; one composed of different alleles is _____.

135. Phenotypes of homozygous traits are either _____ or _____. Phenotypes of heterozygous traits appear _____ and are referred to as _____.

136. The Law of Segregation states that during gamete formation _____
_____. What does "gamete" mean: _____.

137. Gamete formation is properly termed _____.

138. At the end of Meiosis each sperm or ovum posseses _____ strands of chromatin; this is called the _____ count.

139. When the two haploid nuclei merge in fertilization they form _____ pairs for gene expression.

140. There are _____ homologous pairs, each with a _____ and _____ strand.

141. Of the 23 homologous pairs, 1–22 are called _____; pair 23 are called the _____ _____.

142. The sex chromosomes are indicated as _____ and _____ What is the genotype for female: _____ Male: _____

143. The Law of Independent Assortment states that during gamete formation genes are _____
_____.

144. When Mendel crossed a homozygous dominant plant with a homozygous recessive plant it resulted in _____% _____ appearing phenotype.

	A	A
a		
a		

145. These dominant phenotype plants are _____ with _____ genotypes.

146. Heterozygous genotypes are also referred to as _____.

147. What two ratios will result from a monohybrid cross:
Genotype: ____:____:____
Phenotype: ____:____

	A	a
A		
a		

148. What does the phenotype ratio display:
3 _____ to 1 _____.

149. The three dominant progeny of the phenotype ration is mixed. What is the distribution of genotypes in the 1:2:1 ratio: 1 _____ _____ to 2 _____ to 1 _____ _____

150. Crossing individuals with two hybrid traits (Aa × Rr) is called a _____ cross. What would their alleles be:

_____

_____

_____

_____

AR _____ _____ _____

AR				
_____				
_____				
_____				

151. According to Mendel, one would only have to multiply ratios to predict the outcome of dihybrid crosses. The phenotype would be ____:____:____:____.

152. With the 9:3:3:1 ratio, 9 appear _____ for _____ _____, 3 appear _____ for one and _____, 3 appear _____ for the other and _____, and one is _____ _____ for both traits.

153. In human genetics, the majority of normal traits are _____ (A); the majority of abnormal traits are _____(a).

154. A heterozygous/hybrid individual is normal but can pass the trait on; they are referred to as _____.

155. Tay-Sachs Disease is an _____ recessive disorder.
What is the genotype of a carrier: _____ What are
the odds of two carriers having a child with the disease: _____ in _____
or _____:_____

156. Phenotypic sex is determined by X and Y chromosomes. What are the
genotypes for female and male: _____ and _____. What are the
expected odds for couples having either girls or boys: _____:_____

157. Hemophilia is a sex-linked trait that is "passed from mothers to sons";
which chromosome is it linked to? _____ What are the genotypes of:
Normal female: _____
Carrier female: _____
Female with the disease: _____
Normal male: _____
Male with the disease: _____

158. What is the expected outcome of a female carrier and normal male? _____
_____ Can there be male carriers? _____
Why? _____

159. Sickle Cell Anemia is a non-Mendelian form of inheritance referred to as _____.

160. What is meant by Pleiotrophy? _____

161. What are the odds of a heterozygous individual and a
normal individual having a child with some form of
Sickle Cell Anemia? _____ in _____ or _____:_____

162. Blood types are also a non-Mendelian form of
inheritance based on
_____ _____ and _____.

163. What are the three alleles in blood types? _____, _____, and _____. Which two are codominant? _____ and
_____. Which is recessive? _____.

164. With A and B being codominant and O recessive, what are the four phenotypes? _____, _____, _____, and
_____.

165. What are the genotypes for: A: _____ and _____; B: _____ and _____, AB: _____ and O: _____.

166. Blood types express by producing _____ on the surface of the erythrocyte and
_____ as an immune reaction to foreign blood cells.

167. The antigens and antibodies created by each type are:

Phenotype	Genotype	Antigen	Antibodies	Accepts from
A				
B				
AB				
O				

168. Of the four blood types, which is the universal recipient? _____ The universal donor? _____

169. Is it possible for a type A male and type B female to have a type O child? _____

	OO

170. Eye color is the result of polygenic inheritance. What is meant by polygenic? _____

_____

Unit III: The cell: The Structure of Life

Part 1: Membrane Function and Transport

1. Phospholipids
2. fatty acids, phosphate
3. repels, hydrophobic; interacts, hydrophilic
4. tails, heads, amphipathic
5. inward, hydrophobic; bilayer, plasma
6. hydrophilic heads; endomembrane
7. cholesterol and globular proteins
8. stabilize. glycolipids
9. integral, peripheral
10. embedded; channels, pores. carriers
11. 8 angstroms, receptor sites
12. attached, external. enzymes; glycoproteins
13. intercellular communication, glycocalyx
14. flux; fluid mosaic
15. tight; impermeable
16. desmosomes
17. gap, channels
18. electrical
19. selective or semi-permeability
20. diffusion
21. random kinetic motion of particles
22. temperature, pressure, concentration and molecular weight
23. increases the rate
24. increases the rate
25. initial increases rate with gradual reduction
26. the heavier the substance the slower the rate
27. electrochemical gradient, dynamic equilibrium
28. passive diffusion
29. simple, pore
30. lipid, high to low
31. +, non-lipid, 8 angstroms
32. facilitated, cotransporters
33. active transport; ATP
34. Na/K, Calcium, proton
35. Na/K-ATP-ase, Ca^{+2}-ATP-ase. secondary
36. endocytosis. exocytosis
37. pinocytosis. secretion
38. phagocytosis, macrophages
39. solute, solvent
40. dialysis; osmosis
41. isotonic; hypertonic, hypotonic
42. 0. 0.9% NaCl
43. net osmosis out; crenation
44. hypotonic, urea
45. osmotic
46. hydrostatic
47. hydrostatic, osmotic
48. filtration
49. kidney; filtrate
50. excretion, diffusion, facilitated transport and active transport

Part 2: The Cell and Cell Cycle

51. cell is the basic unit of structure and function, cells can only arise from pre-existing cells and cells have similar structures and functions
52. prokaryote and eukaryote
53. bacteria, do not possess membrane-bound organelles
54. endomembrane. cytosol
55. cytoplasm
56. nucleus is concentration of DNA and directs all cell function; nucleolus concentration of RNA and directs protein synthesis
57. chromatin; chromosomes. mRNA
58. oxidation of glucose to produce ATP; cristae, DNA
59. cisternae, lipid, detoxification
60. rough associated with ribosomes. polypeptides
61. secondary and tertiary, enzymes
62. lysosomes, peroxisomes
63. microfilaments and microtubules
64. actin and myosin. tubulins, dimers
65. cellular, organelles
66. centrosome, centrioles
67. spindle apparatus; 9, 3
68. flagella and cilia
69. moving the cell, moving fluids, basal body
70. interphase and mitosis
71. Growth 1, Synthesis, Growth 2
72. organic compounds; DNA; organelles

73. replicated materials are divided-up equally between two new cells
74. diploid
75. 2N. 46, homologous
76. topoisomerase
77. H$^+$, helicase
78. primer
79. RNA Primase, uracil
80. DNA Polymerase III
81. 3' to 5' and 5' to 3'
82. 3' to 5'
83. base by base, Okasaki Fragments
84. leading, lagging
85. H$^+$
86. Phosphodiester, Ligase
87. DNA Polymerase III, Nuclease
88. telomeres
89. cyclins
90. Kinase
91. Prophase, Metaphase, Anaphase and Telophase
92. 92; chromatids, centromere
93. kinetochore
94. nuclear membrane disappears, chromatin condenses into chromosomes, centrioles migrate to the poles, spindle begins forming
95. sister chromatids align along the equator
96. sister chromatids split, and chromosomes migrate to opposite poles
97. Cleavage Furrow; cytokinesis
98. interphase
99. enzymes
100. amino acids
101. nitrogen base
102. 3
103. transcription and translation; Messenger RNA, Transfer RNA and Ribosomal RNA
104. messenger MRA, helicase
105. DNA Polymerase. sense
106. promoter; terminator
107. RNA polymerase, transcript
108. codon
109. introns, exons
110. poly-A-tail; ribosome
111. single, 3 loops
112. amino acid, anti-codon
113. codon; uracil replace thymine
114. 2; large
115. amino-acyl-transferase

116. initiation, elongation and termination
117. methionine, small
118. codon, anticodon, polypeptide
119. elongation. peptide
120. terminator. Golgi apparatus
121. mutation
122. point
123. silent; missense
124. sickle cell anemia, valine. nonsense
125. frameshift, enzyme
126. Tay Sach's, lipid
127. Locus

Part 3: **Human Genetics**

128. Gegor Mendel
129. Gene; Genesis
130. Dominance, Segregation and Independent Assortment
131. Two genes; alleles
132. Always expresses; recedes in the presence of the dominant allele
133. Genotype; phenotype
134. Homozygous; heterozygous
135. Dominant or recessive; dominant, hybrid
136. The two genes separate, one to each gamete;spouse
137. Meiosis
138. 23, haploid
139. Homologous
140. 23, maternal and paternal
141. Autosomes, sex chromosomes
142. X and Y; XX, XY
143. Inherited independently of each other
144. 100% dominant (Aa)
145. Hybrids with heterozygous
146. Monohybrid
147. 1:2:1; 3:1
148. 3 dominant to 1 recessive
149. 1 homozygous dominant to 2 hybrid dominants to 1 homozygous recessive
150. Dihybrid; AR, Ar. aR, ar
151. 9:3:3:1
152. Dominant for both traits; dominant for one and recessive for the other, dominant and recessive, homozygous
153. Dominant; recessive
154. Carriers
155. Autosomal; Tt.1 in 4 or 3:1
156. XX and XY; 1:1

157. X^HX^H, X^HX^h, X^hX^h, X^HY, X^hY
158. One of each X^HX^H, X^HX^h, X^HY, X^hY with 50% of the males having the disease. No. Males have only one allele.
159. Pleiotrophy
160. Any degree of the disease can express in herterozygous individuals
161. 1 in 2 or 1:1
162. Multiple alleles, codominance
163. A, B and O. A and B. O
164. A, B, AB and O
165. AA AO, BB BO, AB, OO
166. Antigens, antibodies

167.

Pheno-type	Geno-type	Anti-gen	Anti-bodies	Ac-cepts from
A	AA AO	A	Anti B	A & O
B	BB BO	B	Anti A	B & O
AB	AB	A & B	None	A, B, AB, O
O	OO	None	Anti A & B	O

168. AB, O
169. Yes (AO x BO)
170. The trait is carried on many genes and not one.

Unit III: Take a Test!

1. Which statements regarding Phospholipids is/are true:
   a) The have hydrophilic heads
   b) They have hydrophobic tails
   c) They are amphipathic
   d) a and b
   e) a, b and c

2. Which of the following helps to stabilize the components of the cell membrane:
   a) integral proteins
   b) peripheral proteins
   c) cholesterol
   d) glycoproteins
   e) microfilaments

3. Which are classified as "antigen markers":
   a) integral proteins
   b) ligand proteins
   c) cholesterol
   d) glycoproteins
   e) microfilaments

4. Forms Ligand receptors for neurotransmitters
   a) integral proteins
   b) peripheral proteins
   c) cholesterol
   d) glycoproteins
   e) microfilaments

5. Forms the Cytoskeleton:
   a) integral proteins
   b) peripheral proteins
   c) cholesterol
   d) glycoproteins
   e) microfilaments

6. Increasing all of the following will increase the rate of diffusion except:
   a) temperature
   b) pressure
   c) molecular weight
   d) concentration
   e) all will increase the rate

7. Which of the following would be considered forms of passive diffusion:
   a) pore diffusion
   b) simple diffusion
   c) facilitated diffusion
   d) a and b
   e) all are passive

8. The Na^+/K^+ Pump is an example of:
   a) dialysis
   b) active transport
   c) facilitated diffusion
   d) pore diffusion
   e) osmosis

9. Non-lipid soluble substances smaller than 1 nanometer will most likely pass through a membrane via:
   a) dialysis
   b) active transport
   c) facilitated diffusion
   d) pore diffusion
   e) osmosis

10. Diffusion by use of cotransporters is also known as:
    a) dialysis
    b) active transport
    c) facilitated diffusion
    d) pore diffusion
    e) osmosis

11. The movement of *solvent* through a membrane is properly known as:
    a) dialysis
    b) active transport
    c) facilitated diffusion
    d) pore diffusion
    e) osmosis

12. A human erythrocyte is placed in a 0.9 % NaCl solution; relative to the RBC the solution is considered to be:
    a) isotonic
    b) hypotonic
    c) hypertonic
    d) ambient

13. A 0.0% NaCl solution, with respect to the same RBC would be considered:
    a) hypotonic
    b) hypertonic
    c) isotonic
    d) ambient

14. Crenation occurs when a cell is placed in which type of solution:
    a) hypotonic
    b) hypertonic
    c) isotonic
    d) ambient

15. Secretion is properly known as:
    a) endocytosis
    b) exocytosis
    c) phagocytosis
    d) lysis

16. Which process defines the use of Ligand receptors in immunity:
    a) endocytosis
    b) exocytosis
    c) phagocytosis
    d) lysis

17. The force by which water is *attracted* from the tissues into the capillaries is called:
    a) turgor pressure
    b) hydrostatic pressure
    c) osmotic pressure
    d) solute pressure

18. Cells which are described as being "electrically coupled are connected by:
    a) Tight Junctions
    b) Gap Junctions
    c) Desmosome
    d) Hemidesmosome
    e) Aquaporins

19. Which is true of "Tight Junctions"
    a) They attach cells to their basal lamina
    b) They allow the free flow of cytoplasm from cell to cell
    c) They connect cells but prevent transmembrane diffusion
    d) They allow water to enter the cell
    e) None of these apply

20. Which connection attaches adjacent cells together while allowing transmembrane diffusion:
    a) Tight Junctions
    b) Gap Junctions
    c) Desmosome
    d) Hemidesmosome
    e) Aquaporins

21. Chromatin is concentrated within the:
    a) nucleus   b) nucleolus
    c) mitochondria   d) centriole   e) golgi apparatus

22. Polypeptides are synthesized in:
    a) mitochondria   b) smooth endoplasmic reticulum
    c) golgi apparatus   d) ribosome   e) centriole

23. Proteins are coiled and folded into enzymes in which structure :
    a) mitochondria   b) smooth endoplasmic reticulum
    c) golgi apparatus   d) ribosome   e) centriole

24. The oxidation of glucose occurs in which organelle::
    a) nucleus   b) nucleolus
    c) mitochondria   d) centriole   e) golgi apparatus

25. Which is composed of microtubules:
    a) nucleolus   b) smooth endoplasmic reticulum
    c) mitochondria   d) lysosome   e) centriole

26. Which best explains why DNA replication is considered to be "semi-conservative":
    a) only half of the chromatin strands are duplicated during any one cycle
    b) each complimentary strand is used as a template to attract a new daughter strand
    c) replication begins at one end and progresses to the opposite end
    d) only the sense strand is replicated
    e) new strands are assembled by breaking Phosphodiester bonds and duplicating the sequence

27. DNA/Chromatin is duplicated during:
    a) mitosis   b) Growth 1
    c) Synthesis   d) Growth 2

28. A human body cell contains:
    a) 46 chromosomes   b) 23 homologous pairs of chromosomes
    c) 23 chromosomes   d) a and b

29. Which is the correct sequence of events:
    1: Anaphase   2: Cytokinesis   3: Interphase
    4: Metaphase   5: Prophase   6: Telophase
    a) 1, 3, 5, 2, 4, 6   b) 3, 5, 4, 1, 6, 2
    c) 6, 3, 5, 2, 4, 1   d) 4, 5, 1, 2, 6, 3

30. Which forms the template for the growing daughter strand:
    a) Helicase   b) DNA polymerase III
    c) RNA primase   d) DNA ligase   e) Topisomerase

31. Which assembles nucleotides into the new daughter strands:
    a) Helicase   b) DNA polymerase III
    c) RNA primase   d) DNA ligase   e) Topisomerase

32. Which spell forms the phosphodiester bonds between nucleotides of the daughter strands:
    a) Helicase
    b) DNA polymerase III
    c) RNA primase
    d) DNA ligase
    e) Topisomerase

33. How is the genetic information in DNA encoded:
    a) by the overall length of the gene
    b) in groups of three nitrogen bases on the sense strand
    c) on both sides of the helix
    d) by the orientation of the Pentose sugars

34. Protein Transcription is carried out by which of the following:
    a) Sense strand
    b) mRNA
    c) tRNA
    d) rRNA

35. Protein Translation is carried out by which of the following:
    a) Sense strand
    b) mRNA
    c) tRNA
    d) rRNA

36. Which of these is associated with the "anticodon"
    a) rRNA
    b) tRNA
    c) mRNA
    d) DNA

37. Which of the following is associated with the "codon":
    a) rRNA
    b) tRNA
    c) mRNA
    d) DNA

38. A base substitution mutation which still codes for the same amino acid is known as:
    a) Silent
    b) Missense
    c) Nonsense
    d) Frameshift

39. In Sickle Cell Anemia a base code change replaces valine with glutamic HCl altering the structure and function of hemoglobin; what type of mutation is this:
    a) Silent
    b) Missense
    c) Nonsense
    d) Frameshift

40. If the sense strand code reads "A T G" the anticodon is:
    a) "A T G"
    b) "A U G"
    c) "T A C"
    d) "U A C"

41. At the start of Mitosis a cell contains:
    a) 92 strands of chromatin
    b) 46 pairs of sister chromatids
    c) 23 pairs of chromosomes
    d) 23 chromosomes
    e) a and b

42. Meiosis results in _____
    a) 4 haploid daughter cells
    b) 2 haploid daughter cells
    c) 4 diploid daughter cells
    d) 2 diploid daughter cells

43. Which describes a nucleus containing different genes for the same trait:
   a) heterozygous
   b) genotype
   c) allele
   d) phenotype
   e) homozygous

44. Traits which requires both maternal and paternal gene to express in the progeny:
   a) dominant
   b) recessive
   c) hybrid
   d) homozygous
   e) heterozygous

45. A variation of a gene for the same trait is known as:
   a) heterozygous
   b) genotype
   c) allele
   d) phenotype
   e) homozygous

46. Traits such as blood types that have more than two variations in their phenotype are the result of:
   a) polygenic
   b) linked genes
   c) multiple alleles
   d) sex linkage

47. Traits that are passed directly from mothers to sons are most likely due to:
   a) polygenic
   b) linked genes
   c) multiple alleles
   d) sex linkage

48. A cross between a man with type A blood and a woman with type B resulted in a child with type O; their genotypes must be:
   a) AB, AB
   b) AO, BB
   c) AO, BO
   d) AA, BO

49. The Czarina Alexandra was a hemophilia carrier; her genotype was:
   a) $X^H X^H$
   b) $X^H X^h$
   c) $X^H Y$
   d) $X^h Y$

50. Her only son, the Czarich Alexi was a hemophiliac; his genotype was:
   a) $X^H X^H$
   b) $X^H X^h$
   c) $X^H Y$
   d) $X^h Y$

Unit IV

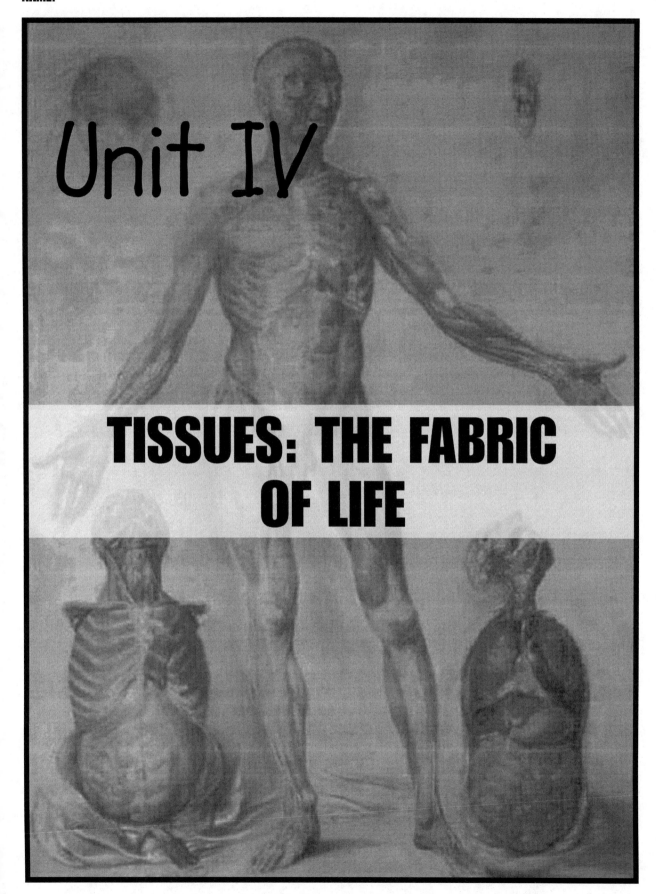

TISSUES: THE FABRIC OF LIFE

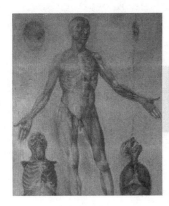

Part 1: Epithelium

1. The fertilization of an ovum produces a _____.

2. The rapid, synchronous divisions of a zygote are referred to as _____.

3. Cleavage produces a tightly packed ball of cells called the _____; these cells are described as _____–_____.

4. Non–differentiated blastula cells are _____ _____ and have the potential to differentiate into any cell line. They are described as being _____.

5. The blastula begins to hollow out, forming the _____; the process by which cells now take on different size and shape is called _____.

6. Differentiation of the gastrula cells gives rise to the three primary (embryonic) germ layers: _____, _____, and _____.

7. The four tissue types that the embryonic tissues differentiate into are _____, _____ _____, _____, and _____.

8. Endoderm gives rise to _____ _____; ectoderm gives rise to both _____ _____ and _____ tissue.

9. Mesoderm gives rise to an embryonic connective tissue called _____, and to _____ and _____.

10. Mesenchyme then differentiates in the _____ _____.

11. Muscle is described as _____ tissue and differentiates from embryonic cells called _____.

12. Mitotically active myoblasts divide by _____ and differentiate into the three muscle fiber types: _____, _____, and _____.

13. Unlike myoblasts, amitotic skeletal, cardiac, and smooth muscle fibers can only increase in mass and size by _____.

14. Nervous tissue is divided into two groups of cells: _____ and _____.

15. Neurons are described as being _____ _____, while glial cells are described as providing a _____ role.

16. Define
    Cell: _____
    Tissue: _____
    Organ: _____
    Organ System: _____

17. Epithelium is derived from which embryonic germ layers? _____, _____, and _____

18. Ectoderm gives rise to _____ and _____ epithelium, and is most noted for the _____ or skin. Endoderm gives rise to _____ epithelium, which functions as _____ tissue. Mesoderm gives rise to _____. What is endothelium noted for? _____

19. All types of epithelium exhibit the same characteristics. Describe "Cellularity": _____ _____.

20. How does cellularity (tightly packed cells) differ from polarity? _____ _____.

21. What are the three surface features of the apical surface? _____, _____, and _____ What structure is associated with the basal surface? The _____ _____, or _____, membrane.

22. Microvilli function by _____ _____ _____, whereas cilia function by _____ of fluids.

23. By increasing surface area microvilli enhance _____ as seen in the small intestine; pores in the apical surface enable _____.

24. In addition to absorption and secretion, other functions of internal lining epithelium include _____ in the glomerulus and _____ in the kidney tubule; the integument functions by providing _____.

25. The Basal Lamina, or basement membrane, is cellular/acellular and is composed of _____ secreted by the _____.

26. Epithelium is vascular/avascular.

27. Avascular epithelium receives nutrients via diffusion through its basal lamina and is dependent on underlying _____ _____. To compensate for dying cells, epithelium has a high _____ rate.

28. Epithelium has three types of specialized junctions: _____, _____, and _____.

29. Gap junctions allow for the _____ of _____ between cells whereas tight junctions prevent it. Desmosomes function by _____
_____.

30. Epithelium can be subdivided into two types or classes: _____ and _____.

31. How does Simple Epithelium differ from Stratified Epithelium? _____
_____.

32. Single–layered Simple and multi–layered Stratified Epithelium are noted for what three cell shape varieties? _____, _____, and _____

33. Squamous cells appear _____; their nuclei appear _____–_____ in shape. Cuboidal cells appear _____; their nuclei are _____ shaped and _____ located. Columnar cells appear _____; their nuclei are _____ shaped and are _____ located.

34. The four varieties of Simple Epithelium include Simple _____, Simple _____, Simple _____, and _____ _____ _____ Epithelium (PSCCE).

35. Simple Squamous is noted as the _____ of blood vessels. It forms the _____ of the lungs and the _____ covering internal organs.

36. Endothelium, like the Simple Squamous of the alveoli, is best suited for _____ of _____ and _____. The Mesothelium forms part of the _____ membrane.

37. The Serous membrane covering the lungs is called the _____, covering the heart, it's called the _____, and covering the lining of the abdominal and pelvic cavities and organs, it's called the _____.

38. Stratified Squamous and Simple Columnar Epithelia form _____ membranes, also referred to as the _____, which overlie the connective tissue (CT) _____
_____.

39. The two functions of Simple Cuboidal Epithelium are _____, as performed in the _____ _____ and _____ in glands.

40. The two functions of Simple Columnar Epithelium are _____ and _____; simple columnar lines the _____ _____.

41. Absorption is enhanced by _____; the secretory cells are referred to as _____ cells and release _____.

42. Columnar cells, which move mucus, possess _____.

43. Pseudostratified Ciliated Columnar Epithelium lines the _____ and is noted for secretory _____ cells.

44. The four varieties of Stratified Epithelium are Stratified _____, Stratified _____, Stratified _____, and _____ Epithelium.

45. Stratified Squamous Epithelium is noted for two types: _____ and _____ – _____.

46. Keratinized Stratified Squamous forms the _____ of the Integument; Non–Keratinized is located lining the _____ cavity, the _____, and the _____.

47. The lining of the Oral Cavity is also known as the _____ _____. Stratified Cuboidal Epithelium forms the secretory tissue of _____ glands and the _____ glands of the breast.

48. Stratified Columnar Epithelium lines the _____ _____. Transitional Epithelium lines the two _____ and the _____ _____ in both sexes.

49. Secretory Glands can be subdivided into two groups: _____ and _____.

50. Endocrine Glands possess/do not possess ducts and secrete _____. Exocrine Glands possess/do not possess ducts.

51. Endocrine glands secrete hormones into the _____ and are known as _____ glands. Examples of endocrine glands include the _____, the _____, and the _____.

52. The _____ cells of exocrine glands always secrete into _____, which empty onto a _____. Examples of exocrine glands include _____ glands of the oral cavity and the _____.

53. The Acini cells of multicellular exocrine glands form either _____ or pocket–like sacs described as _____.

54. Glandular tissue is often surrounded by an external _____ _____ whose CT extensions subdivide the organ into _____.

55. Glandular tissue can also be subdivided by physiologic mode of secretion: either _____ or _____ glands.

56. Merocrine glands function by the process of _____ and are seen in organs such as the _____, _____, and _____ glands.

57. Holocrine glands function by _____ and expelling their _____ _____, as seen in _____ (oil) glands.

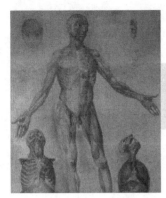

Part 2: Connective Tissues

58. The four major functions of CTs include _____ and _____, _____, _____, and _____ of _____.

59. The three characteristics of all CTs are _____, _____, and _____.

60. After birth, Mesenchyme is referred to as _____ – _____ CT.

61. How does vascularity vary? In cartilage, it is _____, in osseous tissue it is _____ _____.

62. The non–living matrix consists of semi–fluid _____ _____ and _____.

63. List the four classes of connective tissue: _____ _____, _____, _____, and _____.

64. The four principal CT cell types within the non–living matrix are _____, _____, _____, and _____.

65. How does a "–blast" cell differ from a "–cyte"? _____.

66. The three structural elements found in all CTs are _____ _____, _____, and _____.

67. Fibroblasts function in tissue repair by secreting _____ _____; chondroblasts and osteoblasts are noted for secreting their _____ _____.

68. Hematoblasts differentiate into _____, _____, and _____.

69. The ground substance of all CTs contains _____ _____; the ground substance and matrix secreted by chondroblasts also contains _____ _____ and _____ sulfate. The ground substance of bone contains _____.

70. Hyaluronic Acid, Chondroitin Sulfate, and Glucosamine Sulfate are classified as _____ (GAGs). Hydroxyapatite is comprised of the calcium salts _____ and _____.

71. The matrix of blood is called _____. Erythrocytes are also known as _____ Blood Cells and function by _____ of _____.

72. Leukocytes are also known as _____ Blood Cells and function as part of the _____ System.

73. The three fiber types are _____, _____, and _____.

74. The fibers of blood are referred to as _____ proteins, which come out of solution as _____ factors.

75. Collagen fibers are widely dispersed whereas Reticular fibers are confined mainly to _____ tissue. Define Reticular: _____.

76. CT Proper is divided into two subclasses: _____ and _____.

77. The three types of Loose CT are _____, _____, and _____.

78. Define Areola: _____ _____. What is the principal cell type in areolar tissue? _____ How does the ratio of matrix to cells differ between areolar and adipose tissue? _____ _____

79. Functions of tightly packed adipose tissue include _____ _____, _____, and _____. What is the principal cell type in Adipose tissue? _____

80. Adipocytes are avascualar/vascular and amitotic/mitotic.

81. Reticular fibers form an anchoring network for immune cells such as _____ within organs such as _____ _____ and the _____.

82. Three types of Dense CT Proper include _____, _____, and _____.

83. How does Dense Regular CT differ from Irregular CT? _____ _____

84. Dense Regular CT is mostly cells/fibers/matrix and forms _____, _____, and _____.

85. Tendons function by _____, ligaments by _____, and aponeuroses by _____.

86. Dense Irregular CT is found in _____ _____ and forms the _____ of the integument. What is the principal cell type in both Dense Regular and Irregular CT? _____

87. Elastic CT Proper is found in the _____ _____ of the spinal column, the _____ _____, and within the wall of the _____.

88. As chondroblasts mature into chondrocytes, they become encased within _____. Cartilage is vascular/avascular.

89. Avascular cartilage receives nutrition from the surrounding _____.

90. Cartilage grows by two mechanisms: _____ and _____.

91. In interstitial growth, chondroblasts divide within the _____; in appositional growth, chondroblasts divide between the perichondrium and the _____ _____.

92. The three types of cartilage include _____, _____, and _____.

93. Hyaline cartilage is noted for forming the _____ _____ and _____ cartilage covering joint surfaces. Hyaline cartilage is also found in structures such as the _____ _____ and _____ cartilages connecting the ribs and sternum. Hyaline cartilage also forms rings within the wall of the _____.

94. Elastic cartilage forms the _____ and the _____ or external ear. Elastic cartilage is noted for its dark _____ _____.

95. Fibrocartilage forms _____–like structures such as the _____ of the knee and the _____ _____ of the spinal column.

96. Torn Menisci and degenerating IVDs are poor healing structures because they are avascular/vascular and depend on the surrounding _____ for nutrition.

97. The matrix of osseous tissue is solid and is composed of _____.

98. Hydroxyapatite is inorganic and contains the calcium salts _____, _____, and _____.

99. Osseous tissue is found in two forms: compact or _____ bone and spongy or _____ bone.

100. The basic unit of structure of lamellar bone is the _____ or _____ System, and that of cancellous bone is the _____.

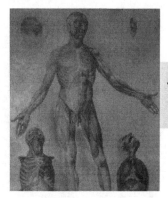

Part 3: The Integument

101. Besides protection, other functions provided by the integument include _____ regulation, prevention of _____ loss, and _____ _____ activation.

102. Temperature regulation by the integument is accomplished via the vascular system by _____ and _____. A principal concern in burn victims with extensive skin loss is _____ and _____. Vitamin D activation is enhanced by exposure to _____.

103. In addition to cushioning against physical trauma, the integument acts as a barrier to _____ and _____.

104. The integument is subdivided into three regions: the outer _____, the underlying _____, and the deeper _____.

105. The epidermis is composed of _____ _____ _____ Epithelium and is derived from _____ of the embryo.

106. Unlike the stratified squamous of the epidermis, the dermis is composed of _____ _____ _____ tissue and is derived from the embryonic tissue _____.

107. The hypodermis is principally composed of _____ tissue, which like the dermis is a _____ tissue derived from _____.

108. The epidermis is subdivided into five layers; the inner most _____ _____, the _____ _____, the _____ _____, the _____ _____, and the outermost _____ _____.

109. The Stratum Basale and Stratum Spinosum are mitotically active and collectively referred to as the Stratum _____. Two cell types predominate: _____ and _____.

110. Keratinocytes originate from mitotically active Basal cells and function by producing _____ _____; Melanocytes produce _____.

111. Keratohyaline granules have a _____ consistency and will accumulate in the Stratum _____. Melanin is classified as a _____.

112. Cells above the Stratum Granulosum die and thin, forming the clear Stratum _____. Cells of the Stratum Corneum consist predominately of _____.

113. The macrophages of the epidermis are known as _____ cells; sensory receptors at the dermal/epidermal junction are called _____ discs.

114. The epidermis is separated from the dermis by the _____ _____.

115. Cancers in which cells of the Stratum Basale migrate inward and penetrate the basal lamina include _____ _____ carcinoma and _____ _____.

116. The Dermis is subdivided into two layers: the _____ layer and the underlying _____ layer.

117. The Papillary layer is noted for projections into the epidermis called _____.

118. Dermal papillae supply nutrition to the overlying epidermis from their _____ _____ and are the site of touch receptors called _____ _____.

119. The Reticular layer is comprised mostly of _____ _____ CT and is the origin of accessory structures such as _____ and _____ glands, and _____ _____. Unlike Meissner's Corpuscles of the Papillary Layer, _____ Corpuscles are pain receptors.

120. Sweat glands, which are composed of _____ _____ epithelium, come in two varieties: _____ and _____ glands.

121. Eccrine glands, also referred to as _____ glands, are located on the _____, _____, and _____, and secrete sweat through _____. Sweat is _____% water.

122. Unlike merocrine glands, holocrine glands are located in the _____ and _____ areas, and empty their secretions into _____ _____. Bacterial activity on these secretions creates _____.

123. Sebaceous glands also empty into hair follicles. Their secretions, however, are _____ and can block ducts, leading to localized infections called _____, or pimples.

124. Carbuncles, which spread to encapsulated pockets within the dermis, are referred to as _____.

125. An abscess, which spreads into subcutaneous tissue layers, forms a _____, more commonly referred to as _____.

126. A break in the continuity of the basal layer of the epidermis is called an _____.

127. Ulcers that do not heal by the replacement of the Stratum Basale instead form _____ tissue, which eventually becomes a _____.

128. Scars that overgrow due to genetic and hormonal factors are called _____.

129. First degree burns are noted for _____ (redness) and _____ (swelling).

130. Second degree burns destroy the _____, producing _____ or blisters, which separate it from the dermis.

131. Third degree burns destroy the _____ and _____, requiring skin _____. The two immediate concerns of widespread third–degree burns are _____ and _____.

132. The rounded base of the hair follicle is called the hair _____; the surrounding sensory nerves form the _____ _____ _____.

133. The outer wall of the follicle is composed of the _____ _____ root sheath; the inner wall is referred to as the _____ root sheath.

134. The epithelial root sheath receives nutrition from the _____ _____, which protrudes upward from the connective tissue sheath. This is covered by a layer of mitotically active cells that produce the _____ _____, or hair shaft.

135. Hair follicles are also associated with _____ _____ muscles, which cause the hair shaft to stand on end.

Unit IV: Tissues

Part 1: Epithelium

1. Zygote
2. cleavage
3. blastula; non–differentiated
4. stem cells, pleuripotent
5. gastrula; differentiation
6. endoderm, mesoderm and ectoderm
7. epithelium, connective tissue, muscle and nervous
8. internal epithelium; nervous and external epithelium
9. mesenchyme, muscle and epithelium
10. The connective tissues
11. contractile tissue, myoblasts
12. hyperplasia, skeletal, cardiac and smooth
13. hypertrophy
14. neurons and glial
15. conductive, supportive
16. basic unit of structure, group of cells of similar size, shape and function, structure composed of two or more tissues combined to perform a specific function; group of organs that perform a general life function
17. endoderm, ectoderm, and mesoderm
18. nerve and internal, epidermis. internal, glandular, endothelium; forms lining of blood vessels
19. highly compacted cells with little interstitial space
20. to different surfaces, basal and apical
21. cilia, microvilli, and pores. basal lamina or basement membane
22. increasing surface area, movement
23. absorption; secretion
24. filtration and excretion; protection
25. acellular, glycoproteins, epithelium
26. avascular
27. connective tissue. mitotic
28. tight, desmosome and gap
29. movement of fluids. binding cells together
30. simple and stratified
31. single layer of cells
32. squamous, cuboidal, and columnar
33. flat; disk–like. Cube shaped; spherical. tall, oblong, and basal
34. squamous, cuboidal, columnar, pseudostratified
35. endothelium, alveoli, mesothelium
36. transport of O_2 and CO_2. serous
37. pleura, pericardium, peritoneum
38. mucous, mucosa, lamina propria
39. fitration, kidney tubule, secretion
40. absorption and secretion; digestive tract
41. microvilli; goblet, mucous
42. cilia
43. trachea, goblet
44. squamous, cuboidal, columnar, and transitional
45. keratinized and Non–keratinized
46. epidermis; oral, anus, and vagina
47. buccal mucosa. salivary, lactiferous
48. male urethra. ureters and urinary bladder
49. Endocrine and Exocrine
50. do not possess ducts, hormones. possess ducts
51. circulatory system, ductless. Pituitary, thyroid, and adrenal
52. acini, ducts, surface. salivary pancreas
53. tubular, alveolar
54. fibrous capsule, lobes
55. merocrine or holocrine
56. exocytosis pancreas, salivary and sweat
57. bursting, cellular contents, sebaceous

Part 2: Connective Tissues

58. Binding and holding, support, protection, transport of substances
59. mesenchymal origin, cells in a non–living matrix, and vascularity
60. non–differentiated
61. avascular, highly vascular
62. ground substance and fibers
63. CT Proper, Cartlage, Osseous, Blood
64. fibroblast, chondroblast, osteoblast, hematobalst
65. blast–cells are mitotically active
66. ground substance, fibers and cells
67. collagen fibers; intercellular matric
68. erythrocytes, leukocytes, and platelets
69. hyaluronic acid; chondroitin sulfate and glucosamine; hydroxyapatite

70. glycosaminoglycans. $CaCO_3$, $CaPO_4$
71. plasma; Red, transport of oxygen
72. White, Immune
73. collagen, elastic and reticular
74. soluble, clotting
75. immune; network–like
76. Loose and Dense
77. Areolar, Adipose, and Reticular
78. open space. fibroblast. Areolar: mostly matrix with few cells and fibers; Adipose: mostly cells with little matrix and fibers
79. nutrient storage, insulation, and protection. Adipocyte/Signet Ring Cell
80. vascular, amitotic
81. macrophages, lymph nodes, spleen
82. Regular, Irregular, and Elastic
83. Regular: fibers run in same direction; Irregular: fibers run in many directions
84. Fibers, tendons, ligaments, and aponeuroses
85. muscle to bone; binding bones together (joints); binding muscles together
86. joint capsule, dermis. Fibroblast
87. ligamentum flava, vocal cords, aorta
88. lacunae. avascular
89. perichondrium
90. Interstitial and appositional
91. matrix; external surface
92. Hyaline, Elastic, and Fibrocartilage
93. fetal skeleton, articular. Nasal septum, costal. Trachea
94. epiglottis, auricle
95. disk–like, menisci, intervertebral discs
96. avascular, perichondrium
97. hydroxyapatite
98. $CaCO_3$, $CaPO_4$, and $CaCl_2$
99. lamellar, cancellous
100. osteon or Haversian, trabeculae

Part 3: The Integument

101. Temperature, water, and Vitamin D
102. vasoconstriction and vasodilation. dehydration and infection. Sunlight
103. toxins and bacteria
104. epidermis, dermis, and hypodermis
105. Kertainized Stratified Squamous. Ectoderm
106. Dense Irregular Connective, mesenchyme
107. adipose, connective, mesoderm
108. stratum basale, stratum spinosum, stratum granulosum, stratum lucidum, stratum corneum

109. Germinatum; Basal Cells and Melanocytes
110. keratohyaline granules; melanin
111. waxy, granulosum; pigment
112. Lucidum. Keratin
113. Dendritic Cells; Merkel's
114. basal lamina
115. Basal cell, Malignant Melanoma
116. Papillary and Reticular
117. dermal papillae
118. capillary bed, Meissner's Corpuscles
119. Dense Irregular, sweat and sebaceous. Pacinian
120. Stratified Cuboidal; Eccrine and Holocrine
121. merocrine, head, palms and soles, pores. 99%
122. axillary and inguinal, hair follicles; body odor
123. oily, carbuncles
124. abscess
125. suppuration, cellulites
126. ulcer
127. granulation, scar
128. keloids
129. hyperemia, edema
130. epidermis, vesiculations
131. dermis and epidermis, grafts. dehydration and infection
132. bulb, root hair plexus
133. connective tissue, epithelial
134. hair papilla, hair matrix
135. arrector pili

Unit IV: Take a Test!

Time allowed: 45 minutes

Part 1:

1. Which layer differentiates into Glandular Tissue:
   a) Endoderm
   b) Mesoderm
   c) Mesenchyme
   d) Ectoderm

2. Which layer differentiates into the Epidermis:
   a) Endoderm
   b) Mesoderm
   c) Mesenchyme
   d) Ectoderm

3. Nervous Tissue is derived from which layer:
   a) Endoderm
   b) Mesoderm
   c) Mesenchyme
   d) Ectoderm

4. Muscle Tissue differentiates from which layer:
   a) Endoderm
   b) Mesoderm
   c) Mesenchyme
   d) Ectoderm

5. The endothelium of capillaries is derived from which layer;:
   a) Endoderm
   b) Mesoderm
   c) Mesenchyme
   d) Ectoderm

6. Which tissue is considered contractile:
   a) Epithelium
   b) Connective
   c) Muscle
   d) Nervous

7. Which tissue is considered conductive:
   a) Epithelium
   b) Connective
   c) Muscle
   d) Nervous

8. Functions of epithelial tissue include all of the following except:
   a) nutrient storage
   b) secretion
   c) protection
   d) filtration
   e) absorption

9. Which of the following is *not* a feature of epithelial tissue:
   a) high cellularity
   b) high mitotic rate
   c) polarity
   d) vascular
   e) basal lamina

10. Which of the following is **not true** of the basal lamina:
    a) it is a demarcation between epithelium and connective tissues
    b) it is composed of cells and fibers within a non–living matrix
    c) it serves as a nutritional source for adjacent epithelium
    d) it is comprised of ground substance–like material

11. Which connection anchors epithelium to its basal lamina:
    a) Tight Junctions   b) Gap Junctions
    c) Desmosome   d) Hemidesmosome   e) Aquapore

12. Osmosis would occur through:
    a) Tight Junctions   b) Gap Junctions
    c) Desmosome   d) Hemidesmosome   e) Aquapore

13. Which of the following is not associated with the apical surface of epithelium:
    a) cilia   b) basal lamina
    c) microvilli   d) pore   e) keratin

14. Which of the following moves mucus over the surface:
    a) cilia   b) lacuna
    c) microvilli   d) pore   e) keratin

15. Which of the following features increases surface area for absorption:
    a) cilia   b) lacuna
    c) microvilli   d) pore   e) keratin

16. Which feature reduces friction:
    a) cilia   b) lacuna
    c) microvilli   d) pore   e) keratin

17. Which is associated with goblet cells:
    a) cilia   b) lacuna
    c) microvilli   d) pore   e) keratin

18. The Connective Tissues all differentiate *directly* from:
    a) Endoderm   b) Mesoderm
    c) Mesenchyme   d) Ectoderm

19. All are considered classes of Connective Tissue except:
    a) CT Proper   b) Cartilage
    b) Osseous   d) Blood   e) all are CTs

20. Which is not a characteristic of all Connective Tissues:
    a) non–living matrix   b) ground substance
    c) cellularity   d) fibers   e) all are characteristics

21. Which of the following is a constituent found in the ground substance of **all** connective tissues:
   a) hydroxyapatite
   b) hyaluronic acid
   c) alkaline phosphatase
   d) metabolic acids
   e) chondroitin sulfate

22. Which is found only in the ground substance of cartilage:
   a) hydroxyapatite
   b) hyaluronic acid
   c) alkaline phosphatase
   d) metabolic acids
   e) chondroitin sulfate

23. Which is found only in the ground substance of osseous tissue:
   a) hydroxyapatite
   b) hyaluronic acid
   c) alkaline phosphatase
   d) metabolic acids
   e) chondroitin sulfate

24. Blood is classified as a Connective Tissue because:
   a) it has cells in a non–living matrix called plasma
   b) it has fibers in the form of soluble proteins
   c) it is derived from mesenchyme
   d) a and b
   e) a, b and c

25. Which tissue is noted for nutrient storage:
   a) adipose
   b) areolar
   c) hyaline cartilage
   d) dense regular CT
   e) reticular

26. Which tissue is generally found forming a vascular lining for epithelium:
   a) adipose
   b) areolar
   c) hyaline cartilage
   d) dense regular CT
   e) reticular

27. Which of the following can be found in lacunae:
   a) fibrocytes
   b) adipocytes
   c) chondrocytes
   d) osteoblasts
   e) none of these

28. Which of the following are spindle–shaped and found crammed in between the collagen fibers of tendons:
   a) fibrocytes
   b) adipocytes
   c) chondrocytes
   d) osteoblasts
   e) none of these

29. Which cell is capable of mitosis:
   a) fibrocytes
   b) adipocytes
   c) chondrocytes
   d) osteoblasts
   e) none of these

30. Which of the following is avascular:
   a) adipose
   b) areolar
   c) fibrocartilage
   d) osseous
   e) all are vascular

31. Red Blood Cells are properly known as:
   a) Leukocytes
   b) Erythrocytes
   c) Thrombocytes
   d) Hematoblast

32. Lymphocytes are classified as:
    a) Leukocytes
    b) Erythrocytes
    c) Thrombocytes
    d) Hematoblast

33. The structural unit of Compact Bone is called the:
    a) Osteon
    b) Trabecula
    c) Perisoteum
    d) Osteoclast

34. Functions of the Integument include all of the following except:
    a) activation of Vitamin D into D_3
    b) water preservation
    c) temperature control
    d) nutrient storage
    e) protection against infection

35. Which layer consists of dead, exfoliating cells:
    a) stratum basalis
    b) stratum spinosum
    c) stratum granulosum
    d) stratum lucidum
    e) stratum corneum

36. Ulcers are a break in continuity in which layer:
    a) stratum basalis
    b) stratum spinosum
    c) stratum granulosum
    d) stratum lucidum
    e) stratum corneum

37. Which is a sensory receptor found in the Epidermis
    a) Melanocyte
    b) Basal Cell
    c) Dendritic Cell
    d) Merkel's Disc
    e) Meissner's Corpuscle

38. Which produce pigment:
    a) Basal Cells
    b) Melanocytes
    c) Keratocytes
    d) Dendritic Cells
    e) Merkel's Discs

39. Which is the macrophage of the epidermis:
    a) Melanocyte
    b) Basal Cell
    c) Dendritic Cell
    d) Merkel's Disc
    e) Meissner's Corpuscle

40. The Papillary Region is composed of:
    a) Stratified Squamous
    b) Areolar CT
    c) Dense Irregular CT
    d) Elastic CT
    e) Dense Regular CT

41. The Reticular Region is composed principally of:
    a) Stratified Squamous
    b) Dense Irregular CT
    c) Areolar CT
    d) Reticular CT
    e) Dense Regular CT

42. Which layer is composed principally of adipose tissue:
    a) epidermis
    b) papillary
    c) reticular
    d) hypodermis

43. The sweat glands of the axilla and inguinal areas are known as:
    a) Eccrine
    b) Holocrine
    c) Sebaceous
    d) Cerumnious

44. The sweat glands found on the palms and soles are known as:
    a) Eccrine
    b) Holocrine
    c) Sebaceous
    d) Cerumnious

45. Which glands are associated with hair shafts:
    a) Eccrine
    b) Holocrine
    c) Sebaceous
    d) Cerumnious

46. A "pus pimple" is more properly known as :
    a) carbuncle
    b) abscess
    c) cellulitis
    d) keloid
    e) an ulcer

47. An encapsulated subcutaneous infection is called:
    a) carbuncle
    b) abscess
    c) cellulitis
    d) keloid
    e) an ulcer

48. Glands which burst releasing secretions and cytoplasm are known as:
    a) Eccrine
    b) Holocrine
    c) Cerminous
    d) Merocrine

49. The outer most surface layer of the hair shaft is called the:
    a) medulla
    b) cortex
    c) cuticle
    d) arector pili
    e) sebum

50. Which layer(s) is/are affected in Second Degree burns
    a) Epidermis
    b) Dermis
    c) Hypodermis
    d) a and b
    e) all three

Part 2: Go to our online Histology Atlas and Identify

Epithelium:

51. Simple Squamous
52. Simple Cuboidal
53. Simple Columnar
54. PSCCE
55. Non Keratinized Stratified
56. Keratinized Stratified
57. Transitional

Connective Tissues:

58. Mesenchyme
59. Areolar
60. Adipose
61. Reticular
62. Dense Regular
63. Dense Irregular
64. Elastic CT
65. Hyaline Cartilage
66. Elastic Cartilage
67. Fibrocartilage
68. Compact Bone
69. Blood/ Cell Types

Muscle:

70. Skeletal
71. Cardiac
72. Smooth

Nervous:

73. Neuron

Integument:

74. Thin Skin
75. Thick Skin/Layers

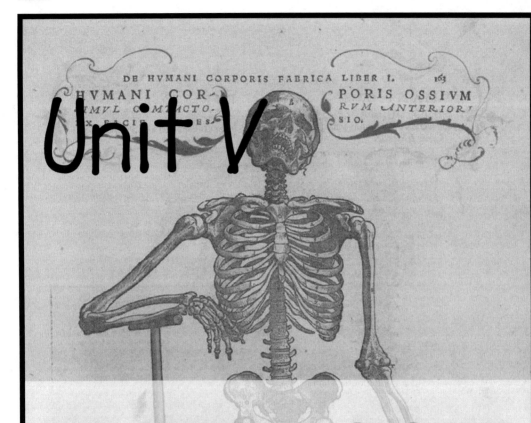

Unit V

THE SKELETAL SYSTEM

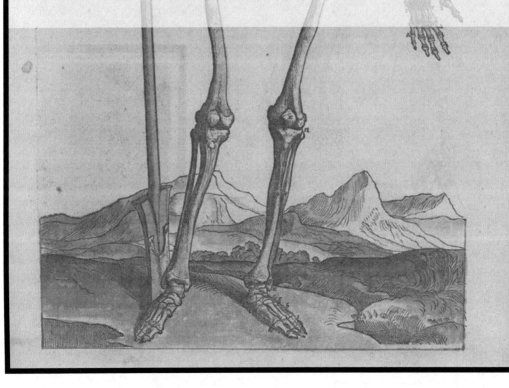

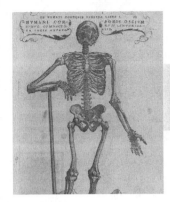

Part 1: Skeletal Tissue

1. Functions of the skeletal system include: _____, _____, _____, _____ _____, _____, and _____.

2. What three regions/organs are protected by the skeletal system? _____, _____ _____, and _____

3. Describe the hematopoietic function of the skeletal system: _____ _____.

4. Describe the respiratory function of the skeletal system: _____ _____.

5. Bone/osseous tissue is used to store _____ _____ (_____, _____, and _____) in its matrix and _____ within the medullary cavity.

6. The making of new bone matrix with the calcium salts $CaCO_3$, $CaCl_2$, and $CaPO_4$ is referred to as _____; the breakdown of bone tissue to release these nutrients is called _____.

7. The six structural types of bones include: _____, _____, _____, _____, _____, and _____.

8. How do the dimensions of long bones differ from short bones? _____ _____.

9. Examples of long bones include the _____ and the _____; Long bones possess _____ secondary ossification centers. Short bones include the _____ of the wrist and the _____ of the ankle.

10. Flat bones are noted for being slightly _____ and possess a central _____. Examples of flat bones include _____ bones, _____ and the _____.

11. Irregular bones are noted for possessing _____ _____ ossification centers and include the _____ and _____ bones of the skull.

12. Sesamoid bones are located within _____ and _____, and function by _____. Wormian bones are located within the _____.

13. The typical long bone is divided into four main regions: the _____, _____, _____, and the _____ _____.

14. The epiphysis is separated from the metaphysis in growing children by the _____ _____; in adults this closes and is visualized radiographically as the _____ _____.

15. The Epiphyseal Plate is composed of _____ _____ and is the site of _____ bone growth.

16. The medullary cavity is located within the _____ and contains _____ _____ in children, most of which is replaced with _____ _____ in adults.

17. Red marrow performs the _____ function of osseous tissue, whereas yellow marrow is _____ tissue and functions in _____ storage.

18. Three areas that red marrow persists in adults include _____, _____, and _____.

19. The three linings of a typical long bone include _____, _____, and _____.

20. The Periosteum is composed of two layers: the outer _____ layer and the inner _____ layer.

21. The Osteogenic layer contains which two cell types? _____ and _____ This layer is also the site of _____ bone growth.

22. Osteoblasts function by performing bone _____, whereas osteoclasts perform bone _____. Osteocytes are located within _____ and function by _____.

23. The Periosteum is attached to bone by _____ _____. The periosteum covers the _____ and _____, but never covers the _____.

24. The epiphyses are covered by _____ _____. All internal surfaces are covered by _____. Major nerves and blood/lymphatic vessels enter the bone through the _____ _____ of the diaphysis.

25. Articular cartilage is composed of _____ cartilage and receives nutrition from its surrounding _____.

26. The two types of bone tissue are _____, also called _____ bone, and _____, also called _____ bone.

27. The basic unit of structure of spongy/cancellous bone is the _____; spongy bone is found in the _____.

28. The basic unit of structure of compact/lamellar bone is the _____, or
    _____. Compact bone is found in the _____ of long bones and on the
    outside of _____ bones.

29. The _____ / _____ Canal runs down the long axis of the Osteon,
    whereas _____ Canal perforates it at a right angle. The concentric rings are called
    _____.

30. During ossification the matrix solidifying around the osteoblasts' cytoplasmic extensions form
    _____. Mature osteocytes maintain the matrix from within their _____.

31. Incomplete Osteons located between complete Haversian systems are called _____
    _____. Lamellae, which ring the shaft of the diaphysis, are called _____
    lamellae.

32. The organic portion of bone is called _____. The inorganic portion is called
    _____ and is composed of _____, _____, and _____.

33. Osteoid consists of _____, _____, and _____
    _____. What portion of bone tissue is inorganic? _____

34. The development of bone tissue is called _____, or _____. Bone
    depositing cells are called _____; bone resorbing cells are called _____.

35. The two mechanisms of osteogenesis/ossification are _____ and _____;
    of the two, _____ occurs first.

36. Intramembranous ossification begins before endochondral and forms the _____. Briefly
    describe/define "Intramembranous ossification": _____
    _____.

37. Endochondral ossification forms the _____ skeleton. Briefly describe/define "endochondral
    ossification": _____
    _____.

38. Intramembranous bone formation begins with the process of _____ within a
    Mesenchymal membrane.

39. The region in which Mesenchyme differentiates into osteoblasts is called the _____
    _____ Center.

40. Primary ossification centers expand and fuse internally forming a network of _____,
    which is referred to as _____ bone.

41. While woven bone is formed internally, the outer surfaces of the membrane differentiate into a
    _____. This allows for the formation of _____ _____
    externally.

42. As the osteogenic layer secretes compact bone externally, woven bone is replaced by _____
    bone and the vascular _____. Intramembranous bone formation is complete at
    _____.

43. The incomplete regions of ossification between cranial bones are known as _____; these will eventually ossify to form _____.

44. Fontanelles function by: _____.

45. Endochondral bone formation uses _____ models as templates; the first step in the process is the differentiation of the cartilage's _____ into a double-layered _____.

46. The _____ layer of the Periosteum secretes matrix, forming the _____ _____, which will support the cartilage model during _____.

47. Cavitation of the model is due to _____ _____

Bone/blood forming elements are brought inside the developing bone/cartilage model by the _____ _____.

48. The Periosteal Bud is responsible for the formation of _____ bone within the cartilage model.

49. The _____ _____ is formed by the resorption of woven bone by _____.

50. Periosteal buds also invade both epiphyses creating _____ _____ centers; the epiphysis is separated from the metaphysis by the _____ _____.

51. Secondary ossification centers form _____ bone within the epiphyses. The Epiphyseal Plates will be the site of _____ bone growth.

52. What occurs in Zone I of the Epiphyseal plate, closest to the epiphysis? _____

53. What is the fate of older chondrocytes in Zone II? _____ This will lead to the formation of _____ bone in Zone III.

54. The Woven Bone of Zone III will be _____ by osteoclasts, expanding the length of the _____ _____.

55. Longitudinal bone growth is dependent upon secretion of _____ hormone by the _____ _____ gland.

56. Growth hormone from the Anterior Pituitary functions in longitudinal bone growth by stimulating the _____ to release the hormone _____.

57. Somatomedins released by the liver stimulate _____ in Zone _____ of the _____ _____ to divide.

58. Excessive growth hormone results in _____; insufficient GH results in _____. In both conditions skeletal proportions appear _____.

59. Thyroid Hormone ensures _____ _____ _____.

60. Deposition of new osteons on the external surface of bone is called _____ bone growth.

61. The adolescent growth spurt and masculinization/feminization of bone structure is brought about by the hormones _____ and _____.

62. Estrogen and testosterone are known as _____, and eventually end _____ bone growth.

63. Appositional bone growth occurs within the _____ layer of the _____, and is stimulated by _____ _____.

64. Bone remodeling is performed by two cells: _____ and _____.

65. Osteoblasts function by secreting _____ _____; osteoclasts resorb bone matrix by secreting _____ _____ and _____ _____.

66. Calcium homeostasis maintains serum calcium at _____.

67. When calcium drops below 9mg/100 ml, the _____ gland secretes _____ Hormone.

68. PTH stimulates _____ activity to increase serum calcium.

69. When calcium rises above 11mg/100 ml, the _____ secretes _____.

70. Calcitonin stimulates _____ activity to decrease serum calcium.

71. Which vitamin is necessary for proper calcium absorption from the small intestine? _____

72. Vitamin D is activated into _____ by what mechanism? _____

73. After activation by sunlight, D$_3$ is then activated into _____ by the _____.

74. What are the effects of Vitamin D deficiency on developing bones? _____
_____

75. Vitamin C is necessary for proper _____ production. The effects of deficiency include
_____.

76. Wolff's Law states:
   a. _____,
   b. _____, and
   c. _____.

77. The first stage in fracture healing involves the formation of the _____ due to rupturing of blood vessels. The interruption of blood supply to an area is referred to as _____ and leads to cellular death, or _____.

78. Heparin functions as an _____; histamine is a _____.

79. The hematoma is soon resolved by growth of new _____ and removal of debris by
_____.

80. New capillaries bring _____ and _____ to the fracture site, which produce the _____ callus.

81. Fibroblasts secrete collagen fiber-based _____ tissue, which bridges the fracture. The cartilage produced will eventually be replaced by _____ _____.

82. Osteoblasts and osteoclasts replace the Fibrocartilaginous Callus with woven bone, forming the

    _____ _____.

83. How does an open/compound fracture differ from a closed/simple fracture? _____
_____

84. How does treatment differ in open and closed reductions? _____
_____

85. Briefly describe the appearance of:
    a. Compression _____
    b. Depressed _____
    c. Greenstick _____

86. Briefly describe the appearance of:
    a. Comminuted _____
    b. Spiral _____
    c. Impacted _____

87. Which disease is characterized by:
    a. reduced number of living osteocytes resulting in reduced matrix/bone density: _____
    b. reduced dietary calcium and Vitamin D (de-mineralized matrix) in adults causing deformity/bowing of weight bearing bones: _____
    c. reduced calcium and D (de-mineralized matrix) in children causing deformity of the Epiphyseal plates:

    _____

88. Osteoporosis affects what portion of the population? _____
Typical treatment includes _____.

89. How do the deformities of Ricketts differ from those of Osteomalacia? _____
_____

90. Which disease is characterized by:
    a. imbalances of osteoblast/-clast activity causing punched-out lesions of the skull and overgrowth of the pelvic bones: _____ Disease
    b. congenitally brittle bone tissue subject to pre- and postnatal fracture: _____

    _____

    c. bacterial infection, especially *staphylococcus*: _____

91. Paget's Disease is also known as _____ _____; Osteomyelitis is best treated with _____.

92. Of the three joint types, in which are bones joined/separated by a
    a. fibrous membrane: _____
    b. cartilage block: _____
    c. fluid-filled cavity: _____

93. By functional classification, which joints are:
    a. immovable: _____
    b. slightly movable: _____
    c. freely movable: _____

94. The three types of fibrous joints include: _____, _____, and
    _____.

95. Sutures connect cranial bones. An example of a syndemoses is _____
    _____. Which bones are involved in a gomphosis? _____ and
    _____

96. The root of the tooth sits within the _____ socket of the maxilla or mandible; the two
    bones are connected by the _____ Ligament.

97. What are the two cartilaginous joint types? _____ (cartilage bar) and
    _____ (fibro-cartilage disc)

98. An example of a synchodroses are the _____-_____ joints. Symphysis
    joints include _____ _____ and the _____ Symphysis.

99. Synovial joints are described as having _____ movement. Unlike the other two types,
    synovial joints are surrounded by a _____ _____ and separated by a
    _____ _____. The ends of the long bones, which make up the joint, are
    covered/lined by _____ _____.

100. The articular capsule is double-layered with an outer _____ layer and an
     inner _____ _____. The articular cartilage is composed of
     _____ cartilage.

101. The fibrous layer of the joint capsule is composed of _____ _____ CT;
     the joint cavity is filled with _____ _____. Synovial membrane covers all
     joint surfaces except those covered by _____.

102. Weight-bearing joints lose synovial fluid on a daily basis due to _____
     _____.

103. Briefly differentiate between the following reinforcing ligaments:
     a. Intrinsic/Capsular _____
     b. Extracapsular _____
     c. Intracapsular _____

104. An example of a fibro-cartilage disc within a synovial joint is the _____ of the knees. A
     flattened "purse" of synovial membrane that accompanies some joints is called a _____.

105. Bursae and tendon sheaths aid synovial joints by: _____.

106. Synovial joints that move in a single plane of motion are termed _____. Those that move in two planes: _____. Three or more: _____.

107. Joints in which articulating bone surfaces are flat to slightly curved are called _____ joints. Those in which one bone rotates about its central axis are _____.

108. Both plane and pivot joints exhibit which type of motion? _____. Plane joints are found as the _____ joints of the hand. An example of a pivot is the _____-_____ joint of the cervical spine.

109. In the Atlanto-Axial joint, C1 rotates around the _____ or _____ process of C2. What motion of the head does this allow? _____. The Atlanto-Occipital joint is a condylar joint. What shape are the articulating surfaces? _____ and _____ What unidirectional motion of the head is created? _____.

110. The elbow is an example of a _____ joint. What opposing motions does it allow? _____ and _____.

111. Unlike the rounded convex-concave surfaces of Condylar joints, those of Elliptical joints are _____ shaped and allow _____ movement. Ellipital joints are found as the _____-_____ joints (knuckles) of the hand.

112. What two planes of motion do metacarpal-phalangeal joints exhibit? _____-_____ and _____-_____ What other biaxial joint is found exclusively in the human hand? _____.

113. The Saddle joint of the human thumb allows which specialized motion? _____ How are the articular surfaces shaped? _____.

114. The joining of a globular head within a cup-shaped receptacle forms which joint type? _____-_____-_____ What type of motion does it allow? _____.

115. Multiaxial ball-in-socket joints are limited to the _____-_____ (shoulder) and _____ (hip) joints. Unlike simple rotation, these joints exhibit _____ (conical).

116. A muscle's anchoring on the "fixed" bone is called the _____; the muscle's attachment to the "moving" bone is its _____.

117. Which disease is characterized by:
    a. metabolic disorder: _____
    b. autoimmune disease: _____
    c. mechanical wear and tear: _____

118. In Gouty Arthritis, individuals genetically cannot break down _____. This elevates _____ _____, which forms _____ crystals.

119. Urate crystals from uric acid form _____ in the tragus of the ear and first metatarsal-phalangeal joint.

120. In Rheumatoid Arthritis (RA), antibodies attack the individual's _____ _____, resulting in _____. The principal joints affected include the _____, _____, and _____. It is uni/bilateral.

121. Bridging of the joint capsules is also called a _____; like many autoimmune diseases, RA is treated with _____.

122. Pannus formation leads to joint immobilization or _____.

123. Unlike RA, osteoarthritis is the mechanical breakdown of the _____ _____. Rather than an Ankylosis, the joint cavity diminishes resulting in fusion or a _____.

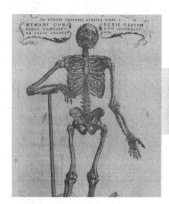

Part 2: The Human Skeleton

124. The human skeleton is divided into two main divisions: _____ and _____.

125. The Axial Skeleton is further subdivided into the _____, _____ _____, and _____ _____.

126. The skull can be divided into the _____, which houses the brain, and the _____.

127. Which type of bones are cranial? _____ Which type are facial? _____

128. What are the joints between cranial and facial bones called? _____ What type of joint are they? _____ What were they formed from? _____

129. Which suture separates the left and right parietal bones? _____ Which suture separates the frontal bone from the parietals? _____

130. The base of the skull is formed by the _____ bone. Which bones forms the sides of the cranium and bears the opening to the external ear? _____

131. Which suture separates the occipital bone from the rest of the cranium? _____ Which separates the temporal bones from the parietals? _____

132. Some irregular bones contain air-filled sinuses. Which are the paranasal sinuses? _____, _____, _____, and _____ bones

133. The "bridge" of the nose is comprised of the two _____ bones. Which bones are referred to as the "cheek" bones? _____

134. Which bones are noted in the nasal cavity? _____ and _____

135. The Ethmoid is noted for the Superior and Inferior _____ and the _____ _____, which projects into the cranium; the Vomer makes up the midline nasal _____.

136. The lateral processes of the Sphenoid are called the _____ _____; it is also noted for the _____ foramen in the back of the orbits and the midline depression, the _____ _____.

137. The roof of the oral cavity is formed by the left and right _____ bones. What is the proper name of the jaw? _____

138. What term is used to describe a convex surface? _____ A concave surface? _____ A pointed projection? _____ process

139. What type of bones are the vertebrae? _____ How many are: Cervical _____; Thoracic: _____; Lumbar: _____. How many segments form the sacrum? _____ fused; the coccyx: _____ fused.

140. The vertebral column presents anterior and posterior curves. What term is used to describe the anterior curve? _____ Posterior? _____

141. Which regions present an anterior lordosis? _____ and _____ A posterior kyphosis? _____ and _____ Which two are secondary curves? _____ and _____

142. Which two vertebrae are considered "atypical"? The _____ or _____, and _____ or _____.

143. What structure found on typical vertebra is missing from the Atlas/C1? _____ or _____ What structure on the Axis/C2 forms a pivot joint with the Atlas? The _____ or _____ process.

144. What foramen is in the transverse process of all cervical vertebrae? _____ Which artery passes through it? _____

145. What is the significance of the vertebral artery? _____

146. What surface feature is found only on the transverse processes and bodies of all thoracic vertebrae? _____

147. What type of joint is formed between the ribs and facets? _____ What type of cartilaginous joints do ribs form with the sternum? _____/_____

148. What type of cartilaginous joint is formed between vertebrae by the intervertebral discs? _____/_____

149. How are the rib pairs classified based on their hyaline cartilage/synchondroses joints? 1–7: _____, 8–10: _____; 11–12: _____

150. What are the segments of the sternum? _____, _____ or _____, and the _____ process. What small U-shaped bone is anterior to the cervical spine? _____

151. What is the superior aspect of the sacrum called? _____ or _____ What is the inferior aspect called? _____ What are the rounded projections on the posterior surface called? _____

152. What opening is found at the sacral apex? _____ What surface feature do the tubercles form? _____ _____

153. The two major divisions of the appendicular skeleton are the _____ and _____ extremities.

154. What are the divisions of the Upper Extremity? The _____ _____, _____, _____, and the _____.

155. What bones comprise the shoulder girdle? _____ and _____; the arm: _____; forearm: _____ and _____; the hand: _____, _____, and _____.

156. What projection of the scapula forms a joint with the clavicle? _____ What other bone does the clavicle form a joint with? _____

157. In addition to the Acromium, the _____ _____ forms a joint with the Humerus. What process only acts as a point of muscular attachment? _____

158. The proper name of the shoulder joint is the _____-_____. What type of joint is this? _____ _____-_____-_____

159. The proximal end of the Humerus is called the _____. What two surface features of muscular attachment are close to it? _____ and _____ _____

160. Distal to the Greater and Lesser Tuberosities, on the lateral aspect, is a projection named for the muscle that inserts there. It's called the _____ _____.

161. The distal end of the Humerus is noted for two convex surfaces: medially the _____ and laterally the _____.

162. What bone articulates with the Trochlear? _____ With the Capitulum? _____ What are the regions superior to each called? _____

163. What fossa is located between the Medial and Lateral Epicondyles on the anterior surface of Humerus? _____ On the posterior surface? _____

164. The proximal end of the Ulna is noted for the _____ _____. What is its distal end called? _____

165. What notch is formed within the Olecranon Process? _____ or _____ What is the "lip" on the anterior surface called? _____ _____ What motion is created here? _____/_____

166. What is the proximal end of the Radius called? _____ What does it articulate with on the Humerus? _____ What two motions are created here? _____/_____ and _____

167. How do the Radius and Ulna appear in anatomical neutral? _____ During full pronation? _____

168. Where does the head of the Radius articulate with the proximal Ulna? _____ notch. The distal Radius with the head of the Ulna? _____ notch. What projection are both bones noted for? _____ _____

169. How many carpal bones make up the wrist? ____; Which one does Radius articulate with? The _____. What are the other bones of the proximal row? _____, _____, and _____.

170. What are the carpals of the distal row, from lateral to medial? _____, _____, _____, and _____.

171. How many metacarpals are there? _____ How many phalanges? _____

172. What are the divisions of the Lower Extremity? The _____ _____, _____, _____, and the _____.

173. What bone(s) makes up the Pelvic Girdle? _____ or _____ The thigh? _____ The leg? _____ and _____ The foot? _____, _____, and _____

174. The Innominate Bone is subdivided into three portions: the _____, _____, and _____.

175. The Ilium, Ischium, and Pubis all meet in the "cup" which forms a joint with the femur called the _____ fossa. The hips are properly known as the _____ _____.

176. What type of joint does the Acetabulum form with the femur? _____-_____-_____ Surface landmarks of the Iliac Crest include the Anterior _____ _____ _____ and Posterior _____ _____ _____.

177. The Posterior Superior Iliac Spine helps locate which joint? _____-_____ What organ is located on the right halfway between the ASIS and the naval? _____ Between the ASIS and the pubis on both sides of the body? _____

178. What joint is formed between the left and right pubic bones? _____ What foramen is formed by the rami of the ischium and pubis? _____ What nerve trunk passes through the large notch superior to the ischial spine? _____

179. The head of the femur is noted for an indentation, the _____ _____. What are the large projections inferior to the neck? _____ and _____ _____.

180. The posterior surface of the femoral shaft is noted by a bony ridge, the _____ _____. What is the back of the distal femur known as? _____ _____ The anterior surface? _____ _____

181. The condyles of the distal femur forms the knee joint with the _____. What projection is between them? _____ _____

182. What projection is noted on the anterior surface of the proximal tibia? The _____ _____. What is the projection of the distal tibia? The _____ _____. What is the distal fibula called? _____ _____

183. Which tendon inserts into the tibial tuberosity? _____ What sesamoid is housed within it? _____

184. Which tarsal bone does the tibia rest on? The _____. Which is known as the heel bone? _____ Which forms the "keystone" of the medial arch of the foot? _____ Of the lateral arch? _____ The other three tarsal bones are the medial, intermediate, and lateral _____.

185. How many metatarsals are there? _____ How many phalanges? _____

Unit V: The Skeletal System

Part 1: Skeletal Tissue

1. Structure, protection, locomotion, nutrient storage, hematopoiesis, respiration
2. brain, spinal cord, heart and lungs
3. red marrow stem cells differentiate into all formed elements
4. expansion and contraction of rib cage creates inspiration and expiration
5. calcium salts ($CaCO_3$, $CaCl_2$, and $CaPO_4$); adipose
6. deposition; resorption
7. Long, Short, Flat, Irregular, Sesamoid, Wormian
8. Long Bones: length exceeds width; Short Bones: equal in all dimesions
9. Humerus and Femur; 2. carpals and tarsals
10. curved, diplöe. cranial, ribs, scapula
11. multiple secondary, vertebra, facial
12. tendons and ligaments, stabilizing joints. sutures
13. epiphysis, metaphysis, diaphysis, and medullary canal
14. epiphyseal plate; epiphyseal line
15. hyaline cartilage, longitudinal
16. diaphysis, red marrow, yellow
17. hematopoietic, adipose, nutrient
18. humerus, femur and sternum
19. periosteum, endosteum, and articular cartilage
20. fibrous, osteogenic
21. osteoblasts and osteoclasts. appositional
22. deposition, resorption. lacunae, maintaining the matrix
23. Sharpey's Fibers. diaphysis and metaphysis, epiphysis
24. articular cartilage, endostuem. nutrient canal
25. hyaline, perichondrium
26. spongy, cancellous; compact, lamellar
27. trabeculae, epiphysis
28. osteon, Haversian. diaphysis, flat
29. Haversian/Central, Volkman's. lamellae
30. canaliculi. lacunae
31. interstitial lamellae, circumferential
32. Osteoid; hydroxyapatite; $CaCO_3$, $CaCl_2$, and $CaPO_4$
33. cells, fibers and ground substance; 2/3
34. Osteogenesis or Ossification; osteoblasts, osteoclasts
35. intramembranous, endochondral; intramembranous
36. Cranium; mesenchymal membrane differentiates into bony tissue
37. fetal; hyaline cartilage models are destroyed and replaced by bone
38. differentiation
39. primary ossification
40. trabeculae, woven
41. periosteum; compact bone
42. spongy, diplöe, 15 weeks
43. fontanelles; sutures
44. allowing head to squeeze through birth canal
45. cartilage; perichondrium into periosteum
46. osteogenic, bony collar, cavitation
47. death of chondrocytes; perisoteal bud
48. woven
49. medullary canal, osteoclasts
50. secondary ossification; epiphyseal plate
51. spongy; longitudinal
52. chondroblasts divide
53. they die; woven
54. resorbed, medullary canal
55. Growth, Anterior Pituitary
56. liver, somatomedins
57. chondroblasts in Zone I, epiphyseal plate
58. giantism, dwarfism; distorted
59. proper bone proportions
60. appositional
61. estrogen and testosterone
62. androgens, longitudinal
63. osteogenic, perisosteum, physical stress
64. osteoblast and osteoclast
65. alkaline phosphatase; lysosomal enzymes and metabolic acids
66. 9–11mg/100 ml
67. Parathyroid, Parathyroid
68. osteoclast
69. Thyroid, calcitonin
70. osteoblast
71. D
72. D_3, exposure to sunlight/UV
73. Calcitriol, kidney

74. poor mineralization results in over-sized growth plates which deform bearing weight
75. collagen; poor wound healing
76. bones are thickest at their anatomical weak point; bones are thickened at muscle insertions; physical stress stimulates appositional growth
77. hematoma; ischemia; necrosis
78. anticoagulant; vasodilator
79. capillaries; macrophages
80. fibroblasts and chondroblasts; fibrocartilaginous callus
81. granulation; woven bone
82. bony callus
83. Closed/Simple does break through skin
84. Closed/Simple reduction does not require surgery
85. a. crushed, vertebral bodies in elderly
    b. broken inward on one side, cranial
    c. broken outward on one side, children
86. a. fragmented
    b. bone is fractured in spiral due to torque forces
    c. part shaft telescopes into other
87. Osteoporosis; Osteomalacia; Rickets
88. post-menopausal females; exercise, calcium supplementation, HRT
89. Rickets deformity is permanent
90. Paget's; Osteogenesis Imperfecta; Osteomyelitis
91. Osteitis Deformans; antibiotics
92. Fibrous; Cartilaginous; Synovial
93. Synarthrosis; Amphiarthrosis; Diarthrosis
94. Sutures, Syndemoses; Gomphosis
95. tibiofibular ligament; tooth and maxillary or mandible
96. alveolar; Periodontal
97. Synchodroses; Symphysis
98. costal-sternal; Intervertrbral discs; Pubic
99. diarthrotic; joint capsule, joint cavity; articular cartilage
100. fibrous, synovial membrane. hyaline
101. dense irregular. synovial fluid. cartilage
102. weeping lubrication
103. a. a thickened part of the capsule
     b. a separate, external structure
     c. a separate, internal structure
104. menisci; bursa
105. reducing friction
106. Uniaxial, Biaxial, Multiaxial
107. Plane; Pivot
108. Uniaxial; Intercarpal; Atlanto-Axial

109. Dens or Odontoid; side to side "No"; Convex and Concave; nodding "Yes"
110. Hinge; Flexion and Extension
111. Oval; Biaxial; Metacarpalphalangeal
112. Flexion-Extension and Abduction-Adduction; Saddle
113. Opposition; each surface is both concave then convex
114. Ball-in-Socket; Multiaxial
115. Glenohumeral and Acetabular; Circumduction
116. origin; insertion
117. Gouty arthritis; Rheumatoid; Osteoarthritis
118. purines; uric acid, urate
119. Tofi
120. joint capsule, bridging. knees, wrists, knuckles; bilateral
121. pannus; cortisone
122. ankylosis
123. articular cartilage; synostosis

Part 2: The Human Skeleton

124. Axial and Appendicular
125. skull, vertebral column and rib cage
126. cranium, face
127. flat, irregular
128. sutures, fibrous, fontanelles
129. sagittal, coronal
130. Occipital, Temporal
131. Lambdoidal, squamosal
132. Frontal, Ethmoid, Sphenoid and Maxillary
133. nasal, Zygomatic
134. Ethmoid and Vomer
135. conchae, crista galli; spetum
136. greater wings, optic, sella tursica
137. Maxillary; Mandible
138. Condyle, fossa, Styloid
139. irregular; 7, 12, 5, 5, 4
140. Lordosis, Kyphosis
141. cervical and lumbar; thoracic and sacral
142. Atlas or C1, Axis or C2
143. Body or Centrum; Dens or Odontoid
144. transverse; vertebral
145. forms the Circle of Willis
146. rib facets
147. synovial; hyaline/synchondroses
148. fibrocartilage/symphysis
149. true, flase, floating
150. manubrium, body or gladiolus, xiphoid; hyoid
151. body or promontory; apex; tubercles
152. hiatus; sacral crest

153. Upper and Lower
154. shoulder girdle, arm, forearm, hand
155. scapula and clavicle; Humerus; radius and ulna; carpals, metacarpals and phalanges
156. acromium; sternum
157. glenoid fossa; coracoid
158. gleno-humeral; false ball-in-socket
159. head; greater and lesser Tuberosities
160. deltoid Tuberosity
161. trochlear; capitulum
162. Ulna; Radius; epicondyles
163. coronoid; olecranon
164. olecranon process; head
165. trochlear or Semilunar; coronoid process; flexion/extension
166. head; capitulum; flexion/extension and pronation
167. parallel; radius crossed over the ulna
168. radial; ulnar; styloid processes
169. 8; scaphoid; lunate, triquetal and piceform

170. trapezium, trapezoid, capitate and hamate
171. 5; 14
172. pelvic girdle, thigh, leg and foot
173. innominate or coxal; femure, tibia and fibula; tarsals, metatarsals and phalanges
174. illium, ischium and pubis
175. acetabular; iliac crests
176. ball-in-socket; anterior superior iliac spine and posterior superior iliac spine
177. sacro-iliac; appendix; ovary
178. symphysis; Obturator; sciatic
179. fovea Capitus; greater and lesser trochantors
180. linea aspera; popliteal fossa; patellar fossa
181. tibia; intercondylar eminence
182. tibial Tuberosity; medial Malleolus; lateral Malleolus
183. quadriceps; patella
184. talus; calcaneus; navicular; cuboid; cuneiforms
185. 5, 14

Unit V: Take a Test!

Time allowed: 45 minutes

1. All of the following are functions of the Skeletal System *except:*
   a) Protection
   b) Movement
   c) Ventilation
   d) Hematopöeisis
   e) all are functions

2. How do bones perform nutrient storage:
   a) as hydroxyapatite
   b) as adipose tissue
   c) as red marrow
   d) a and b
   e) a, b and c

3. Bones which possess multiple secondary ossification centers are called:
   a) long bones
   b) short bones
   c) flat bones
   d) irregular bones
   e) sesamoid bones

4. A bone located within a tendon to stabilize a joint is classified as:
   a) long bones
   b) short bones
   c) flat bones
   d) irregular bones
   e) sesamoid bones

5. The proximal and distal ends of the long bone are called the:
   a) Metaphysis
   b) Epiphysis
   c) Diaphysis
   d) Epiphyseal Plate
   e) Medullary Cavity

6. The Epiphyseal Plates:
   a) increase in thickness throughout life
   b) separate the diaphysis and metaphysis
   c) are the site of longitudinal growth
   d) a and b
   e) a, b and c

7. The Epiphyseal Plates are formed from:
   a) Hyaline cartilage
   b) Fibrocartilage
   c) Elastic cartilage
   d) Fibrous membranes

8. The Periosteum:
   a) has an inner osteogenic layer
   b) is the site of appositional bone growth
   c) supplies nutrition to the Epiphyseal plates
   d) a and b
   e) a, b and c

9. Which of the following is not lined by endosteum:
   a) volkman's canal
   b) epiphysis
   c) medullary cavity
   d) haversian canal
   e) all are lined

10. Articular cartilage lines the surface of the:
    a) Diaphysis   b) Medullary Cavity
    c) Epiphysis   d) Epiphyseal Plate   e) Metaphysis

11. Hematopöeisis occurs in which area:
    a) red marrow   b) epiphyseal plate
    c) yellow marrow   d) endosteum   e) osteon

12. Compact Bone is generally found in the:
    a) Epiphysis   b) Metaphysis
    c) Diaphysis   d) a and b   e) all areas

13. Cancellous Bone is generally found in the:
    a) Epiphysis   b) Metaphysis
    c) Diaphysis   d) a and b   e) all areas

14. Which is the structural unit of spongy bone:
    a) lacuna   b) lamella
    c) trabeculae   d) osteon   e) canaliculi

15. Osteoid consists of all of the following except:
    a) hyaluronic acid   b) collagen fibers
    c) hydroxyapatite   d) osteoblasts   e) osteocytes

16. Which cell is responsible for bone resorption:
    a) Osteoclast   b) Osteocyte
    c) Osteoblast   d) all of these

17. Which cell is responsible for bone deposit:
    a) Osteoclast   b) Osteocyte
    c) Osteoblast   d) all of these

18. Which is true of Intramembranous bone formation:
    a) osseous tissue differentiates directly from mesenchyme
    b) the bones formed have a diplöe
    c) regions of incomplete ossification are called fontanelles
    d) suture joints are formed at the end of growth
    e) all are true

19. Which is the correct sequence of events:
    1) Periosteal Bud introduces Bone and Marrow elements
    2) Cavitation
    3) Secondary Ossification Centers form
    4) Formation of the Medullary Cavity
    5) Perichondrium differentiates into a Periosteum
    6) Formation of the Bony Collar
    a) 3,6,2,1,5,4   b) 6,2,3,5,4,1   c) 5,6,2,1,4,3   d) 2,6,3,1,4,5

20. Cavitation in endochondral ossification is due to death of:
   a) chondrocytes   b) osteocytes
   c) osteoblasts   d) fibrocytes   e) osteoclasts

21. The Medullary cavity is formed by the action of:
   a) chondrocytes   b) osteoblast
   c) osteoclast   d) osteocyte   e) chondroblasts

22. Osteoblast activity can be monitored by measuring serum levels of:
   a) metabolic acids   b) hyaluronic acid
   c) osteoid   d) hydroxapatite   e) alkaline phosphatase

23. Which event precedes the others in longitudinal bone growth:
   a) osteoid is secreted   b) osteoid is calcified
   c) chondroblasts divide   d) woven bone is formed
   e) osteoclasts extend medullary cavity

24. Chondroblasts of the Epiphyseal plate are stimulated by:
   a) physical stress   b) calcitonin
   c) PTH   d) thyroid hormone   e) somatomedins

25. Which hormone both initiates a "growth spurt" and ends longitudinal growth:
   a) Growth Hormone   b) Calcitonin
   c) Thyroid Hormone   d) Testosterone   e) PTH

26. The purpose of calcium homeostasis is to maintain:
   a) uniform bone development
   b) blood calcium levels at 9-11mg/100ml
   c) health of bone tissue
   d) thickness of compact bone
   e) all of these

27. Which is the most likely response to serum calcium dropping below 9mg/100 ml:
   a) the Kidney secretes Calcitriol to increase calcium absorption
   b) the Thyroid secretes Calcitonin to increase osteoblast activity
   c) the Parathyroid secretes PTH to increase osteoclast activity
   d) the Anterior Pituitary secretes Growth Hormone to increase chondroblast activity

28. Which of the following occurs in appositional bone growth:
   a) chondroblasts increase in numbers
   b) chondrocytes become woven bone
   c) osteons are formed by the osteogenic layer of the periosteum
   d) osteoblasts secrete new osteoid in the epiphyseal plate
   e) osteoclasts resorb woven bone making the diaphysis thinner

29. Why is proper daily intake of Vitamin D important to both children and adults:
    a) increases calcium resorption
    b) stimulates osteoclast activity
    c) stimulates osteoblast activity
    d) forms collagen fibers

30. Which of the following would be associated in Osteomalcia in adults:
    a) osteoid is poorly mineralized
    b) weight bearing bones bow out causing pain
    c) reduced bone density leads to fractures
    d) a and b
    e) all of the above

31. What are the consequences of Ricketts:
    a) Epiphyseal plates overgrow and deform
    b) The joint capsule calcifies
    c) Articular cartilage degenerates
    d) Reduced Growth Hormone causes Dwarfism
    e) bones become brittle and fracture

32. According to Wolff's Law:
    a) Bones are thickest where they are structurally weakest
    b) Bones are thicker at muscular attachments
    c) Bones get thinner in response to increased weight
    d) a and b
    e) a, b and c

33. Which fracture is most associated with vertebral bodies in patients with osteoporosis:
    a) comminuted
    b) compression
    c) depression
    d) greenstick
    e) spiral

34. In which of the following fractures does the diaphysis appear broken outward:
    a) comminuted
    b) compression
    c) depression
    d) greenstick
    e) spiral

35. The fibrocartilaginous callus:
    a) forms the pubic symphysis
    b) forms the embryonic skeleton
    c) forms the bridge between fractures
    d) forms the menisci of the knee

36. Which of the following is noted by decreased bone density due to reduced numbers of living osteocytes:
    a) osteitis deformans
    b) osteomyelitis
    c) ostemalacia
    d) osteogenesis imperfecta
    e) osteoporosis

37. Which implies a normal joint without movement:
    a) synarthrotic
    b) amphiarthrotic
    c) diarthrotic
    d) ankyloses
    e) synostosis

38. Multi-axial joints would be classified as:
    a) synarthrotic
    b) amphiarthrotic
    c) diarthrotic
    d) ankylosis
    e) synostosis

39. Joints formed by hyaline cartilage such as the Costal-sternals are classified as a:
    a) Gomphosis
    b) Symphysis
    c) Sutures
    d) Synovial
    e) Synchondroses

40. A 'gomphosis' is classified as:
    a) fibrous joint
    b) cartilaginous joint
    c) synovial joint
    d) diarthroses
    e) freely movable

41. Intervertebral Discs form which type of joints:
    a) Synchondroses
    b) Symphysis
    c) Syndemoses
    d) Synovial

42. IVD's have a poor healing rate because:
    a) they are not adapted for weight-bearing compression
    b) they are dependent upon their single nutrient canal
    c) they must depend on the periosteum for nutrition by diffusion
    d) they are avascular
    e) none of these are true

43. The outer Joint Capsule is formed from:
    a) dense regular CT
    b) dense irregular CT
    c) hyaline cartilage
    d) elastic cartilage
    e) fibrocartilage

44. Which would be considered an accessory structure to synovial joints:
    a) joint cavity
    b) synovial membrane
    c) menisci
    d) reinforcing ligaments
    e) joint capsule

45. Tendons and ligaments are formed from:
    a) dense regular CT
    b) dense irregular CT
    c) hyaline cartilage
    d) elastic cartilage
    e) fibrocartilage

46. Which of the following is classified as a genetic disease:
    a) osteoarthritis
    b) osteoporosis
    c) gouty arthritis
    d) rheumatoid arthritis
    e) osteomyelitis

47. Which of the following is best treated by antibiotics:
    a) osteitis deformans
    b) osteoporosis
    c) ostemalacia
    d) osteogenesis imperfecta
    e) osteomyelitis

48. In which disease does the patient's immune system attack the joint capsule:
    a) osteoarthritis
    b) osteoporosis
    c) gouty arthritis
    d) rheumatoid arthritis
    e) osteomyelitis

49. Which is noted by degeneration of the articular cartilage leading to a synostosis:
    a) rheumatoid arthritis
    b) osteoporosis
    c) gouty arthritis
    d) osteoarthritis
    e) osteomyelitis

50. Which implies the immobilization of a joint by calcification of its joint capsule:
    a) Symphysis
    b) Ankylosis
    c) Synostosis
    d) Synchondroses
    e) Synarthrosis

Part 2: Allow 30 minutes

1. The bones of the cranium are which type:
   a) flat
   b) irregular
   c) long
   d) short
   e) sesamoid

2. The bones of the face are which type:
   a) flat
   b) irregular
   c) long
   d) short
   e) sesamoid

3. The base of the skull is formed by the:
   a) Temporal
   b) Zygomatic
   c) Parietal
   d) Sphenoid
   e) Occipital

4. The left and right Parietal Bones are joined by which suture:
   a) Coronal
   b) Lambdoidal
   c) Sagittal
   d) Squamosal

5. Which suture separates the Occiput from the rest of the cranium:
   a) Coronal
   b) Lambdoidal
   c) Sagittal
   d) Squamosal

6. A needle-like bony projection is known as a _____ process:
   a) condyle
   b) fossa
   c) styloid
   d) tubercle
   e) trochanter

7. A convex articular surface is generally called a:
   a) condyle
   b) fossa
   c) styloid
   d) tubercle
   e) trochanter

8. Which bone helps form the nasal septum:
   a) Palatine
   b) Nasal
   c) Vomer
   d) Lacrimal
   e) Maxillary

9. The anterior portion of the hard palate is formed by the:
   a) Temporal
   b) Maxillary
   c) Vomer
   d) Lacrimal
   e) Mandible

10. Which is not considered a paranasal pneumatic/sinus bone:
    a) Maxillary
    b) Ethmoid
    c) Temporal
    d) Sphenoid
    e) Frontal

11. Teeth are associated with which bone:
    a) Maxillary
    b) Ethmoid
    c) Vomer
    d) Sphenoid
    e) Frontal

12. The optic foramen passes through which bone:
    a) Maxillary
    b) Ethmoid
    c) Vomer
    d) Sphenoid
    e) Frontal

13. Which process of the ethmoid projects into the cranial cavity:
    a) mastoid
    b) crista galli
    c) conchae
    d) pterygoid
    e) coronoid

14. The sella tursica is located within which bone:
    a) Maxillary
    b) Ethmoid
    c) Temporal
    d) Sphenoid
    e) Frontal

15. Vertebra are which class of bone:
    a) flat
    b) irregular
    c) long
    d) short
    e) sesamoid

16. There are _____ Cervical Vertebra:
    a) 2   b) 4   c) 5   d) 7   e) 12

17. The bony projection of the axis which forms a pivot joint with the atlas is called the:
    a) styloid
    b) odontoid
    c) mastoid
    d) coronoid
    e) olecranon

18. The sacrum is formed by _____ fused segments:
    a) 2   b) 4   c) 5   d) 7   e) 12

19. Which is only present in cervical vertebra:
    a) Rib Facets
    b) Transverse Foramen
    c) Articular Facets
    d) Transverse Processes
    e) Lamina

20. Which are only associated with Thoracic vertebra:
    a) Rib Facets
    b) Transverse Foramen
    c) Articular Facets
    d) Transverse Processes
    e) Lamina

21. Which of the following statements is true:
    a) all ribs articulate with the sternum
    b) ribs 1-7 form bony joints with the sternum
    c) ribs 8-10 have a common costal cartilage
    d) ribs 11 and 12 do not articulate with the spinal column
    e) all are true

22. The opening at the apex of the sacrum is called its:
    a) ala   b) base   c) tubercle
    d) hiatus   e) coccyx

23. The small process extending from the inferior aspect of the sternum is called:
    a) manubrium   b) gladiolus   c) xiphoid
    d) neck   e) facet

24. Which part of the scapula articulates with the clavicle:
    a) glenoid   b) acromion   c) coracoid
    d) coronoid   e) olecranon

25. The proper name of the shoulder joint is:
    a) gleno-humeral   b) acromial-clavicular   c) trochlear
    d) acetabular   e) popliteal

26. The _____ is the proximal end of the ulna:
    a) glenoid   b) acromion   c) coracoid
    d) capitulum   e) olecranon

27. The radius articulates with which process of the humerus:
    a) glenoid   b) trochlear   c) coracoid
    d) capitulum   e) olecranon

28. Which bone articulates with the radius at the wrist:
    a) pisiform   b) trapezoid   c) hamate
    d) scaphoid   e) cuneiform

29. The carpal bones are which type:
    a) flat   b) irregular   c) long
    d) short   e) sesamoid

30. There are _____ carpal bones:
    a) 6   b) 7   c) 8   d) 9   e) 10

31. On which region of the pelvic bone would one rest their hands when told to put them on their hips:
    a) ilium   b) ischium   c) pubis
    d) obturator   e) acetabulum

32. On which region would one properly 'sit':
   a) ilium
   b) ischium
   c) pubis
   d) obturator
   e) acetabulum

33. Which forms the os coxa with the femur:
   a) ilium
   b) ischium
   c) pubis
   d) obturator
   e) acetabulum

34. The thickened region of the femoral diaphysis is known as the:
   a) greater trochanter
   b) popliteal fossa
   c) linea aspera
   d) neck
   e) condyle

35. The posterior-inferior surface of the femur is known as the:
   a) patellar fossa
   b) popliteal fossa
   c) linea aspera
   d) neck
   e) condyle

36. Which is the point-of-attachment of the quadriceps tendon:
   a) greater trochanter
   b) medial malleolus
   c) lateral malleolus
   d) tibial tuberosity
   e) intercondylar eminence

37. The distal end of the fibula is called the:
   a) greater trochanter
   b) medial malleolus
   c) lateral malleolus
   d) tibial tuberosity
   e) intercondylar eminence

38. The tibia articulates with which bone:
   a) talus
   b) calcaneus
   c) cuboid
   d) navicular
   e) cuneiform

39. Which bone forms the heel:
   a) talus
   b) calcaneus
   c) cuboid
   d) navicular
   e) cuneiform

40. There are _____ tarsal bones:
   a) 6
   b) 7
   c) 8
   d) 9
   e) 10

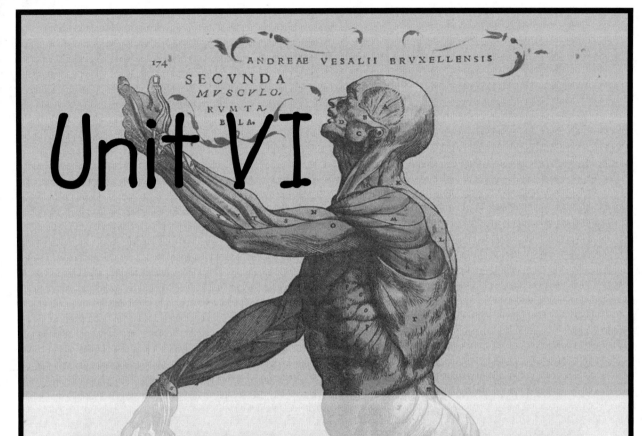

Unit VI

THE MUSCULAR SYSTEM

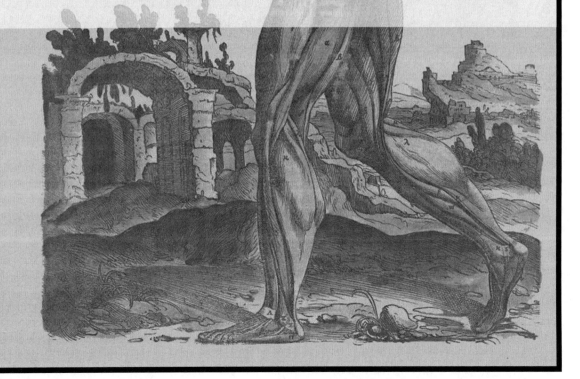

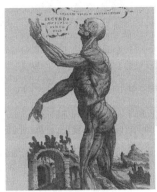

Part 1: Muscle Physiology

1. Muscle tissue is derived directly from embryonic _____; due to their elongate shape, muscle cells are referred to as _____.

2. All muscle fibers are amitotic, which means _____.
    List the three muscle fiber types: _____, _____, and _____.

3. Define:
    Excitability: _____
    Contractility: _____
    Extensibility: _____
    Elasticity: _____

4. Indicate if the fiber is uni-/multi-nucleate, invol-/voluntary and non-striated/striated:
    Skeletal: _____ _____ _____
    Cardiac: _____ _____ _____
    Smooth: _____ _____ _____

5. The striations of skeletal and cardiac muscle are formed by _____
    _____.

6. Multinucleate skeletal fibers are formed by the fusion of many embryonic cells which now function as one unit; this is called a _____. Skeletal fibers are voluntary because each fiber has its own
    _____ _____.

7. Although separate cells, all the cardiac fibers in an individual chamber act as a functional syncytium because of the _____ _____, which acts as an electrical connection.

8. Define peristalsis: _____
    _____.

9. The shortening of muscle fibers is accomplished by the movement of the microfilaments
    _____ and _____; because they are associated with muscle, these
    micro-filaments are also referred to as _____.

10. Blood pressure is measured during systole, then diastole (120/80). What type of muscular activity is measured during systole? _____.
During diastole? _____.

11. In terms of the muscle tissue, systemic hypertension is due to _____
_____.

12. Vasoconstriction by the smooth muscle walls of blood vessels also conserves body heat. How does the muscular system generate heat? _____
_____

13. Shivering is initiated by the _____ What mechanism reduces body heat?
_____

14. The specialized cell/plasma membrane of a skeletal muscle fiber is called the _____.
Individual fibers are wrapped within a CT sheath called the _____.

15. Fibers and their surrounding endomysium are bundled into _____; these are surrounded by the CT _____.

16. Fasicles and their surrounding perimysium are bundled together to form the _____
_____, which is surrounded by the _____.

17. Some skeletal muscles and their surrounding epimysiums form functional groups surrounded by
_____.

18. What specialized characteristic does the sarcolemma exhibit? _____ This means that it can be _____ when adequately stimulated.

19. Cytoplasm refers to cytosol and accompanying organelles. What term is used to describe the contents of skeletal fibers? _____

20. What two compounds make sarcoplasm different than cytoplasm? _____ and
_____

21. What is the function of Myoglobin? _____
What is glycogen? _____

22. What three structures/organelles are found only in the sarcoplasm of skeletal fibers?
_____-_____, _____ _____, and
_____

23. The sarcolemma conducts the depolarization wave to the _____-_____.

24. The T-tubule is the conductive pathway from the sarcolemma to the _____
_____.

25. What is the function of the sarcoplasmic reticulum? _____
What structures does it surround? _____

26. What compound holds calcium within the sarcoplasmic reticulum? _____

27. Myofibrils are also known as _____ _____. Each myofibril is composed of a string of contractile units called _____.

28. Individual sarcomeres are attached at their _____ _____. The striations of skeletal fibers are created by the alignment of the contractile proteins _____ and _____.

29. Thin actin myofilaments create light regions referred to as the _____ Bands. Thick myosin myofilaments create the darker _____ Bands. The middle of the myosin filament is noted for the _____ Line.

30. The "M Line" is composed of which regulatory protein? _____ Which regulatory protein attaches the "M Line" to the "Z Disc"? _____

31. Titin gives which characteristic to muscle tissue? _____

32. During relaxation, actin fibers extending into the A Band are separated by the _____ Zone. The globular ends of myosin are known as _____.

33. During contraction myosin crossbridges attach and pull actin into the H zone up to the M line. What compound inhibits crossbridge attachment during relaxation? _____

34. What environmental change in the sarcomere inhibits tropomysin? _____

35. By what mechanism does Ca^{+2} move from the sarcoplasmic reticulum to the sarcomere? What compound holds calcium inside the sarcomere? _____

36. Why is it important for calcium to bind to troponin? _____
_____

37. a: _____
38. b: _____
39. c: _____
40. d: _____
41. e: _____
42. f: _____
43. g: _____
44. h: _____
45. i: _____

46. The meeting of nerve and muscle is called the _____-_____ Junction. The swollen ends of the telodendria are called the _____ _____.

47. The specialized region of the sarcolemma at the neuromuscular junction is called the
_____ _____ _____; it is separated from the
telodendria's synaptic bulb by the _____ _____.

48. The sarcolemma's motor end plate is noted for its creased _____ _____.
The synaptic gutter is filled with _____ _____.

49. The motor end plate's junctional folds have specific _____ _____. The
synaptic bulb contains _____ _____.

50. Synaptic vesicles contain the neurotransmitter _____(_____). How does a nerve
impulse stimulate its release? _____
_____.

51. After increased calcium permeability stimulates exocytosis, ACh crosses the fluid-filled synaptic gutter by
_____.

52. Prior to ACh stimulation, the end plate and sarcolmma are said to be polarized. What does this mean?
_____

53. How is the resting potential of the sarcolemma maintained by ion balance? _____
_____

54. When ACh binds to a receptor site it creates an _____ _____
_____.

55. During an end plate potential _____ permeability increases. This allows _____
_____.

56. When Na^+ rushes inside the fiber during the end plate potential, it changes the charge inside from
_____ to _____; this is called a _____.

57. Define threshold: _____
_____

58. End plate potentials are individual depolarizations that accumulate to reach threshold and stimulate an
action potential. What is an action potential? _____
_____

59. The action potential is also referred to as the Ca^{+2} signal. Why? _____
_____

60. After the AP is conducted from the sarcolemma to the t-tubule to the sarcoplasmic reticulum, Ca^{+2} is
released and moves into the sarcomere along an electrochemical gradient. What prevents it from flowing
back when the gradient reverses? _____. How does Ca^+ bring about contraction/
shortening in the sarcomere? _____

61. A single muscle fiber contraction is called a _____.

62. What is meant by the "all or none" effect of muscle fiber contraction? _____
_____

63. If skeletal fibers contract 100% or not at all, why are skeletal muscle contractions graded?

_____

64. What must occur in order for a contracted fiber to relax/return to resting length?

_____

65. What enzyme breaks the Troponin-Ca^+ bond? _____-_____-_____

66. Ca^{+2}-ATP-ase is released in response to what "new" signal? _____

67. Repolarization is initiated immediately after the start of the _____ _____.

68. The start of the action potential stimulates the motor end plate to secrete the enzyme

_____.

69. Acetylcholinesterase degrades ACh into _____ and _____, breaking the
bond with the receptor sites. This allows the motor end plate to _____.

70. What changes to the ion/charge balance take place during repolarization?

_____

71. What specific event ends the Ca^{+2} signal? _____

_____

72. Define refractory: _____

_____

73. What occurs after Ca-ATP-ase breaks the Ca-Troponin bonds? _____

_____

74. Which events occur faster: electrical or chemical?
    Which occurs faster: Repolarization or Ca^{+2} diffusion back to the SR?

75. Must all the Ca^{+2} leave the sarcomere before a fiber is ready to contract again? _____

76. What effect is created when Ca^{+2} return lags behind repolarization? _____

77. Describe the Treppe effect: _____

_____

78. As higher levels of Ca^{+2} remain in the sarcomere, contractions become stronger and longer leading to

_____.

79. Tetany is defined as _____.

80. When a muscle is in tetany and cannot relax, it is called a _____, or muscle

_____.

81. Contractures are due to _____.

82. Contractions in which muscle tension increases but muscle length remains unchanged are called
    _____. Those in which muscle length shortens but tension remains unchanged are

_____.

83. The principal source of energy for aerobic cells is _____.

84. ATP cannot be stored; the principal source of energy for coupling ADP and P is _____.

85. The process by which free energy for ATP coupling is obtained by the dismantling of glucose is called _____.

86. The oxidation of glucose is also called _____ _____.

$$C_6H_{12}O_6 + 6H_2O + 6O_2 \rightarrow 6CO_2 + 12H_2O + 38ATP\ (38ADP + 38\ P)$$

87. What is the source of CO_2 in the above equation? _____
    What is the source of energy for the coupling of ADP and P? _____
    What is the function of oxygen? _____

88. Aerobic respiration is subdivided into 4 stages. The first stage occurs in the _____ and is called _____.

89. Glycolysis means "_____ _____" and requires an input of _____ _____.

90. With the input of 2 ATPs enzymes split glucose in "half" yielding two molecules of _____, as well as coupling _____ ATPs and bonding _____ H^+ to NAD.

91. The two pyruvates can each now enter Stage 2, which is called _____-_____- _____. This occurs in the _____.

92. Each pyruvate requires _____ _____ in order to enter the mitochondria of skeletal fibers and begin Stage 2 Acetyl-Co-A. These are supplied by _____. Once inside, these reactions occur on the _____.

93. Stage 2 is brief and is noted for the removal of _____ and the bonding of _____ H^+ to NAD. Stage 2 ends with each pyruvate's conversion to _____-_____-_____.

94. Each Acetyl-Co-A enters the _____ _____ or _____ Cycle. Each binds to the compound _____, which is recycled at the end.

95. Acetyl-Co-A combines with oxaolacetate to form _____.

96. During the Citric Acid/Kreb's Cycle, citrate is decarboxylated and H^+ is bound to _____ and _____. What compound is left at the end of the cycle? _____

97. NAD and FADH are called _____ _____. When bonded to H^+, they are known as _____ and _____, respectively.

98. NADH and $FADH_2$ carry their electrons into Stage 4, which is known by four descriptive processes that occur: the _____ _____ system, _____ _____, _____ _____, and _____.

99. The Electron Transport System implies that _____ _____.

100. What type of chemical reaction occurs as electrons are passed from carrier to carrier? _____

101. When is a compound reduced? _____
     When is it oxidized? _____

102. The Cytochrome Sink describes _____
     _____.

103. Chemiosmosis describes _____
     _____.

104. What enzyme is activated by the Proton Pump? _____ What reaction does it catalyze?
     _____ _____

105. Oxidative Phosphorylization describes _____
     _____.

106. What is the source of free energy for ATP synthesis? The _____ _____
     System.

107. What is O_2's role in Stage 4 of aerobic respiration? _____

108. What occurs if there is insufficient O_2 to bond with the used H^+ ions to form H_2O? _____
     _____

109. Without sufficient O_2, ATP coupling halts and pyruvates can no longer enter the mitochondria. What
     stage of aerobic respiration still continues? _____

110. Glycolyis continues without O_2 and is called _____. The pyruvates produced, however,
     ferment into _____ _____.

111. Lactic Acid buildup creates _____ _____.

112. Fatigue is defined as _____
     _____.

113. How is oxygen debt created? _____
     _____

114. What happens to lactic acid after activity stops and O_2 levels rise? _____
     _____

115. Anaerobic respiration requires 2 ATP and produces 4 ATP. Why is this of little help during muscle
     activity? _____
     _____

116. In addition to aerobic and anaerobic respiration, cells can obtain ATP from _____
     _____.

117. Creatine Phosphate combines with _____ to produce _____ ATP + Creatine + P.

118. What is the direct effect of rigor mortis in the sarcomere? _____ _____ _____

119. Why do the myosin crossbridges remain permanently attached? _____
     _____

120. Muscle rigidity begins within _____ hours and peaks after _____ hours. Muscle tissue begins to soften after 60 hours. What does this indicate? _____

121. Define Paralysis: _____

122. What is spastic paralysis? _____

123. What is flaccid paralysis? _____

124. How does curare cause flaccid paralysis? _____

_____

125. Define Atrophy: _____
     Atrophy can be caused by _____ or _____ .

126. Disuse Atrophy is reversible and is commonly due to _____ .

127. Define Hypertrophy: _____
     Hypertrophy is caused by _____ .

128. How does hypertrophy compare in skeletal versus cardiac fibers? _____

_____

129. Reduced or lack of blood supply to cardiac muscle is called _____ .

130. During ischemia, muscle fibers are deprived of _____, resulting in necrosis. This leaves an area of dead tissue called an _____ .

131. Increased smooth muscle activity is called _____ .

132. A common ailment associated with hypermotility of the large intestinal wall is _____ . A life-threatening amoebic infection of the intestine is _____ .

133. The life-threatening effects of dysentery are _____ and _____

_____ .

134. How is hypermotility related to ulcerative colitis? _____

_____

135. Decreased smooth muscle activity is called _____ .

136. What common ailment is associated with hypomotility of the colon? _____
     What is an ileus? _____

137. Tetanus produces a _____, which causes _____ paralysis. Botulism's neurotoxin causes _____ paralysis.

138. Spastic paralysis eventually causes death by _____ . How is this brought about?

_____

139. Botulism victims also die of asphyxiation, but by flaccid paralysis. How is this brought about?

_____

140. How is trichinosis most commonly contracted? _____
     Why is it referred to as the "muscle worm"? _____
     _____

141. What is fibromyalgia? _____
     _____

142. Define Strain: _____.
     Define Sprain: _____.

143. Define Congenital: _____.

144. What are the two principal causes of Cerebral Palsy? _____ and _____
     _____

145. The Upper Motor Neurons (UMNs) damaged during birth from hypoxia or trauma results in
     _____
     _____.

146. Define Iatrogenic: _____.

147. Epilepsy is characterized by _____.

148. Epileptic seizures are created by _____.
     Epilepsy can be the result of _____ _____ and sustained
     _____ _____

149. Muscular Dystrophy (MD) is classified as what type of disease? _____. MD generally
     leads to the metabolic _____.

150. The result of the metabolic breakdown of the neuromuscular junction is _____; MD
     generally causes death by _____.

151. Myasthenia gravis is classified as what type of disease? _____

152. The autoimmune antibodies produced in myasthenia gravis attack and destroy the _____
     _____ of the _____ _____ _____.

153. The result of reduced receptor sites on the motor end plate leads to _____
     _____.

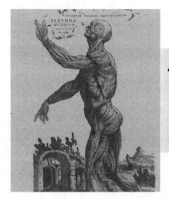

Part 2: The Skeletal Muscle System

154. The anchoring of a muscle to its fixed bone is called the _____; the attachment of a muscle's tendon to the moving bone is called the _____.

155. Describe the actions of the origin and insertion during contraction: _____
_____.

156. What are muscles of opposing function called? _____

157. What occurs to muscle's antagonist when it contracts? _____

158. What happens to a muscle's antagonist when it is stretched? _____

159. What is the clinical/therapeutic value of passive contraction? _____
_____

160. Define flexion: _____.
What is its antagonist motion? _____

161. In addition to increasing the angle between bones, extension is also defined by: _____
_____.

162. What regions of the body exhibit hyperextension? _____ and _____
_____ What formations of the bones of joints such as the elbow prevent hyperextension?
_____ _____ What term describes the bending of the side of the head to the shoulder? _____ _____

163. What other region displays lateral flexion? _____ _____

164. What specialized motion decreases the angle between the foot and the tibia? _____
What is the "top" surface of the foot called? _____

165. Describe how one walks during dorsiflexion: _____.
What is the antagonist motion to dorsiflexion? _____

166. Describe how one walks during plantarflexion: _____.
What is the sole of the foot also known as? _____ _____

167. How do the palms face when in the anatomical neutral position? _____

168. Bringing the palms to face anterior/forward is the properly known as: _____.

169. What is the antagonist action to supination? _____ What term describes the "back"/posterior surface of the hand? _____

170. Define abduction: _____.
What is its antagonist action? _____

171. Spreading out of the fingers is known as adduction/abduction. Bringing the fingers together is called: _____. What exclusive motion of the human thumb allows for grasping? _____

172. What motion is the antagonist to opposition? _____

173. Define rotation: _____.
How is rotation described in the humerus? _____ or _____

174. How does circumduction differ from rotation? _____

175. What type of joint exhibits Rotation? _____ Which type exhibits Circumduction? _____-_____-_____

176. What are the two Ball-in-Socket joints (proper names)? _____ and _____

177. What motion describes drawing back of the scapulae? _____

178. What is the antagonist to Retraction? _____

179. Although the mandible protracts and retracts, what motion describes chewing? _____

180. Define "Eversion": _____.
What is its antagonist motion? _____

181. Muscles are often named for the alignment of their fascicles; what is the proper term for: straight (superior to inferior): _____; across (left to right): _____; at an angle: _____.

182. Muscles are often named for their shape. Draw a:

Trapezoid: Rhombus: Delta:

183. What shape is an "Orbicularis" muscle? _____

184. What term describes a muscle with two origins/heads? _____; three: _____; four: _____

185. Which muscle raises the upper lip? _____ _____ _____

186. Which muscle produces the smile? _____

187. Which muscle squints the eye? _____ _____

188. Which muscle raises the eyebrows? _____

189. Which muscle forms the cheek and is the principal of mastication? _____

190. Which muscle purses the lips? _____

191. Which muscle compresses the cheeks and allows whistling? _____ _____

192. Head/Neck extension and lateral flexion are the function of the _____.

193. Head/Neck rotation is a function of the _____.

194. Which muscle draws the lip downward into a frown? _____ _____ _____

195. Which is a sheet-like muscle covering the anterior neck? _____

196. Which muscle, named for its cranial origin, assists in mastication? _____

197. Which muscle forms the posterior element of the epicranious? _____.

198. Which deep muscles connect the cervical spine to the upper ribs like guy-wires on an antenna? _____

199. The Scalenes perform which motions: _____ and _____.

200. Which bone acts as an origin for the deep muscles of the anterior neck? _____

201. Which muscle laterally flexes adjacent vertebrae? _____

202. Which muscle originates on the transverse process and inserts into the lamina above it? _____

203. Which muscle extends adjacent vertebrae? _____

204. Which muscle originates on the transverse process and inserts into the spinous above it? _____

205. Which is the primary Abductor of the shoulder? _____.

206. Which two antagonists to the Deltoid form the borders of the axilla? _____ _____ and _____ _____

207. Besides Adduction, what other shoulder action is performed by the Pectoralis Major? _____ _____; by the Latissimus dorsi? _____ _____

208. Which muscle, named for its knife-edge appearance, pulls the scapula forward and acts as a secondary respirator? _____ _____

209. What word is also used for "humerus"? _____

210. Which muscle, named for its origin on the scapula and insertion on the humerus, flexes the arm? _____

211. Which pair of muscles, named for their shape and respective sizes, retract the scapula? _____ _____ and _____ _____

212. What are the four muscles of the Rotator Cuff? _____, _____, _____ and _____ _____

213. What bone do all four muscles insert into? _____ What motion do they create? _____ What other function do they provide to the shoulder girdle? _____

214. Which muscle, named for its number and location of origins/heads, crosses both the shoulder and elbowti? _____ _____

215. What two actions are performed by the Biceps Brachii? _____ _____ and _____ _____

216. Which similarly named muscle also crosses two joints, is the primary forearm extensor and assists the Latissimus in arm extension: _____ _____

217. What is the common origin of all wrist flexors? _____ Wrist extensors? _____

218. Which muscle, named for the humerus, is deep to the Biceps and flexes the forearm? _____

219. Based on its name, what are the origin and insertion of the "Flexor Carpi Radialis"? _____ and _____

220. Based on its name, what are the origin and insertion of the "Extensor Carpi Ulnaris"? _____ and _____

221. Which muscle turns the palms face-down/posterior? _____ _____

222. Muscles of the thumb are collectively called _____. What word also means "thumb"? _____

223. Which muscle allow for grasping? _____ _____

224. What muscle acts as the antagonist to Opposition? _____ _____

225. Which muscles of the hand Flexes the fingers? _____ Which groups Adduct and Abduct the fingers? _____

226. Which muscle flexes the trunk? _____ _____

227. Which muscles rotate and laterally flex the trunk? _____ _____ and _____ _____

228. What three muscles comprise the "Erector Spinae" group? _____, _____ and _____

229. What are the three primary muscles of respiration? _____ and _____ _____, and the _____ _____

230. Describe the musculo-skeletal actions of Inspiration: _____ _____.

231. Describe the musculo-skeletal actions of Expiration: _____ _____.

232. What constitutes a secondary muscle of respiration? _____ _____

233. Which two muscles flex the trunk onto the thigh? _____ and _____

234. Which muscle is the primary hip/thigh extensor? _____ _____

235. Which muscle is the primary hip/thigh abductor? _____ _____

236. Which action is performed by both the Pectineus and Gracilis? _____

237. List the four muscles of the Quadriceps Femoris group: _____ _____, _____ _____, _____ _____, and _____ _____.

238. What action do they perform? _____ _____

239. List the three primary muscles of knee flexion: _____ _____, _____, and _____.

240. What name is given to this knee flexor group? _____

241. Which is the Lateral Hamstring? _____ _____

242. Which muscle flexes the knee and crosses the leg? _____

243. Which deep muscle originates on the anterior surface of the sacrum, inserts into the posterior greater trochantor, and externally rotates the femur? _____

244. Which muscle is the primary dorsiflexor? _____ _____

245. Which two muscles assist the Tibialis Anterior? _____ _____ _____ and _____ _____ _____

246. What term means "big toe"? _____

247. Which muscles evert the foot? _____ _____ and _____

248. Which three muscles perform plantarflexion? _____, _____, and _____

249. What common tendon do these plantar muscles form? _____

Unit VI: The Muscular System

Part 1: Physiology

1. Mesoderm; fibers
2. they do not divide. Skeletal, Cardiac and Smooth
3. Ability to detect and respond to stimuli; ability to shorten forcibly when adequately stimulated; ability to stretch beyond resting length; ability to recoil back
4. multi-, vol, striated;
   uni-, invol, striated;
   uni-, invol, non-striated
5. alignment of actin and myosin
6. Syncytium; nerve supply
7. intercalated disc
8. Rhythmic, wave-like contractions of smooth muscle
9. actin and myosin; myofilaments
10. cardiac muscle contraction; smooth muscle resistance of aorta
11. increased smooth muscle constriction of vascular tree
12. friction generated by actin and myosin and skeletal muscles
13. hypothalamus; vasodilation of peripheral vessels
14. sarclemma; endomysium
15. fasicles; perimysium
16. skeletal muscle, epimysium
17. fascia
18. excitable; depolarized
19. sacroplasm
20. myoglobin and glycogen
21. binds to oxygen; animal starch
22. T-Tubule, Sarcoplasmic Reticulum, myofibrils
23. T-tubule
24. sarcoplasmic reticulum
25. calcium storage; myofibril
26. calsequestrin
27. contractile elements; sarcomeres
28. Z Lines; actin and myosin
29. I Bands; A Bands; M Line
30. Myomesin. Titin
31. Elasticity
32. H Zone; crossbridges
33. Tropomysin
34. increased calcium in the sarcomere
35. by diffusion along a gradient; Troponin

36. prevent calcium from diffusing back out before inactivating Tropomysin
37. I Band
38. A Band
39. H Zone
40. Crossbridge
41. Z Line
42. M Line/Myomesin
43. Myosin/Thick Filament
44. Titin
45. Actin/Thin Filament
46. neuro-muscular junction; synaptic bulb
47. motor end-plate; synaptic gutter
48. junctional folds; interstitial fluid
49. receptor sites; synaptic vesicles
50. acetylcholine (ACh); increases calcium permeability which stimulates exocytosis of synaptic vesicles
51. diffusion
52. the outside of the embrane bears a (+) charge, the inside (−)
53. Na$^+$ outside, weaker K$^+$ inside
54. end-plate potential
55. Na$^+$; Na$^+$ to rush in and K$^+$ to rush out
56. (−) to (+); depolarization
57. minimum number of end-plate potentials/ depolarizations required to initiate an action potential
58. wave of depolarizations that sweeps across the entire sarcolemma
59. when conducted by T-tubule to sarcoplasmic reticulum it stimulates calcium release
60. troponin; inhibits tropomysin allowing crossbridges to attach
61. twitch
62. a fiber contracts 100% or not at all
63. degree of contraction dependent on number of individual fibers recruited
64. calcium levels must drop allowing tropomysin to reactivate and block crossbridges
65. Ca-ATP-ase
66. repolarization
67. action potential
68. acetylcholinesterase

69. choline and acetone; repolarize
70. K⁺ rushes out changing the charge inside the membrane (−)
71. the degradation of ACh
72. the period of time repolarization that a fiber is immune to stimulus
73. Calcium diffuses out of the sarcomere and into the sarcoplasmic reticulum
74. electrical, repolarization
75. no
76. treppe
77. consecutive contractions occur sooner, last longer and are stronger
78. tetany
79. inability to relax
80. contracture, spasm
81. sustained high calcium in the sarcomere
82. isometric; isotonic
83. ATP
84. glucose
85. oxidation
86. aerobic respiration
87. glucose ($C_6H_{12}O_6$); hydrogen; remove waste hydrogen as water
88. cytosol, glycolysis
89. sugar-splitting, 2 ATP
90. pyruvate, 4 ATPs, 2H⁺
91. Acetyl-Co-Enzyme-A; mitochondria
92. 1 ATP; the net 2 ATPs from Glycolysis; cristae
93. CO_2, 2H⁺; Acetyl-Co-Enzyme-A
94. Citric Acid or Krebs. oxaloacetate
95. citrate
96. NAD and FADH; oxaloacetate
97. electron carriers; NADH and FADH₂
98. Electron Transport; the Cytochrome Sink; Chemiosmosis; Oxidative Phosphorylization
99. Hydrogen electrons are passed from carrier to carrier
100. Redox
101. When it accepts an electron; when it gives up an electron
102. Hydrogen electrons release less and less energy with successive cytochrome redox reactions
103. the movement of Hydrogen protons through pores of cristae along a gradient/the Proton pump
104. ATP-Synthetase; ATP synthesis
105. P coupling to ADP when oxygen is present/ATP synthesis
106. electron transport system
107. bonds with waste Hydrogen to form water

108. oxidation halts after glycolysis; pyruvates cannot enter mictochondria
109. glycolysis
110. Anaerobic Respiration; Lactic Acid
111. fatigue
112. inability to contract due to insufficient Oxygen
113. performing muscle activity which exceeds oxygen-ventilation ability
114. reverts back to pyruvate and re-enters aerobic pathway
115. it only produces enough ATP to split another glucose
116. Creatine Phosphate
117. P, 1 ATP
118. permanent crossbridge attachment
119. calcium remains bound to troponin without Ca-ATP-ase
120. 6, 12; decomposition of tissue
121. inability to control a voluntary muscle
122. muscle remains contracted, cannot relax it
123. muscle remains relaxed, cannot contract it
124. inhibits the motor end plate from responding to ACh
125. loss of mass or substance; disuse or neurological disorders
126. splitting/immobilization of limbs
127. increased mass beyond "normal" body limits; increased work demands on muscle tissue
128. strengthening effect in skeletal; weakens cardiac, associated with disease
129. ischemia
130. Oxygen; infarct
131. hypermotility
132. diarrhea; dysentery
133. dehydration and electrolyte imbalance
134. erosion of intestinal lining down to capillary bed
135. hypomotility
136. constipation; paralyzed section of colon, generally following long surgeries
137. neurotoxin, spastic; flaccid
138. asphyxiation; respiratory muscles go into tetany preventing inspiration
139. respiratory muscles will not contract
140. eating poorly cooked contaminated pork; parasite worm forms cysts on diaphragm; leads to respiratory failure
141. viral related (EBV, Mononucleosis) inflammation of fibers and CT sheaths
142. stretching of muscle fiber beyond extensibility limit without damage; stretching with fiber damage and hemorrhage

143. born with; developmental or birth related
144. hypoxia and birth trauma (forceps delivery)
145. paralysis of voluntary muscles affected by involved region of cerebral cortex
146. physician induced
147. seizures
148. uncontrolled cortical stimulation; head trauma, high fevers
149. sex-linked genetic; breakdown of the neuromuscular junction
150. paralysis; asphyxiation
151. autoimmune
152. receptor sites, motor end plate
153. junctional fatigue

Part 2: The Skeletal Muscle System

154. Origin; Insertion
155. The origin "pulls" the insertion towards it
156. Antagonists
157. Passively stretched
158. Passively contracts
159. Maintains muscle mass
160. Reduction in the angle between two bones; Extension
161. Restoring the joint/body part to neutral
162. Neck and Lumbar Spine; Lateral Flexion
163. Lumbar spine
164. Dorsiflexion; Dorsum
165. On their heels; Plantarflexion
166. On their toes; plantar surface
167. Anterior/forward
168. Supination
169. Pronation; Dorsum
170. Movement of body part away from the midline; Adduction
171. Abduction; Adduction; Opposition
172. Abduction
173. Turning of a bone around its central axis; Internal or External
174. Conical motion around a central point requiring the actions of many muscles
175. Pivot; Ball-in-Socket
176. Glenohumeral (shoulder) and Acetabular (hip)
177. Retraction
178. Protraction
179. Mastication
180. Turning of the plantar surface outward; Inversion
181. Rectus; Transverse; Oblique

182.
183. Circular
184. Biceps; Triceps; Quadriceps
185. Levator Labii Superioris
186. Zygomaticus
187. Orbicularis Oculi
188. Temporalis
189. Masseter
190. Orbicularis Oris
191. Buccinator
192. Trapezius
193. SCM
194. Depressor Labii Inferioris
195. Platysma
196. Temporalis
197. Occipitalis
198. Scalenes
199. Rotation and Flexion
200. Hyoid
201. Intertransversarii
202. Rotatores
203. Interspinalis
204. Multifidus
205. Deltoid
206. Pectoralis Major and Latissimus Doris
207. Arm Flexion; Arm Extension
208. Serratus Anterior
209. Brachi
210. Coracobrachialis
211. Rhomboid Major and Rhomboid Minor
212. Subscapularis, Infraspinatus, Supraspinatus and Teres Minor
213. Humerus; Circumduction; Stabilizes
214. Biceps Brachii
215. Arm flexion and Forearm flexion
216. Triceps Brachii
217. Medial Epicondyle of Humerus; Lateral Epicondyle
218. Brachialis
219. O: Medial Epicondyle; I: Radial side of wrist
220. Lateral Epicondyle; Ulnar side of wrist
221. Pronator Teres
222. Thenar; Pollicis
223. Opponens Pollicis
224. Abductor Pollicis
225. Lumbricales; Interossei

226. Rectus Abdominus
227. Internal Oblique, External Oblique
228. Iliocostalis, Longissimus, Spinalis
229. Diaphragm, Internal Intercostal, External Intercostal
230. External Intercostals pull ribs up and out, Diaphragm moves down
231. Internal Intercostals pull ribs down and in, Diaphragm moves up
232. Any muscle which originates or inserts on the rib cage which can assist in increasing thoracic volume
233. Psoas and Iliacus
234. Gluteus Maximus
235. Gluteus Medius
236. Adduction
237. Rectus Femoris, Vastus Medialis, Vastus Intermedialis, Vastus Lateralis
238. Knee/Leg Extension
239. Biceps Femoris, Semimebranosus, Semitendinosus
240. Hamstrings
241. Biceps Femoris
242. Sartorius
243. Piriformis
244. Tibialis Anterior
245. Extensor Digitorum Longus, Extensor Hallucis
246. Hallucis
247. Fibularis Longus, Fibularis Brevis
248. Gastrocnemius, Plantaris, Soleus
249. Calcaneal/Achille's

Unit VI: Take a Test!

1. Which of the following statements concerning muscle tissue are true:
    a) it converts chemical energy into kinetic
    b) embryonic cells divide by hyperplasia
    c) mature fibers divide by mitosis
    d) a and b are true
    e) a, b and c

2. The growth in both size and mass of a muscle fiber is called:
    a) Hyperplasia   b) Hypertrophy
    c) Atrophy   d) Mitosis   e) Meiosis

3. Which of the following is defined as a fiber's ability to recoil after stretching:
    a) excitability   b) contractility
    c) extensibility   d) elasticity   e) irritability

4. Which is true of skeletal muscle fibers:
    a) they are multinucleate   b) they are striated
    c) they are branched   d) a and b   e) a, b and c

5. Intercalated discs:
    a) anchor fibers with a desmosome
    b) electrically couple fibers with a gap junction
    c) insure simultaneous contraction of all cardiac fibers
    d) a and b
    e) a, b and c

6. Smooth muscles propel food and fluids by which type of contractions:
    a) isotonic   b) isometric
    c) paralytic   d) peristalsis   e) flaccid

7. Contractions in which muscle tension increases but muscle length remains the same are called:
    a) isotonic   b) isometric
    c) paralytic   d) peristalsis   e) flaccid

8. The sarcolemma:
    a) surrounds a fascicle
    b) surrounds the skeletal muscle
    c) is the excitable membrane of the muscle fiber
    d) surrounds a functional group of muscles

9. Which is the Connective Tissue sheath that surrounds a skeletal fiber:
   a) sarcolemma
   b) endomysium
   c) perimysium
   d) epimysium
   e) fascia

10. Which is defined as the contractile unit:
   a) sarcolemma
   b) sacroplasmic reticulum
   c) myofibril
   d) T-tubule
   e) sarcomere

11. Myoglobin functions by:
   a) inhibiting Tropomysin
   b) inhibiting actin and myosin from crossbridging
   c) binding O_2 inside the sarcoplasm
   d) binding Ca^{+2} inside the Sarcoplasmic reticulum
   e) binding with Ca^{+2} and preventing it from diffusing out of the sarcomere

12. The Action Potential is conducted inside the muscle fiber by which structure:
   a) sarcoplasmic reticulum
   b) myofibril
   c) myomesin
   d) transverse tubule
   e) titin

13. Upon entering the fiber the Action Potential will stimulate the release of:
   a) Ca^{+2}
   b) Ca^{+2}-ATP-ase
   c) ACh
   d) Acetylcholinesterase
   e) Acetyl-CO-A

14. Which of the following is noted for its receptor sites for ACh:
   a) the synaptic boot
   b) Actin
   c) the sarcoplasmic reticulum
   d) the motor end plate
   e) the T-Tubule

15. The all or none principle applies to:
   a) ACh release
   b) skeletal fiber contraction
   c) end plate potentials
   d) skeletal muscle contraction
   e) all of these

16. What is the effect of ACh at the neuromuscular junction :
   a) opens the Ca^{+2} gates
   b) opens the K^+ gates
   c) opens the Na^+ gates
   d) it releases Ca^{+2}-ATP-ase
   e) a and b are true

17. When at rest the sarcolemma is described as being "polarized"; why?
   a) Na^+ creates a net (+) charge in the ECF
   b) K^+ creates a net (+) charge in the ICF
   c) K^+ creates a net (-) charge in the ICF
   d) a and b are true
   e) a and c are true

18. Repolarization increases the sarcolemma's membrane permeability to:
   a) K^+
   b) Na^+
   c) Cl^-
   d) Ca^{+2}
   e) O_2

19. Depolarizations increases the sarcolemma's membrane permeability to:
   a) K^+
   b) Na^+
   c) Cl^-
   d) Ca^{+2}
   e) O_2

20. Nerve impulses increase the synaptic boot's membrane permeability to:
    a) K^+ b) Na^+ c) Cl^- d) Ca^{+2} e) O_2

21. Which forms the "light" bands in striated muscle fibers:
    a) Z-line b) M-line
    c) H-zone d) A-band e) I-band

22. Which of the following is closed during contraction:
    a) Z-line b) M-line
    c) H-zone d) A-band e) I-band

23. Which is the correct sequence of events:
    1) Threshold
    2) Ca^{+2} diffuses into sarcomere
    3) Na^+ permeability increases
    4) Myosin binding sites are exposed
    5) Ca^{+2} permeability increases
    6) Shortening of Fiber
    a) 2,1,3,5,4,6 b) 2,3,5,4,1,6
    c) 3,2,5,4,1,6 d) 5,3,1,2,4,6 e) 5,2,3,1,4,6

24. Threshold is defined as:
    a) the closing of Na^+ gates
    b) the opening of K^+ gates
    c) the opening of the voltage Na^+ gates
    d) the period of time during repolarization that a fiber is immune to stimulus
    e) the restoration of the resting length

25. An Action Potential is best defined as:
    a) the closing of Na^+ gates
    b) a graded muscle contraction
    c) the opening of K^+ gates
    d) the period of time during repolarization that a fiber is immune to stimulus
    e) a wave of depolarization that sweeps across the sarcolemma

26. Which best describes the action of Tropomyosin:
    a) binding with Ca^{+2} and preventing it from diffusing out of the sarcomere
    b) holding Ca^{+2} inside the Sarcoplasmic reticulum
    c) degrading ACh into acetate and choline
    d) inhibiting actin and myosin from cross-bridging
    e) inhibiting Troponin

27. Which best describes the action of Troponin:
    a) binding with Ca^{+2} and preventing it from diffusing out of the sarcomere
    b) holding Ca^{+2} inside the Sarcoplasmic reticulum
    c) degrading ACh into acetate and choline
    d) inhibiting actin and myosin from cross-bridging
    e) inhibiting Tropomyosin

28. How is Calcium involved in a muscle twitch:
    a) Ca^{+2} inhibits Tropomysin
    b) it binds to ACh
    c) Ca^{+2} repolarizes the motor end plate
    d) a and b
    e) a, b and c

29. The Motor End Plate secretes _____ to begin repolarization:
    a) Acetylcholinesterase   b) Calsequestrin
    c) ATP-Synthase   d) ACh   e) Ca^{+2}-ATP-ase

30. Which is the correct sequence of events:
    1) $Ca+^2$-ATP-ase is secreted
    2) Acetylcholinestersase is secreted
    3) Threshold
    4) K+ permeability increases
    5) $Ca+^2$ diffuses out of sarcomere
    6) Fiber relaxes
    a) 3,4,1,2,5,6   b) 2,4,3,1,5,6
    c) 5,3,2,1,4,6   d) 3, 2, 4, 1, 5, 6   e) 1,2,3,5,4,6

31. What is the effect of Acetylcholinesterase at the neuromuscular junction :
    a) opens the Ca^{+2} gates   b) opens the K^+ gates
    c) opens the Na^+ gates   d) it releases Ca^{+2}-ATP-ase   e) a and b are true

32. What substance is released by the sarcoplasmic reticulum in response to repolarization:
    a) Acetylcholinesterase   b) Calsequestrin
    c) ATP-Synthase   d) ACh   e) Ca^{+2}-ATP-ase

33. Refractory is defined as:
    a) the closing of Na^+ gates
    b) the period of time during repolarization that a fiber is immune to stimulus
    c) the closing of K^+ gates
    d) a wave of depolarization that sweeps across the sarcolemma
    e) the minimum number of depolarizations needed for an action potential

34. The process by which successive muscle fiber contractions start sooner, are stronger and last longer is called:
    a) treppe   b) twitch
    c) tetany   d) graded   e) fasiculation

35. Tetany is best defined as:
    a) permanent crossbridge attachment
    b) the time during repolarization that a fiber is immune to stimulus
    c) the inability to contract a fiber
    d) the inability to relax a fiber
    e) metabolic breakdown of the neuromuscular junction

36. Contractures such as writer's cramp are due to:
   a) calcium accumulation within the sarcomere
   b) insufficient calcium secretion
   c) prolonged repolarization
   d) excessive ACh
   e) reduced oxygen availability

37. In which stage does acetyl-Co-A combine with oxaloacetate:
   a) chemiosmosis   b) citric acid cycle
   c) glycolysis   d) oxidative phosphorylation   e) Electron Transport

38. 2ATP as activation energy is required for which stage:
   a) chemiosmosis   b) citric acid cycle
   c) glycolysis   d) oxidative phosphorylation   e) electron Transport

39. Which process releases free energy for ATP couplings:
   a) chemiosmosis   b) citric acid cycle
   c) glycolysis   d) oxidative phosphorylation   e) electron Transport

40. The formation of ATP (ADP + P = ATP) is also known as:
   a) chemiosmosis   b) citric acid cycle
   c) glycolysis   d) oxidative phosphorylation   e) Electron Transport

41. The activation of ATP-Synthase occurs during:
   a) chemiosmosis   b) citric acid cycle
   c) glycolysis   d) oxidative phosphorylation   e) Electron Transport

42. Which is the only stage that continues during periods of O_2 debt:
   a) chemiosmosis   b) citric acid cycle
   c) glycolysis   d) oxidative phosphorylation   e) electron Transport

43. On entering the mitochondria pyruvate is converted into:
   a) Acetyl-CO-A   b) ATP- Synthase   c) Ca^{+2}-ATP-Ase
   d) Creatine Phosphate   e) Lactic acid

44. Which of the following accumulates during O_2 debt:
   a) Acetyl-CO-A   b) ATP- Synthase   c) Ca^{+2}-ATP-Ase
   d) Creatine Phosphate   e) Lactic acid

45. The symptoms of muscle fatigue during exercise are due to:
   a) reduced oxygen availability
   b) lactic acid accumulation
   c) calcium accumulation within the sarcomere
   d) a and b
   e) a, b and c

46. "Flaccid Paralysis" can be defined as:
    a) the inability to use a voluntary muscle
    b) the inability to contract a muscle
    c) the inability to relax a muscle
    d) a and b
    e) a and c

47. Which is used to describe injuries in which fibers loss mass or substance:
    a) strain   b) sprain
    c) ileus   d) paralysis   e) atrophy

48. Destruction of Upper Motor Neurons due to birth trauma may result in:
    a) atrophy   b) epilepsy
    c) cerebral palsy   d) myasthenia gravis   e) muscular dystrophy

49. The Bacterium of Tetanus produces s neurotoxin which will result in:
    a) permanent crossbridge attachment
    b) uncontrolled cortical stimulation and seizures
    c) spastic paralysis and asphyxiation
    d) flaccid paralysis and asphyxiation
    e) junctional fatigue

50. The effects of rigor mortis are due to:
    a) permanent crossbridge attachment
    b) metabolic breakdown of the N-M junction and fiber
    c) reduced ACh secretion
    d) a and b
    e) a, b and c

1. Reducing the angle between two bones:
    a) flexion   b) extension
    c) abduction   d) adduction   e) opposition

2. Moving an extremity away from the body midline:
    a) flexion   b) extension
    c) abduction   d) adduction   e) opposition

3. Moving the shoulder or hip in a conical motion:
    a) circumduction   b) rotation
    c) pronation   d) supination   e) dorsiflexion

4. Walking on one's heels:
    a) circumduction   b) rotation
    c) pronation   d) supination   e) dorsiflexion

5. Drawing the scapula together:
    a) protraction   b) extension
    c) abduction   d) adduction   e) retraction

6. Grasping with the thumb:
    a) flexion   b) extension
    c) abduction   d) adduction   e) opposition

7. Turning the palms to face posterior
    a) circumduction   b) rotation
    c) pronation   d) supination   e) dorsiflexion

8. Standing on one's toes:
    a) dorsiflexion   b) elevation
    c) inversion   d) eversion   e) plantar flexion

9. Turning the sole to face outward
    a) dorsiflexion   b) elevation
    c) inversion   d) eversion   e) plantar flexion

10. Moving an extremity towards the body midline:
    a) flexion   b) extension
    c) abduction   d) adduction   e) opposition

11. Chewing is performed by the:
    a) Orbicularis oris   b) Zygomaticus
    c) Masseter   d) SCM   e) Frontalis

12.	Smiling would be performed by which muscle:
	a) Orbicularis oris	b) Zygomaticus
	c) Masseter	d) SCM	e) Temporalis

13.	Squinting is accomplished by contracting which muscle:
	a) Orbicularis oculi	b) Frontalis
	c) Temporalis	d) Zygomaticus	e) Buccinator

14.	Which of the following rotates the head left or right:
	a) Deltoid	b) SCM
	c) Trapezius	d) Platysma	e) Pectoralis

15.	Which of the following ABducts the arm/shoulder:
	a) Biceps brachii	b) Triceps brachi
	c) Deltoid	d) Latissimus dorsi	e) Coracobrachialis

16.	Which ADDucts the arm/shoulder:
	a) Biceps brachii	b) Triceps brachii
	c) Deltoid	d) Latissimus dorsi	e) Coracobrachialis

17.	Which flexes the arm:
	a) Brachialis	b) Triceps brachi
	c) Deltoid	d) Latissimus dorsi	e) Coracobrachialis

18.	Which extends the arm:
	a) Biceps brachii	b) Triceps brachi
	c) Deltoid	d) Latissimus dorsi	e) Coracobrachialis

19.	Which flexes the forearm:
	a) Biceps brachii	b) Triceps brachi
	c) Deltoid	d) Latissimus dorsi	e) Coracobrachialis

20.	Which extends the forearm:
	a) Biceps brachii	b) Triceps brachi
	c) Deltoid	d) Latissimus dorsi	e) Coracobrachialis

21.	Retraction of the scapula is performed by:
	a) Levator Scapulae	b) Subscapularis
	c) Rhomboid Major	d) Supraspinatus	e) Teres Minor

22.	Shrugging the shoulders is done by the:
	a) Levator Scapulae	b) Subscapularis
	c) Rhomboid Major	d) Supraspinatus	e) Teres Minor

23.	Which of the following allows one to grasp objects:
	a) Abductor pollicis	b) Opponens pollicis
	c) Extensor hallicus	d) Flexor hallicis	e) Flexor digitorum

24. Which flexes the trunk:
    a) Rectus abdominalis
    b) Oblique abdominalis
    c) Transverse abdominalis
    d) Serratus anterior

25. Which muscle is considered a "secondary muscle of respiration":
    a) External Intercostal
    b) Internal Intercostal
    c) Serratus anterior
    d) Diaphragm

26. Which laterally flexes adjacent vertebrae:
    a) Interspinalis
    b) Mutifidus
    c) Intertransversarii
    d) Rotatore

27. Which flexes the hip/thigh:
    a) Gluteus medius
    b) Gluteus maximus
    c) Psoas
    d) Piriformis
    e) Gracilis

28. Which extends the hip/thigh:
    a) Gluteus medius
    b) Gluteus maximus
    c) Psoas
    d) Piriformis
    e) Gracilis

29. Which ABducts the hip/thigh:
    a) Gluteus medius
    b) Gluteus maximus
    c) Psoas
    d) Piriformis
    e) Gracilis

30. Which ADDucts the hip/thigh:
    a) Gluteus medius
    b) Gluteus maximus
    c) Psoas
    d) Piriformis
    e) Gracilis

31. Which externally rotates the hip/thigh:
    a) Gluteus medius
    b) Gluteus maximus
    c) Psoas
    d) Piriformis
    e) Gracilis

32. Which flexes the knee/leg:
    a) Rectus femoris
    b) Biceps femoris
    c) Tibialis anterior
    d) Gastrocnemius
    e) Fibularis longus

33. Which extends the knee/leg:
    a) Rectus femoris
    b) Biceps femoris
    c) Tibialis anterior
    d) Gastrocnemius
    e) Fibularis longus

34. Which dorsiflexes the foot:
    a) Rectus femoris
    b) Biceps femoris
    c) Tibialis anterior
    d) Gastrocnemius
    e) Fibularis longus

35. Which plantarflexes the foot:
    a) Rectus femoris
    b) Biceps femoris
    c) Tibialis anterior
    d) Gastrocnemius
    e) Fibularis longus

36. Which everts the foot:
   a) Rectus femoris
   b) Biceps femoris
   c) Tibialis anterior
   d) Gastrocnemius
   e) Fibularis longus

37. The Calcaneal tendon is formed by all of the following except:
   a) Gastrocnemius
   b) Semimembranous
   c) Plantaris
   d) Soleus
   e) All are part

38. Which is not part of the Rotator Cuff group:
   a) Teres Major
   b) Supraspinatus
   c) Infraspinatus
   d) Subscapularis
   e) Teres Minor

39. The "Hamstrings" include all of the following Except:
   a) Biceps Femoris
   b) Semimembranosus
   c) Semitendinosus
   d) Rectus Femoris
   e) all are part

40. Which is not part of the Quadriceps Group:
   a) Rectus Femoris
   b) Vastus Medialis
   c) Vastus Lateralis
   d) Vastus Intermedialis
   e) all are part

1: a, 2: c; 3: a, 4: e; 5: e, 6: e; 7: c, 8: e; 9: d, 10: d, 11: c; 12: b, 13: a, 14: b, 15: c, 16: d, 17: e, 18: b, 19: a, 20: b, 21: c, 22: a, 23: a, 24: a, 25: c, 26: c, 27: c, 28: b, 29: a, 30: e, 31: d, 32: b, 33: a, 34: c, 35: d, 36: e, 37: b, 38: a, 39: d, 40: e

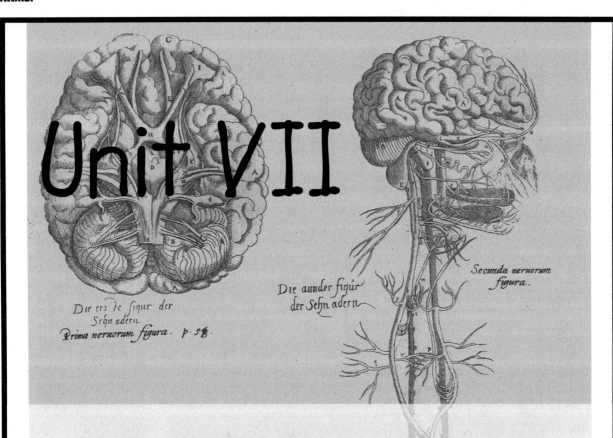

Die ers de figur der
Seha adern
Prima neruorum figura. p. 58.

Die ander figur
der Sehn adern

Secunda neruorum
figura.

Unit VII

THE NERVOUS SYSTEM

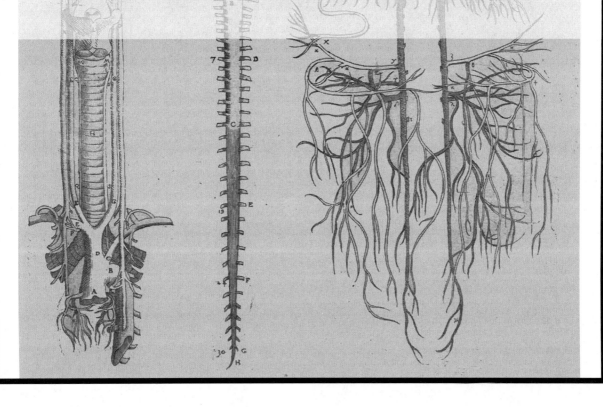

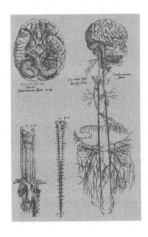

Part 1: **Nerve Physiology**

1. The Nervous System is divided into two main portions: the _____ and _____ Nervous Systems.

2. The Central Nervous System consists of the _____ and _____ _____. The Peripheral Nervous System is composed of _____ and _____ nerves.

3. The Spinal and Cranial nerves of the Peripheral Nervous System are subdivided into the incoming _____/_____ division and the outgoing _____/_____ division.

4. Somatic Afferent fibers bring sensory information from the _____ and _____ to the _____ Nervous System.

5. Visceral Afferent fibers bring sensory information from _____ and _____ to the _____ Nervous System.

6. The Motor or Efferent Division of the PNS can be further divided into the _____ and _____ Nervous Systems.

7. Somatic Efferent fibers carry motor output from the Central Nervous System to _____ _____. The Somatic NS is also referred to as the _____ NS.

8. Visceral Efferent fibers carry motor output from the Autonomic Nervous System to _____ and _____. The ANS is also referred to as the _____ NS and is subdivided into the _____ and _____ Nervous Systems.

9. The Sympathetic Nervous System stimulates the "_____ or _____" response; the Parasympathetic stimulates the "_____ and _____" response.

10. Define Integration: _____ _____.

11. The two principal cell types of nervous tissue are _____ and _____ cells.

12. Neurons function as _____ cells; Glial cells are also known as _____ cells.

13. The four glial cells of the CNS are: _____, _____, _____, and _____ Cells.

14. Astrocytes possess cytoplasmic extensions called _____, which function as part of the _____ _____ _____.

15. Microglia engulf debris and function as the _____ of the CNS. Oligodendrocytes function by _____.

16. Ependymal Cells line the _____ of the CNS; they possess _____, which help circulate the _____ Fluid.

17. The two glial/supportive cells of the PNS are the _____ Cell and the _____ Cell.

18. Schwann Cells, like Oligodendrocytes, function by _____. Schwann Cells also function like Microglia and act as the _____ of the PNS. Satellite Cells have a _____ role.

19. What three characteristics are associated with conductive neurons? _____, high _____, and high _____ _____.

20. The neuron can be divided into four function regions: _____, _____, _____, and _____.

21. The Biosynthetic region, the cell body, is also known as the _____ and its nucleus, the _____. The Receptive, Conductive and Secretory Regions are _____ _____, which extend from the Cell Body.

22. In addition to their large perikaryon, the soma is noted for its rough endoplasmic reticulum, the _____ _____. The amitotic neuron lacks a _____.

23. Collections of cell bodies in the CNS are called _____; those in the PNS are called _____ ("knot on a string").

24. Receptive processes are called _____; conducting processes are called _____. The secretory portion consists of _____.

25. Materials produced by the soma are transported to the telodendria by _____ _____ _____.

26. The return flow, called Retrograde Axoplasmic Streaming, is responsible for inadvertently delivering _____ and viruses such as _____ to the cell bodies.

27. Collections of conducting axons in the CNS are called _____; those in the PNS are called _____.

28. Dendrites conduct electrical signals _____; axons conduct nerve impulses _____.

29. The signals conducted by the dendrites are called _____ _____ since they lose intensity as they travel.

30. Unlike Graded Potentials, the nerve impulses generated by the axons are _____-distance _____ _____.

31. Action Potentials/Nerve Impulses originate on the _____ _____ and are conducted along the axon's plasma membrane, the _____ to the _____.

32. The axolemma of peripheral nerves are covered by myelin sheaths secreted by _____ Cells.

33. Schwann cells form myelin beads by _____; the outer most layer of the bead is called the _____.

34. The neurilemma is the plasma membrane of the Schwann Cells. Myelin functions by providing _____ and increasing _____ _____.

35. Myelin beads are separated by exposed patches of axolemma called the _____ of _____.

36. The Nodes of Ranvier allow for the exit of branches called _____ _____ and also provide for Internodal or _____ Conduction.

37. Unlike Schwann cells, a single Oligodendrocyte can myelinate up to _____ axons in the CNS. Myelinated tracts of the CNS form the _____ Matter; unmyelinated cell bodies form the _____ Matter.

38. List the three structural neuron types: _____, _____, and _____.

39. All embryonic neurons begin as Bipolar neurons; after development is complete they are only found as special senses in the _____ of the eye, the _____ nerve, and the _____ mucosa.

40. Unipolar neurons are noted for the incoming dendrite, the _____ process, and its outgoing axon, the _____ process.

41. Multipolar neurons are the most abundant, comprising _____% of all neurons. Most have _____'s of dendrites and a single axon with _____'s of telodendria.

42. The three functional neuron types are: _____, _____, and _____/_____.

43. Which is the principal motor neuron? _____ Which is the principal sensory neuron? _____ Which is the principal association/interneuron? _____

44. What function is performed by association/interneurons? _____ Unipolar sensory cell bodies are located in the _____ _____ _____.

45. When opposite charges are separated, they create an electric _____; the flow of charges between these two points is called _____.

46. An electric potential is measured as _____; any hindrance to the flow of current creates _____.

47. Substances creating little or no resistance are called _____; those that resist current are _____.

48. The axolemma possesses two principal types of channels: _____ and _____ channels.

49. Passive channels are also called _____ channels as they allow substances to diffuse along an _____ gradient. Gated channels are either _____-gated or _____-gated.

50. Na$^+$ and K$^+$ passively diffuse along their electrochemical gradients through _____ channels; Chemically-gated Channels open in response to _____.

51. The Rest Potential of a nerve fiber indicates that it is _____ _____

52. The Rest Potential is measured at _____ mV; this potential is created by separating high amounts of _____ outside the membrane and high amounts of _____ inside.

53. Sodium's (Na$^+$) strong positive charge is balanced by extracellular _____; Potassium's (K$^+$) weaker positive charge is balanced by intercellular _____.

54. The diffusion of Na$^+$ and K$^+$ across the membrane is counteracted by the _____.

55. The Na$^+$/K$^+$ functions by pumping out _____ Na$^+$ for every _____ K$^+$ pumped in. Pumps are mechanisms of _____ Transport and require energy in the form of _____.

56. A _____ is a reduction in membrane potential (negativity) bringing it closer to 0 mV; a _____ increases the electro-negativity of the membrane.

57. Depolarizations increase/decrease the probability of initiating a nerve impulse; hyperpolarizations increase/decrease the probability.

58. Dendrites have _____-gated receptors that respond to _____.

59. Neurotransmitters open chemically-gated channels and initiate a _____ potential.

60. Graded Potentials are _____-distance electric signals that lose intensity as they travel to the _____ _____.

61. Graded Potentials can depolarize the axon hillock by opening _____-gated _____ channels.

62. By opening voltage-gated Na^+ channels, Na^+ rushes _____, making the membrane less/more negative.

63. Depolarizations increase/decrease Na^+ permeability, decreasing negativity until reaching _____.

64. Threshold, _____ mV is the value at which all Na^+ gates open. Define Threshold: _____ _____.

65. Na^+ continues to rush in until the membrane potential is reduced to _____ mV.

66. At 0 mV Na^+ gates _____ decreasing/increasing Na^+ permeability. Membrane potential continues rising until it reaches _____ mV.

67. At +30 mV K^+ gates open/close, increasing/decreasing K^+ permeability, allowing K^+ to rush in/out.

68. As K^+ rushes out of the fiber it increases/decreases electronegativity, allowing the fiber to _____.

69. During repolarization, electronegativity can increase to _____ mV; this is called a _____.

70. After hyperpolarizing at −90 mV the rest potential is restored by the _____ _____.

71. Once threshold is reached, the action potential initiated depolarizes the adjacent membrane propagating a _____ _____.

72. Nerve Impulses are waves of _____ _____, which are propagated towards the _____.

73. Define Refractory: _____.

74. Absolute Refractory occurs during the time that Na^+ gates are _____ and implies that _____.

75. Relative Refractory occurs when K^+ gates are _____ and Na^+ are _____. How does Relative Refractory differ from Absolute? _____ _____.

76. Rest Potential:

_____

77. Threshold:

_____

78. Na⁺ gates close:

_____

79. K⁺ gates open:

_____

80. Hyperpolarization:

_____

81. Repolarization begins:

_____

82. Action Potential begins:

_____

83. EPSP: _____

84. IPSP: _____

85. Action Potential: _____

86. Repolarization: _____

87. Hyperpolarization: _____

88. Absolute Refractory: _____

89. Relative Refractory: _____

90. Chemical Na⁺ gates opened: _____

91. Voltage Na⁺ gates opened: _____

92. Voltage Na⁺ gates closed: _____

93. K⁺ gates opened: _____

94. K⁺ gates closed: _____

95. Cl⁻ gates opened: _____

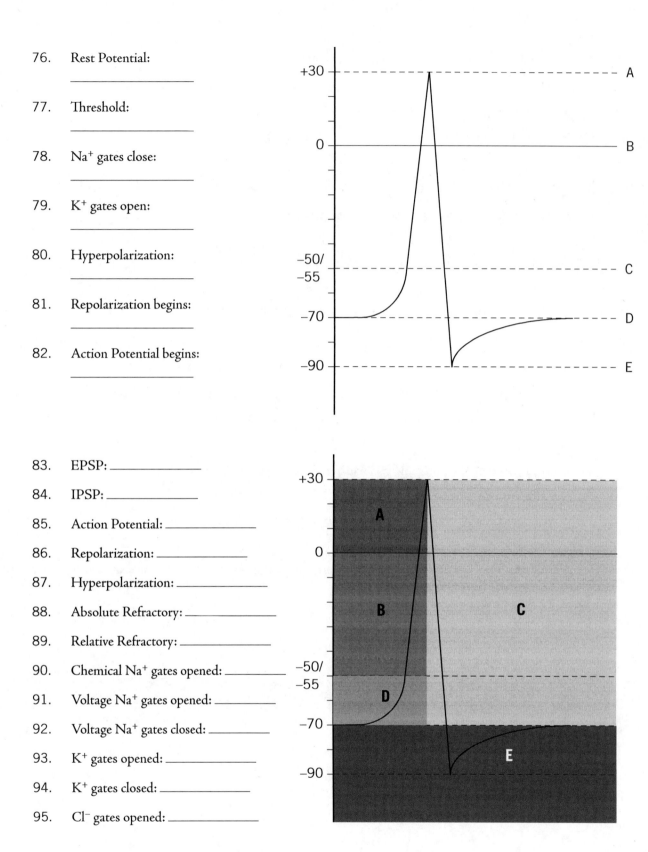

96. The magnitude of a nerve's effect is based on the magnitude/volume of _____ _____.

97. The volume of neurotransmitter secretion is dependent on the _____ of nerve transmission/impulses. _____ Refractory allows for increased frequency of nerve impulses.

98. The velocity of nerve impulses is determined by two factors: _____ diameter and the _____.

99. Describe type A fibers as per axon diameter, thickness of myelin, speed, and targets: _____ _____.

100. Describe type B fibers: _____.

101. Describe type C fibers: _____.

102. The two types of synapses are _____ and _____.

103. Electrical synapses are actually _____ junctions, which allow the passage of electrolytes such as _____ and _____.

104. Cells connected by Gap junctions are described as being _____ _____ and are found in neurons mediating _____ movement, the _____ _____ in cardiac muscle and in _____ muscle.

105. Chemical synapses have three structural components: the _____-_____ _____, the _____ _____, and the _____- _____ _____.

106. The pre-synaptic neuron conducts impulses towards/away from the synaptic gutter; the post-synaptic neuron conducts impulses towards/away from the synaptic gutter.

107. The pre-synaptic neuron secretes _____ for which the post-synaptic neuron possesses specific _____ _____.

108. The three chemical events in nerve transmission are: _____, _____, and _____.

109. Which events occur faster—chemical or electrical?

110. The change over from electrical conduction to the chemical events of secretion, diffusion and reception create the phenomena of _____ _____. Chemical synapses are bi-/uni-directional.

111. Nerve Impulses increase _____ permeability of the synaptic boot.

112. Increased intracellular calcium in the synaptic boot stimulates _____ of synaptic vesicles, resulting in _____ of neurotransmitters.

113. The three characteristics of all neurotransmitters include:

_____,

_____, and

_____.

114. The Ion Fluxes created by neurotransmitters change the _____ of the post-synaptic

_____.

115. Excitatory neurotransmitters increase _____ permeability of the post-synaptic membrane;
Inhibitory neurotransmitters increase _____ and _____ permeability.

116. An EPSP increases Na^+ permeability, which _____ the membrane; EPSP's
increase/decrease the probability of a nerve impulse.

117. An IPSP increases K^+ and Cl^- permeability, which _____ the membrane; IPSPs
increase/decrease the probability of a nerve impulse.

118. The three mechanisms by which neurotransmitters clear the synapse include:

_____,

_____, and

_____.

119. The four traditional categories of neurotransmitters include: _____,

_____ _____, _____ _____, and

_____.

120. Acetylcholine is cleared from the synapse by _____ _____. ACh targets
include the _____ Junction and _____.

121. Biogenic Amines include two groups of neurotransmitters: _____ and

_____.

122. Catecholamines are based on the amino acid _____; Indolamines are based on the amino
acid _____.

123. The Catecholamines derived from L-Tyrosine include: _____, _____, and
_____ (NE).

124. Dopamine and Norepinephrine are described as "_____ _____"
neurotransmitters; Epinephrine is produced by the _____ _____ and
acts as a hormone during _____ Responses.

125. The Indolamine derived from L-Tryptophane is _____, and from Histidine is

_____.

126. How does Serotonin function? _____
How is Serotonin cleared from the synapse? _____

127. Catecholamines are Inhibitory/Excitatory.
Indolamines are Inhibitory/Excitatory.

128. Amino Acids which act as neurotransmitters, include _____, _____, and
_____.

129. GABA and L-Glycine are Inhibitory/Excitatory. Excessive Glutamate is released in response to
_____, which leads to death of neighboring neurons by excitotoxicity.

130. Neuropeptides include _____ and _____.

131. Endorphins and Enkephalins are Inhibitory/Excitatory. Endorphins are the body's natural
_____ and control/reduce _____.

132. Neurons are organized into functional groups called _____ _____.

133. Post-synaptic fibers of neuron pools are directly in the _____ Zone and reach threshold,
or in the _____ Zone where they are depolarized but not to threshold.

134. Neuronal circuits in which a single UMN can trigger thousands of muscle fibers are called
_____ Circuits. Circuits in which many different stimuli bring about the same effect/
reaction are called _____ Circuits.

135. Circuits that facilitate rhythmic and repetitive movements such as cross-crawling are called
_____/_____ Circuits; those involved in cognitive problem solving
are called _____ _____-_____ Circuits.

136. The two types of neural processing are _____ as in reflex arcs, and _____
as used in cognitive activities.

137. How does plasticity differ from neurogenesis? _____
_____

138. Why are axons of the PNS capable of regeneration whereas those of the CNS are not? _____
_____

139. After a PNS axon is damaged, what happens to the Nissl Bodies? _____. What term
describes the breakdown of the axon and myelin? _____ _____

140. Despite Chromatolysis and Wallerian degeneration, the neurilemma remains intact. What structure do the
remaining Schwann cells produce? _____ _____

141. What is the significance of the regeneration tube? _____
_____

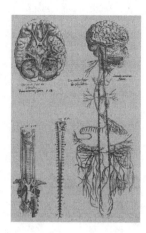

Part 2: Anatomy of the CNS and PNS

142. Which embryonic layer differentiates into nervous tissue? _____

143. Ectoderm thickens in the three-week embryo forming the _____ _____.

144. The developing Neural Plate invaginates forming the _____ _____, which is flanked by the _____ _____.

145. The fusing of the neural folds around the neural groove forms the _____ _____.

146. The neural tube forms vesicles, which is divided into three regions: _____, _____, and _____.

147. The Prosencephalon is referred to as the _____, the Mesencepahlaon as the _____, and the Rhombencephalon as the _____. The remaining portion becomes the _____ _____.

148. The Prosencephalon differentiates into the _____ and the _____.

149. The Mesencephalon differentiates into the _____.

150. The Rhombencephalon differentiates into the _____ and the _____.

151. The fluid-filled swellings of the neural tube will develop into _____.

152. Non-myelinated cell bodies are collectively referred to as _____ _____. Myelinated axons are referred to as _____ matter.

153. The Telencephalon will differentiate into the _____ _____.

154. The Cerebral Hemispheres, or Cerebrum, include the _____ _____, white matter _____ and the _____ _____, and house the _____ ventricles.

155. The Diencephalon will differentiate into the _____, the _____, the _____, and house the _____ ventricle.

156. The Mesencephalon, or midbrain, houses the _____ _____, connecting the Third and Fourth ventricles.

157. The Metencephalon will differentiate into the _____, the _____, and the _____ ventricle.

158. The Myelencephalon will differentiate into the _____ _____.

159. The Midbrain, Pons, and Medulla Oblongata are collectively referred to as the _____ _____.

160. The CNS is covered by what three different protective layers?

_____

_____

_____

161. The three layers of the Meninges, from outer to innermost are the _____ _____, the _____ Mater, and the _____ _____.

162. The dura of the brain differs from that of the spinal cord in that it _____

_____.

163. The two layers of the brain's dura are the outer _____ and the inner _____.

164. The dura of the spinal cord does not have a _____ layer with osseous attachment.

165. Separations between the layers of the brain's dura form dural _____, which drain deoxygenated blood into the _____ _____.

166. The _____ layer of the dura forms folds or _____; the _____ _____, which separates the cerebral hemispheres; the _____ _____, which separates the cerebellar hemispheres; and the _____ _____, which separates the cerebrum from the cerebellum.

167. The Falx cerebri is located within the _____ fissure. The Tentorium cerebelli is located within the _____ fissure.

168. Unlike the brain and cranium, the meninges and the spinal column are separated by the _____ space.

169. The dura and the arachnoid are separated by the _____ space.

170. The arachnoid mater is separated from the pia by the _____ space. What circulates through this space? _____

171. Projections of the brain's arachnoid called _____ _____ protrude into the _____ _____ for used CSF to reach venous blood.

172. The spinal pia is attached to the dura by _____ _____.

173. CSF is formed by non-neural _____ cells of the _____
_____, which hangs from the roof of the _____.

174. Ciliated _____ cells of the Choroid Plexus line the ventricles to circulate the
_____.

175. CSF differs from blood in that CSF has no _____, less (list 2) _____,
and more (list 2) _____.

176. CSF drains from the fourth ventricle into the _____ _____ of the spinal
cord and the two _____ _____ of the subarachnoid space.

177. The CSF drains from the Central canal and Lateral Aperatures into the _____
_____ before being pumped upward to the brain.

178. CSF is absorbed by the _____ _____; the total adult volume at any time
is _____. The choroid plexus secretes approximately _____ per day.

179. The three layers of the blood brain barrier include _____ of the capillary, its surrounding
_____ _____, and the _____ of astrocytes.

180. Areas of the brain not shielded by the blood brain barrier include the _____ and the
_____ centers.

181. The spinal cord is demarcated from the brain at the _____ _____.

182. The spinal cord tapers to an end at the level of _____ and is known as the
_____ _____.

183. The collection of spinal nerves exiting from the Conus Medullaris are known as the _____
_____ or "Horse's Tail." The fused end of the meninges that anchors the cord to the coccyx
is called the _____ _____.

184. There are _____ cervical nerves, _____ thoracic/dorsal, _____ lumbar, _____ sacral and
_____ coccygeal, for a total of _____ spinal nerves.

185. The spinal cord is divided into left and right halves by the _____ _____
_____ and the _____ _____ _____.

186. The left and right regions of gray matter are subdivided into three _____: the
_____, carrying _____; the _____, carrying
_____; and the _____, carrying _____.

187. The left and right regions are connected by the _____ _____.

188. The Gray Commissure is the site of _____ _____ synapsing and the
_____ of ascending pathways.

189. The Lateral Horn is located between what levels? _____

190. The white matter is subdivided into three pairs of _____ or _____; the _____, _____, and _____.

191. Funiculi are subdivided into myelinated axon tracts called _____; ascending carry _____/_____ and descending carry _____/ _____.

192. Pain and temperature is carried by the _____ to the thalamus and then directed to the _____ gyrus.

193. Two-point discrimination, vibration and proprioception, are carried by the _____ _____.

194. Unconscious proprioception is carried by the _____.

195. The crossing from left to right of descending UMNs to the extremities is known as _____, which occurs in the _____ tracts of the _____.

196. UMNs of the axial skeleton descend in the _____ _____ Tract and do/do not decussate.

197. UMNs of the extremities descend in the _____ _____ Tract and do/do not decussate.

198. Equilibrium is mediated by the _____ Tract whose fibers do/do not decussate.

199. Head/neck/eye movement is coordinated by the _____ tract from the superior colliculi.

200. In deep tendon reflexes, sensory neurons synapse with motor in the _____ _____ and do/do not ascend to the thalamus.

201. The Horns of the Spinal Cord receive and send fibers through pathways called _____.

202. The _____ Root carries motor/efferent fibers from cell bodies of the _____ Horn.

203. The _____ Root carries sensory/afferent fibers from cell bodies of the _____ _____ _____ to the _____ Horn.

204. Autonomic motor fibers have cell bodies in the _____ _____ and exit by the _____ Root.

205. The Ventral and Dorsal Roots combine to form _____ _____.

206. Upon exiting the spinal cord, spinal nerves divide into three branches: the _____ _____, the _____ _____, and the _____ Branch.

207. The Dorsal Ramus carries sensory/motor/both fibers from somatic/visceral/both receptors; the Ventral Ramus carries sensory/motor/both fibers to somatic/visceral/both targets.

208. What structures are innervated by the Meningeal Branch? _____
_____

209. The CT sheath surrounding an individual axon within a peripheral or cranial nerve is called the
_____. The CT sheath surrounding a fascicle of axons is called the _____,
and that surrounding the entire peripheral nerve, the _____.

210. Nerves of the Dorsal Rami go directly to their receptors and targets whereas those of Ventral Rami of the
Cervical and Lumbo-Sacral region first form _____. Dorsal and Ventral Thoracic Rami
form the _____ Nerves.

211. The two major plexuxes of the cervical region are _____ and _____.
Those of the Lumbo-Sacral are the _____ and _____.

212. The Cervical Plexus is comprised of nerves originating at levels _____–_____; the nerves formed by
their unions are divided into _____ and _____ Branches.

213. The Superficial Branches of the Cervical Plexus are Sensory/Motor; those of the Deep Branch are
predominantly Sensory/Motor.

214. Superficial Sensory Branches include the _____ Nerve from the skin covering
_____ and the _____ Nerve from the skin covering
_____

215. The Deep Motor Branches include the _____ _____ innervating the
deep hyoid muscles and the _____ Nerve to the diaphragm.

216. The Brachial Plexus is comprised of nerves originating at levels _____–_____ and are referred to as
the _____ of the plexus; these in turn merge to form three _____.

217. The Trunks formed are the _____ (C5, C6), _____ (C7),
and _____ (C8, T1). Each Trunk will divide into _____ and
_____ Divisions.

218. The Posterior Division of all three trunks merge to form the Posterior _____.

219. Cords are also formed by the Anterior Divisions: those of the Upper and Middle Trunk form the
_____ Cord, that of the Lower Trunk forms the _____ Cord.

220. Cords in turn form peripheral nerves that service the shoulder and upper extremity; the five major nerves
include: _____, _____, _____, _____,
and _____.

221. The Axillary Nerve supplies the _____ for Abduction and the _____
_____.

222. The Musculocutaneous Nerve provides arm flexion by supplying the _____ and
_____ _____.

223. The Radial Nerve innervates muscles of the _____ arm and forearm, providing
_____ of both.

224. The Median Nerve supplies most of the muscles of the _____ arm and provides for _____ of the forearm.

225. The Ulnar Nerve supplies most of the muscles of the _____.

226. The Roots of the Lumbar Plexus originate from levels _____–_____.

227. L1 splits into _____ and _____ Branches.

228. The Upper Branch of L1 forms the _____ and _____ Nerves. The Lower Branch joins with a slip from L2 forming the _____ Nerve.

229. The Iliohypogastric Nerve supplies the _____.
The Ilioinguinal Nerve supplies the _____,
as well as the _____.
The Genitofemoral Nerve supplies the _____ and _____.

230. Roots L2, L3, and L4 split into _____ and _____ Divisions.

231. The Dorsal Division further divides and forms the _____ _____ and _____ Nerves.

232. The Lateral Cutaneous Nerve supplies the _____; the Femoral Nerve innervates the _____ muscles of the thigh and the _____ muscles of the leg.

233. The Ventral Division forms the _____ Nerve.

234. The Obturator Nerve innervates the muscles of hip _____.

235. The Sacral Plexus is formed by roots from levels _____–_____, all of which divide into _____ and _____ Divisions.

236. Roots L4 and L5 combine to form the _____ Trunk.

237. The Dorsal/Posterior Division forms the Superior and Inferior _____ Nerves and the _____ _____ Nerve.

238. The Superior Gluteal Nerve innervates the _____ _____ and _____ _____ providing hip abduction. The Inferior Gluteal innervates the Gluteus Maximus providing _____. The Common Fibular Nerve divides into _____ and _____ branches.

239. The Superficial Fibular innervates the Fibularis Longus and Brevis providing foot _____. The Deep Fibular branch innervates the Tibialis anterior, Extensor Hallucis, and Extensor Digitorum providing _____.

240. The Ventral/Anterior Division of the Sacral Plexus forms the _____ and _____ Nerves.

241. The Pudendal Nerve supplies the muscles of the _____ and sensory to the _____. The Tibial Nerve further divides into Medial and Lateral _____ Nerves.

242. The Medial and Lateral Plantar Nerves innervate the muscles of _____. The Tibial and Common Fibular Nerves combined form the _____ Nerve.

243. The region of skin providing sensation to the CNS is known as a _____.

244. Abnormal sensations such as "pins and needles" are known as _____. Loss of sensation is called _____.

245. In a spinal cord injury there is anesthesia and flaccid paralysis below the level of injury because _____.

246. DTRs are preserved because _____.

247. Sympathetic innervation to visceral targets is unaffected because _____.

248. Injuries above C2 are generally fatal because _____.

249. Injuries at C5 affect all four extremities, the result of which is termed _____. Why is speech, chewing, and swallowing preserved? _____.

250. Those at L2 or lower affect only the lower extremeties and are termed _____.

251. Which disease is characterized by viral destruction of anterior horn motor nuclei resulting in paralysis? _____ _____

252. Genetic destruction of anterior horn and pyramidal tracts causing paralysis of vocal, esophageal, and respiratory muscles: _____ _____ _____.

253. Bacterial destruction/demyelination of posterior columns causing loss of proprioception: _____ _____.

254. Auto-immune disease causing demyelination of somatic and visceral motor fibers: _____ _____.

255. The folds of the cerebrum are created by _____ (rises) and _____ (depressions), and are collectively called _____.

256. The five lobes of the cerebral hemisphere are: _____, _____, _____, _____, and inner _____.

257. The _____ fissure separates the cerebral hemispheres; the _____ of _____ separates the parietal and frontal lobes; the _____ of _____ separates the temporal lobe from the rest of the hemisphere.

258. Each hemisphere is divided into three regions: the outer _____ _____, the underlying _____ _____, and the inner _____.

259. The Basal Nuclei include the _____ nucleus, the _____, and the _____ _____.

260. The Putamen and Globus Pallidus form the _____ Nucleus. The Caudate Nucleus is associated with the _____, which is part of the Limbic System.

261. In addition to the Amygdaloid, the Limbic System includes the _____ gyrus and _____, and is interconnected by the _____. The Limbic System is referred to as our _____ brain.

262. The Amygdaloid recognizes _____. What emotional response does it elicit? _____

263. The Cingulate Nucleus expresses emotion via _____ _____. The Hippocampus is involved with _____. Which special sense has the greatest influence on the Limbic System? _____

264. The major myelinated tracts include: the _____ _____, integrating the right and left hemispheres; the _____ _____, integrating lobes of the same hemisphere; the _____ _____, integrating gyri and nuclei of the same lobe; and the _____ _____, connecting the motor cortex to the basal nuclei.

265. The functional regions of the cortex are divided into/located:
Motor: _____
Sensory: _____
Conscious Behavior: _____
Visual: _____
Auditory: _____

266. The Precentral Gyrus is noted for Upper Motor Neurons. What is the Premotor Cortex noted for? _____ _____ _____. What is Broca's area noted for? _____

267. How does Wernicke's Area differ from Broca's? _____

268. UMN of the Precentral Gyrus/Motor Cortex form the _____ _____, which enters the Internal Capsule to reach the basal nuclei.

269. Describe the function of the basal nuclei: _____

What disease is associated with dysfunction of the nuclei? _____

270. Which nuclei make up the Corpus Striatum? _____ and _____
From which area do they receive input? _____ via the _____

271. The output nuclei of the Basal Nuclei, the _____ _____, with the _____ _____ of the Midbrain, extend to which cortexes? The _____ and _____.

272. The three regions of the Diencephalon are the _____, the _____, and the _____.

273. Describe the functions of the Pineal: _____

274. The Thalamus is composed of two large oval masses of gray matter interconnected by the _____, or _____ _____.

275. Describe the function of the thalamus: _____

276. The thalamus consists of seven nuclei: the Anterior Nucleus connects the _____ to the _____ System and functions in _____ and _____. The Medial Group connects to the _____ and deals with _____.

277. Which structure is located inferior to the Thalamus? _____

278. The Hypothalamus consists of four major regions: _____, _____, _____ and _____.

279. The Tuberal region is noted for the _____, which connects it to the _____ and _____ _____. Axons of the Supraoptic region form the _____ Tract to the Posterior Pituitary.

280. List the seven principal functions of the Hypothalamus: _____, _____, _____, _____, _____, _____, and _____.

281. The three regions of the brain stem include: the _____, the _____, and the _____.

282. The anterior surface of the Midbrain is noted for the the left and right _____; the posterior surface is noted for the region known as the _____.

283. The paired Cerebral Peduncles contain the descending _____ tracts. The Tectum is noted for the paired _____.

284. Why are the Corticospinal Tracts are also called Pyramidal Tracts? _____ _____ What dark staining nucleus lies deep to these tracts? _____ _____

285. The Substantia Nigra inhibits which two functional regions: the _____ and the _____ _____.

286. What are the two paired nuclei of the Corpora Quadrgemina called? _____ and _____

287. What is the function of the Superior Colliculi? _____ _____ What reflex is associated with the Inferior Colliculi? _____ _____

288. The main mass of the Midbrain is also called the _____.

289. What colored nucleus and associated tract is within the Tegmentum? _____ Nucleus and _____ Tract

290. What does the Red Nucleus control? _____ _____ The Rubrospinal Tract are Upper Motor Neurons, which descend to the _____.

291. What term is used to describe the network-like collection of gray and white matter that extends from the Midbrain through the rest of the brain stem? _____ _____

292. What three columns form and extend through the Reticular Formation: the midline _____ Nuclei and _____ and _____ Groups.

293. Which four areas do the reticular neurons extend to? _____, _____, _____, and the _____ _____

294. From the Thalamus, reticular neurons are directed to the cerebral cortex forming the _____ _____ System.

295. The Reticular Activating System is responsible for _____ and _____. Its descending motor pathway, the _____ Tract, mediates _____ tone.

296. The Midbrain is also the origin of Cranial Nerves _____ (_____) and _____ (_____).

297. The Pons serves as a bridge between the (_____) and the (_____). It is also the origin of Cranial Nerves _____ (_____), _____ (_____), _____ (_____), and _____ (_____).

298. The pathway between the Cerebellum and the Cortex is the Middle _____ _____. Within the Pons are two Respiratory Nuclei: the _____ and _____ Centers.

299. The Medulla is noted for _____ of the Corticospinal tracts, which travel within the _____. It is also the origin of Cranial Nerves _____ (_____), _____ (_____), _____ (_____ _____), and _____ (_____).

300. Lateral to the pyramids are oval swellings called the _____, which house the _____ Nuclei.

301. Olivary Nuclei inform the cerebellum of _____ _____.

302. The Medulla is also the site of visceral nuclei: the _____ and _____ Centers and mediates _____.

303. Describe the function of the Cerebellum: _____

_____.

304. The cerebellar hemispheres are connected by the _____ _____; the
folds of the cerebellum are known as _____, and the white matter is referred to as the

_____ _____.

305. The three lobes of the cerebellar hemisphere are: _____, _____, and
the _____.

306. The Cerebellum is noted for three white matter tracts, the _____ _____.

307. The Superior Cerebellar Peduncle connects the cerebellum to the _____, the middle to
the _____, and the inferior to the _____ _____.

308. Cortical atrophy, possibly familial, due to amyloid plaque is called _____.

309. How does a concussion differ from a contusion? _____

_____

310. How does a CVA differ from TIA? _____

_____

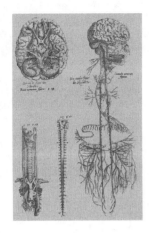

Part 3: The ANS

311. The two divisions of the Autonomic Nervous System are the _____ and
     _____.

312. Both Sympathetic and Parasympathetic are composed of two neurons which synapse in
     _____.

313. Pre-Ganglionic Sympathetic fibers synapse in ganglia which are close to/far from their origin; the
     Post-ganglionic fibers travel to target organs which are close to/far from the ganglia.

314. Pre-Ganglionic Parasympathetic fibers synapse in ganglia which are close to/far from their origin; the
     Post-ganglionic fibers travel to target organs, which are close to/far from the ganglia.

315. The Sympathetic Nervous System is also referred to as the _____-_____
     output; Sympathetic motor nuclei originate in the _____ _____ of the
     spinal cord, at levels _____.

316. The Parasympathetic NS is also referred to as the _____-_____ output;
     Parasympathetic motor nuclei originate in Cranial Nerves _____, _____, _____ and _____, and
     Spinal Nerves _____, _____, and _____.

317. The Sympathetic NS creates the "_____ or _____" response by:
     dilating/constricting pupils, dilating/constricting bronchioles, increasing/decreasing respiratory rate,
     increasing/decreasing heart rate, increasing/decreasing, blood pressure, dilating/constricting arteries to
     the abdominal organs, dilating/constricting arteries to the liver, heart, extremities and brain, inhibiting/
     promoting peristalsis, inhibiting/promoting secretions and glycogenolysis/glycogen synthesis.

318. The Parasympathetic NS creates the "_____ and _____" response by:
     dilating/constricting pupils, dilating/constricting bronchioles, increasing/decreasing respiratory rate,
     increasing/decreasing heart rate, increasing/decreasing, blood pressure, dilating/constricting arteries to
     the abdominal organs, dilating/constricting arteries to the liver, heart, extremities and brain, inhibiting/
     promoting peristalsis, inhibiting/promoting secretions and glycogenolysis/glycogen synthesis.

319. In addition to digestion, what three other functions are mediated by the Parasympathetic N.S.?
     _____, _____ and _____ _____.

320. Pre-ganglionic Sympathetic motor fibers leave the lateral horn and travel with somatic axons within the _____ _____ and as part of the spinal nerve. After exiting the IVF the Pre-ganglionic fiber enters the myelinated _____ _____ _____.

321. White Rami Communicans exit from the Spinal Nerve and first enter the _____ Chain Ganglia.

322. After entering the Paravertebral Chain Pre-ganglionic fibers may synapse within the chain or may exit as _____ _____.

323. Splanchnic Nerves may then travel to the three _____ Ganglia or the _____ _____.

324. The Pre-Vertebral Ganglia are located on the _____ and include the _____, _____ _____ and _____ _____.

325. Post-Ganglionic fibers from the Celiac Ganglion travel to organs of the epigastric and hypochondriac regions such as the _____, _____, _____, _____ and portions of the _____ _____. Those from the Superior Mesenteric Ganglion travel organs of the umbilical region such as portions of the _____ _____ and _____. Post-Ganglionic fibers from the Inferior Mesenteric Ganglion travel to organs of the Hypogastric and pelvic regions such as the _____, _____ and the _____.

326. The Post-Ganglionic Fibers of the Adrenal Medulla secrete the Catecholamines _____ and _____ into the circulatory system.

327. Because Epinephrine and Norepinephrine travel to their targets in the blood they at now desecribed as being _____.

328. Pre-Ganglionic Sympathetic fibers that do not exit the Paravertebral chain may synapse in what three ways: by _____, _____ or _____.

329. Because Pre-Ganglionics can ascend and descend before synapsing the Paravertebral Chains each have _____ ganglia. Post-Ganglionic fibers then exit the chain by _____ _____ _____ and then travel within _____ _____.

330. All pre-ganglionic Sympathetic fibers secrete: _____; most post-ganglionic sympathetic fibers secrete _____, except those to _____, _____, and _____.

331. The Cranial Nerves III, VII, and IX of the Parasympathetic NS form four ganglia: the _____, _____, _____, and _____.

332. The Ciliary Ganglion receives Pre-Ganglionic fibers from CN III and performs _____ _____; the Pterygopalatine from CN VII and performs _____ and stimulates _____ secretions.

333. The Submandibular Ganglion also receives Preganglionic Fibers from CN VII; the Otic Ganglion receives fibers from CN IX and both Post-Ganglionics stimulate _____. The Otic Ganglion stimulates the _____ Gland.

334. Cranial Nerve X supplies _____% of the Parasympathetic output and help form major plexuses. These include the _____ in the neck, and _____ and _____ in the thorax, all of which are named for the organs they supply.

335. In the abdominal cavity, Vagal Trunks form the _____ Plexus from which smaller plexuses then form: the _____ to the stomach and upper abdominal organs, the Superior and Inferior _____, and Superior _____ to the small and large intestines.

336. Sacral Nerves 2, 3, and 4 form _____ _____ Nerves, which form the Inferior _____ Plexus. This serves the _____, _____, and _____.

337. All pre-ganglionic and post-ganglionic parasympathetic fibers secrete _____.

338. Fibers that secrete and receptors that respond to AcetylCHOLINE are called _____; those that secrete or respond to NE are referred to as _____ (ADRENAL medulla).

339. Which three fibers are Cholinergic? _____ _____, _____ _____, and _____ _____.

340. There are two types of Cholinergic receptors: _____ and _____.

341. Nicotinic receptors in the ANS include all _____ _____ and the _____ _____, and the _____ _____ of skeletal muscle. The effect on nicotinic receptors is always inhibitory/excitatory.

342. Muscarinic receptors include _____ _____ targets and the ACh targets of the Sympathetic N.S.: _____ _____, _____ _____, and the _____.

343. Adrenergic fibers are _____ _____. Adrenergic receptors are either _____ or _____.

344. The beta receptors of the heart are inhibited/excited by NE.

345. Despite its name, which CNS centers ultimately regulate the functions of the Autonomic Nervous System: the _____ System and _____.

Unit VII: The Nervous System

Part 1: Physiology

1. Central and Peripheral
2. Brain and Spinal Cord; Cranial and Spinal
3. Sensory/Afferent; Motor/Efferent
4. skin and muscles, Central
5. organs and glands, Central
6. Somatic and Autonomic
7. skeletal muscles; Voluntary
8. organs and glands; Involuntary, Sympathetic, and Parasympathetic
9. "Fight or Flight"; "Rest and Digest"
10. new sensory data is compared to past experience to effect a response
11. neurons and glial
12. conductive; supportive
13. Astocytes, Oligodendrocytes, Microglia, and Ependymal Cells
14. pseudopodia, Blood Brain Barrier
15. Macrophage; myelinating axons
16. ventricles; cilia, Cerebral Spinal
17. Schwann, Satellite
18. secreting myelin sheath; macrophage; supportive
19. amitotic, great longevity, high metabolic rate
20. Receptive, Biosynthetic, Conductive, Secretory
21. soma, perikaryon; cytoplasmic processes
22. Nissl Bodies; centriole
23. Nuclei; Ganglia
24. dendrites; axons; telodendria
25. anterograde axoplasmic streaming
26. toxins, rabies
27. tracts; nerves
28. to the soma; away from the soma
29. graded potentials
30. long-distance nerve impulses
31. axon hillock; axolemma, terminus
32. Schwann
33. raveling around the axon; neurilemma
34. insulation; conduction velocity
35. Nodes of Ranvier
36. axon collaterals; Saltatory
37. 60; white; gray
38. bipolar, unipolar, multipolar

39. retina, auditory, olfactory
40. peripheral, proximal
41. 99%, 100's, 10,000
42. Sensory, Motor, and Association/Interneuron
43. multipolar; unipolar; multipolar
44. Integration; Dorsal Root Ganglia
45. potential; current
46. voltage; resistance
47. conductors; insulators
48. Passive and Gated
49. Leakage, electrochemical/concentration; chemically or voltage
50. leakage; neurotransmitters
51. in a state of electrical readiness to conduct a nerve impulse
52. $-70mV$; Na^+, K^+
53. Cl^-; proteins
54. Na^+/K^+ Pump
55. $3Na^+$, $2K^+$; Active, ATP
56. depolarization; hyperpolarization
57. increase; decrease
58. chemically-gated; neurotransmitters
59. graded potential
60. short, axon hillock
61. voltage-gated, Na^+
62. in, less
63. increase, threshold
64. $-55/-50$ mV; the minimum amount of depolarization (reduction in negativity) required to initiate an action potential
65. 0 mV
66. close, decreasing; $+30$ mV
67. open, increasing, out
68. increases, repolarize
69. -90 mV; hyperpolarization
70. Na^+/K^+ pump
71. Nerve Impulse
72. action potentials, terminus
73. the period of time during repolarization that the nerve fiber is immune to further stimulus
74. open, absolutely no response to further stimuli
75. open, closed; a relatively strong stimulus can re-open the Na^+ gates

76. −70 mV (D)
77. −50/−55 mV (C)
78. 0 mV (B)
79. +30 mV (A)
80. −90 mV (E)
81. +30 mV (A)
82. −50/−55 mV (C)
83. −70 to −55 mV (D)
84. −70 to −90 mV (E)
85. B, A and C
86. +30 to −70 mV (C)
87. −70 to −90 mV (E)
88. −55 to 0 mV (B)
89. −70 to −90 mV (E)
90. −70 to −55 mV (D)
91. −55/-50 to 0 mV (B)
92. 0 mV; A, C and E
93. +30 to −90 mV; C and E
94. −70 to +30 mV; D, B and A
95. −70 to −90 mV (E)
96. neurotransmitter secretion
97. frequency; Relative
98. axon, degree of myelination
99. thickest diameter, thickest myelination, fastest speed; skin and skeletal muscle
100. moderate diameter, myelination, speed; viscera
101. thinnest, no myelination, slowest speed; light touch and pressure
102. electric and chemical
103. gap, Na$^+$ and Cl$^-$
104. electrically coupled, eye, intercalated disc, smooth
105. pre-synaptic neuron, synaptic cleft, post-synaptic neuron
106. towards, away
107. neurotransmitters, receptor sites
108. secretion, diffusion and reception
109. Electrical
110. Synaptic Delay; unidirectional
111. calcium
112. exocytosis, secretion
113. synthesized by pre-synaptic neuron, creates ion fluxes in post-synaptic neuron, natural way of clearing from synapse
114. permeability, membrane
115. Na$^+$; K$^+$ and Cl$^-$
116. depolarizes; increase
117. hyperpolarizes; decrease
118. enzyme degradation, re-uptake by the pre-synaptic neuron, diffusion from cleft

119. ACh, Biogenic Amines, Amino Acids, Neuropeptides
120. enzyme degradation; neuromuscular, ANS
121. Catecholamines and Indolamines
122. L-Tyrosine; L-Tryptophan
123. Dopamine, Epinephrine Norepinephrine
124. "feel good"; Adrenal Medulla, Sympathetic
125. Serotonin; Histamine
126. induces sleep; re-uptake
127. Excitatory; Inhibitory
128. GABA, L-Glycine, Glutamate
129. Excitatory; ischemia
130. Endorphins and Enkephalins
131. Inhibitory; opiates, pain
132. Neuronal Pools
133. Discharge; Facilitated
134. Diverging, Converging
135. Oscillating/Reverberating; Parallel After Discharge
136. Series, Parallel
137. Plasticity: neuron changes with experience; Neurogenesis: new neurons
138. Regeneration requires Neurilemma of Schwann cells
139. Chromatolysis; Wallerian Degeneration
140. Regeneration Tube
141. New axon grows within tube towards target

Part 2: Anatomy of the CNS and PNS

142. Ectoderm
143. Neural Plate
144. Neural groove, Neural Crest
145. Neural Tube
146. Prosencephalon, Mesencephalon, Rhombencephalon
147. Forebrain, Midbrain, Hindbrain, Spinal Cord
148. Telecephalon and Diencephalon
149. Midbrain
150. Metencephalon and Myelencephalon
151. Ventricles
152. Gray Matter; White Matter
153. Cerebral Hemispheres
154. Cerebral Cortex, tracts, Basal Nuclei, Lateral
155. Epithalamus (Pineal), Thalamus, Hypothalamus, Third Ventricle
156. Cerebral Aqueduct
157. Pons, Cerebellum, Fourth
158. Medulla Oblongata
159. Brain Stem
160. Osseous: Cranial Bones; Soft Tissue: Meninges; Fluid: CSF
161. Dura Mater, Arachnoid, Pia Mater
162. two layers with separations forming sinuses

163. periosteal and meningeal
164. perisoteal
165. sinuses, venous system
166. meningeal, septa; Falx Cerebri, Falx Cerebelli, Tentorium Cerebelli
167. Longitudinal; Transverse
168. Epidural
169. Subdural
170. Subarachnoid; CSF
171. granulation villi, dural sinuses
172. denticulate ligaments
173. epithelial, Choroid Plexus, ventricles
174. Ependymal, CSF
175. no cells, K^+ and proteins, more Na^+ and Cl^-
176. Central Canal, Lateral Aperatures
177. Lumbar Cistern
178. dural sinuses; 150 ml; 900–1200 ml/day
179. endothelium, basal lamina, pseudopodia
180. Hyppthalamus, vomiting
181. foramen magnum
182. L1–L2, Conus Medularis
183. Cauda Equina; Filum Terminale
184. 8, 12, 5, 5, 1, 31
185. Posterior Median Sulcus, Anterior Median Fissure
186. Horns: Posterior—Sensory; Anterior—Motor; Lateral—Sympathetic Output
187. Gray Commissure
188. Reflex arc, decussation
189. T1–L2
190. Columns or Funiculi; Posterior, Lateral and Anterior
191. Fasiculi; Sensory Afferents, Motor Efferents
192. Spinothalamic, Post-central gyrus
193. Fasiculis gracilis
194. Spinocerebellar
195. Decussation, Pyrimidal, Medulla Oblogata
196. Anterior Corticospinal, do not
197. Lateral Corticospinal, decussate
198. Vestibulospinal, do not
199. Tectospinal
200. Gray Commissure; does not
201. Roots
202. Ventral, Anterior
203. Dorsal, Dorsal Root Ganglion, Horn
204. Lateral Horn, Anterior
205. Spinal Nerves
206. Dorsal Ramus, Ventral Ramus, Meningeal
207. Both, Both; Both, Both
208. Vertebra, ligaments, blood vessels and meninges
209. endoneurium, perineurium, epineurium
210. Plexuses; Intercostal
211. Cervical and Brachial; Lumbar and Sacral
212. C1–C4; Superficial and Deep
213. Sensory; Motor
214. Auricular, ear and parotid; Supraclavicular, upper chest and shoulder
215. Ansa Cervicalis, Phrenic
216. C5–T1, roots; Trunks
217. Upper, Middle and Lower; Anterior and Posterior
218. Cord
219. Lateral, Medial
220. Axillary, Musculocutaneous, Radial, Median, Ulnar
221. Deltoid, Teres minor
222. Coracobrachilais, Biceps Brachii
223. Posterior, Extension
224. Anterior, Flexion
225. Hand
226. L1–L4
227. Upper and Lower
228. Iliohypogastric and Ilioinguinal; Genitofemoral
229. Muscles of Anterolateral abdominal wall; Muscles Anterolateral abdominal wall and genitals
230. Dorsal and Ventral
231. Lateral Cutaneous and Femoral
232. Skin of the thigh; Flexor, Extensor
233. Obturator
234. Adduction
235. L4–S4, Dorsal and Ventral
236. Lumbosacral
237. Gluteal, Common Fibular
238. Gluteus Medius and Gluteus Minimus; Extension; Deep and Superficial
239. Eversion; Dorsiflexion
240. Pudendal and Tibial
241. Perineum, genitals; Plantar
242. Plantarflexion; Sciatic
243. Dermatome
244. Paraesthesia, anesthesia
245. sensory afferents cannot ascend past the injury to the thalamus; motor efferents cannot descend past the injury to reach LMN
246. they do not acend to the thalamus
247. the originate at their level of exit and do not ascend or descend
248. disrupts the motor output to the diaphragm
249. Quadriplegia; innervated by cranial nerves
250. Paraplegia
251. Poliomyelitis
252. Amyotrophic Lateral Sclerosis

253. Tabes Dorsalis
254. Multiple Sclerosis
255. Gyri and Sulci; convolutions
256. Frontal, Parietal, Temporal, Occipital, Insula
257. Longitudinal, Fissure of Rolando, Fissure of Sylvius
258. Cerebral Cortex, White Matter, Basal Nuclei
259. Caudate, Putamen, Globus Pallidus
260. Lentiform, Amygdaloid
261. Cingulate and Hippocampus; Fornix; Emotional
262. Angry and fearful facial expression, danger; fear
263. Physical gestures; Memory. Olfaction
264. Corpus Callosum, Anterior Commissure, Arcuate Fasiculi, Internal Capsule
265. Frontal; Parietal; Prefrontal; Occipital; Temporal
266. Learned Motor Skills. Speech
267. Spoken language recognition
268. Corona Radiata
269. mediate voluntary motor control and cognition; Parkinson's
270. Lentiform and Caudate; Cortex via the Internal Capsule
271. Globus Pallidus, Substantia Nigra; Prefrontal and Premotor
272. Epithalamus (pineal) Thalamus and Hypothalamus
273. control Circadian Rhythms, Sleep/ Wake cycle; inhibit precocious puberty
274. Intermediate or Interthalamic Adhesion
275. edits and sorts sensory afferents to appropriate cortex
276. Hypothalamus to Limbic; emotions and memory. Cortex, cognition
277. Hypothalamus
278. Mammillary, Tuberal, Supraoptic and Preoptic
279. Infundibulum, Anterior and Posterior Pituitary. Hypothalamic Hypophyseal
280. ANS control, Endocrine control, Emotional center, Temperature, Thirst, Hunger, Sleep/Wake cycle
281. Midbrain, Pons, Medulla Oblongata
282. Cerebral Peduncles; Tectum
283. Corticospinal Tracts. Corpora Quadrigemina
284. Formed from Pyramidal Multipolar Neurons. Substantia Nigra
285. Thalamus and Basal Nuclei
286. Superior and Inferior Colliculi
287. Coordiante head and eye movement; Startle Reflex
288. Tegmentum
289. Red Nucleus and Rubrospinal Tract
290. Muscle Tone; Extremities
291. Reticular Formation
292. Raphe, Medial and Lateral

293. Hypothalamus, Thalamus, Cerebellum and Spinal Cord
294. Reticular Activating
295. Arousal and Alertness. Reticulospinal Tract, muscle
296. III Oculomotor, IV Trochlear
297. Cerebrum and cerebellum; V Trigeminal, VI Abducens, VII Facial and VIII Vestibulo-cochlear
298. Middle Cerebellar Peduncle
299. Decussation, Pyramids; IX Glosspharyngeal, X Vagus, XI Spinal Accessory and XII Hypoglossal
300. Olives, Olivary
301. muscle stretch
302. Cardiovascular and Respiratory, heart and respiratory rate
303. create blueprint for smooth, coordin-ated skeletal muscle contractions
304. Central Vermis; folia, Arbor Vitae
305. Anterior, Posterior, Floculonodular
306. Cerebellar Peduncles
307. Cerebrum, Pons, Medulla Oblongata
308. Alzheimer's
309. Concussion: no neurological damage; Contusion: damage with coma and possibly death
310. TIA: transient ischemic attack, reversible effects; CVA: cerebro-vascular accident: usually with hemorrhage leading to permanent neurological deficit/loss of function

Part 3: The ANS

311. Sympathetic and Parasympathetic
312. Ganglia
313. Close to; far from
314. Far from; close to
315. Thoraco-Lumbar; Lateral Horn T1–L2
316. Cranial-Sacral; III, VII, IX, and X; S2, S3 and S4
317. "Fight or Flight": dilating pupils, dilating bronchioles, increasing respiratory/cardiac/BP, constricting arteries to the abdominal organs, dilating arteries to the liver/ heart/extremities/brain, inhibiting peristalsis, inhibiting secretions, Glycogenolysis
318. Rest and Digest; constricting pupils,constricting bronchioles, decreasing respiratory/heart/BP, dilating arteries to the abdominal organs. constricting arteries to the liver, heart, extremities and brain, promoting peristalsis/secretions and glycogen synthesis.
319. Urination, Defecation and Sexual Arousal
320. Anterior Root; White Rami Communicans
321. Paravertebral
322. Splanchnic Nerves

323. Pre-Vertebral or Adrenal Medulla

324. Aorta, Celiac, Superior Mesenteric and Inferior Mesenteric

325. Stomach, Spleen, Liver, Kidneys and Small Intestine. Small Intestine and Colon. Bladder, Rectum, and the Genitals

326. Epinephrine and Norepinephrine

327. Hormones

328. Ascending, descending or at their level of entry

329. 23. Gray Rami Communicans, Spinal Nerves

330. Acetylcholine; Norepinephrine, Sweat Glands, Blood Vessels and the Genitals

331. Ciliary, Pterygopalatine, Submandibular and Otic

332. Pupil constriction; Lacrimation and Nasal

333. Salivation. Parotid

334. 90%; Esophageal, Cardiac and Pulmonary

335. Aortic; Celiac, Mesenteric, Hypogastric

336. Pelvic Splanchnic, Hypogastric, Bladder, rectum and genitals

337. Acetylcholine

338. Cholinergic, Adrenergic

339. Pre-Ganglionic Parasympathetic, Post-Ganglionic Parasympathetic and Pre-Ganglionic Sympathetic

340. Nicotinic and Muscarinic

341. Post-Ganglionic Fibers, Adrenal Medulla, Motor End Plates. Excitatory

342. Post-Ganglionic Parasympathetic, Sweat Glands, Blood Vessels and the Genitals

343. Post-Ganglionic Sympathetic; Alpha α or Beta β

344. Excited

345. Limbic System and Hypothalamus

Unit VII: **Take a Test!**

Part 1: Time allowed: 50 minutes

1. The processing and interpretation of sensory data to effect a response is:
    a) communication
    b) integration
    c) discrimination
    d) initiation

2. Which of the following *is not* classified as a "general sense":
    a) pain
    b) pressure
    c) proprioception
    d) kinesthesia
    e) all are general senses

3. The Peripheral Nervous System includes all of the following except:
    a) Cranial Nerves
    b) Spinal cord
    c) Sympathetic
    d) Parasympathetic
    e) all are part

4. "Afferent" implies
    a) incoming
    b) motor
    c) a response
    d) a and b
    e) a, b and c

5. "Visceral" implies which of the following:
    a) from skeletal muscles
    b) from the integument
    c) from organs
    d) a and b
    e) a, b and c

6. **Somatic~Efferent** fibers bring data from:
    a) the ANS to skeletal muscles
    b) the ANS to organs and smooth muscles
    c) the CNS to skeletal muscles
    d) organs and smooth muscle to the CNS
    e) skin and skeletal muscles to the CNS

7. Which of the following is not characteristic of neurons:
    a) high metabolic rate
    b) extreme longevity
    c) high mitotic rate
    d) electrically conductive

8. "Plasticity" can be defined by all of the following *except:*
    a) neurons grow in size to accommodate growth of the individual
    b) neurons can replicate to replace old ones in adults
    c) axon collaterals form and reconnect severed peripheral nerves to their targets
    d) axon collaterals make new connections in response to learning

9. Which is described as the neuron's Receptive region:
    a) axon
    b) axon hillock
    c) dendrite
    d) soma
    e) terminus

10. Which is described as the neuron's Secretory region:
    a) axon   b) axon hillock
    c) dendrite   d) soma   e) terminus

11. Nerve impulses are propagated along the neuron's:
    a) axon   b) axon hillock
    c) dendrite   d) soma   e) terminus

12. An Action Potential usually originates from the:
    a) dendrite   b) soma
    c) axon hillock   d) axon   e) terminus

13. Neurotransmitters are synthesized by:
    a) Nucleus   b) Nissl Bodies
    c) Telodendria   d) Neurilemma   e) Synaptic Vesicles

14. Which represents the plasma membrane of the Schwann cell:
    a) neurilemma   b) myelin sheath
    c) axolemma   d) soma   e) none of these

15. The soma can be infected by rabies via:
    a) antereograde axoplasmic streaming   b) demyelination
    c) retrograde axoplasmic streaming   d) glioma formation

16. Which is true regarding the Nodes of Ranvier:
    a) they are exposed patches of Axolemma
    b) they allow Axon collaterals to exit
    c) they are the sites of Saltatory Conduction
    d) the further apart their spacing the faster the conduction velocity
    e) all are true

17. Which cell's pseudopodia form part of the Blood Brain Barrier:
    a) astrocyte   b) satellite
    c) ependymal cell   d) oligodendrocyte   e) schwann

18. Myelin is secreted in the CNS by:
    a) astrocyte   b) satellite
    c) ependymal cell   d) oligodendrocyte   e) schwann

19. Which is cell is associated with the Choroid Plexus and the production of CSF:
    a) astrocyte   b) satellite
    c) ependymal cell   d) oligodendrocyte   e) schwann

20. Gray Matter consists of which of the following elements:
    a) soma   b) non-myelinated telodendria
    c) tracts   d) a and b   e) a, b and c

21. Which describes a collection of cell bodies in the PNS:
    a) ganglion   b) tract
    c) nucleus   d) plexus   e) nerve

22. Which describes a collection of axons in the CNS:
    a) ganglion   b) tract
    c) nucleus   d) plexus   e) nerve

23. Which of the following are most likely to give rise to brain tumors:
    a) multipolar neurons   b) bipolar neurons
    c) unipolar neurons   d) glial cells   e) all could

24. Which sensory neurons have their soma located in Dorsal Root Ganglia:
    a) multipolar neurons   b) bipolar neurons
    c) unipolar neurons   d) pyramidal neurons

25. Motor neurons are classified/described as:
    a) multipolar neurons   b) bipolar neurons
    c) unipolar neurons   d) satellite cells   e) microglia

26. Which best explains why Peripheral Nerve Axons regenerate successfully whereas CNS tracts do not:
    a) CNS tracts are non-myelinated
    b) the axolemma of the PNS nerves heal
    c) PNS Satellite Cells repair the damage
    d) the neurilemma forms a regeneration tube

27. The Na^+/K^+ pump is necessary due to the presence of:
    a) chemically gated channels   b) voltage-gated channels
    c) passive/leakage ion channels d) carrier-gated channels

28. The initiation of a Graded Potential is accomplished by the opening of:
    a) chemically gated channels   b) voltage-gated channels
    c) passive/leakage ion channels d) carrier-gated channels

29. Graded potentials:
    a) are long distance signals   b) maintain their full charge as they travel
    c) are considered nerve impulses d) if strong enough can initiate an action potential

30. Nerve Impulses are propagated by the opening of:
    a) chemically gated channels   b) voltage-gated channels
    c) passive/leakage ion channels d) carrier-gated channels

Questions 31–36 refer to the graph on the right:
Which value represents:

31. Repolarization begins:

32. Na⁺ gates close:

33. K⁺ gates open:

34. Hyperpolarization:

35. Rest Potential:

36. Threshold:

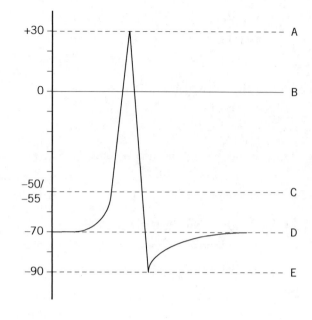

37. Which fast fiber type conduct impulses from pain receptors to the CNS and from the CNS to skeletal muscles:
    a) Type A   b) Type B
    c) Type C   d) Non-Myelinated

38. An amino acid such as Glycine is considered a neurotransmitter because:
    a) it creates ion fluxes in the post-synaptic membrane
    b) it is synthesized/secreted by the pre-synaptic neuron
    c) it can be cleared naturally from the synapse
    d) a and b are correct
    e) a, b and c are correct

39. Which is not a mechanism of neurotransmitter clearing:
    a) absorption by the post-synaptic membrane   b) enzymes
    c) reuptake by the pre-synaptic terminal   d) diffusion from cleft

40. ACh is cleared from the synapse by:
    a) absorption by the post-synaptic membrane   b) enzymes
    c) reuptake by the pre-synaptic terminal   d) diffusion from cleft

41. Which neurotransmitter is based on L-Tyrosine:
    a) histamine   b) serotonin
    c) Norepinephrine   d) ACh   e) endorphin

42. Which is considered a Indolamine:
    a) Enkephalin   b) Serotonin
    c) Norepinephrine   d) ACh   e) Endorphin

43. Which is considered a neuropeptide:
    a) histamine   b) serotonin
    c) Norepinephrine   d) ACh   e) endorphin

44. An Inhibitory neurotransmitter will:
    a) cause hyperpolarization of the post-synaptic neuron membrane
    b) cause depolarization of the post-synaptic neuron membrane
    c) increase the chances of its target reaching an action potential
    d) decrease the negativity of the post-synaptic neuron membrane

45. Excitatory neurotransmitters:
    a) increase K^+ permeability   b) increase Cl^- permeability
    c) increase Na^+ permeability   d) increase Ca^+ permeability   e) a and b

46. Inhibitory neurotransmitters:
    a) increase K^+ permeability   b) increase Cl^- permeability
    c) increase Na^+ permeability   d) increase Ca^+ permeability   e) a and b

47. Nerve Impulses/action potentials increase _____ permeability of the synaptic boot:
    a) K^+ b) Ca^+ c) Na^+ d) Cl^- e) a and b

48. Temporal Summation implies that:
    a) many neurons fire on the same membrane to reach Threshold
    b) one neuron fires many times on the same membrane to reach threshold
    c) the longer an axon the faster it fires on its target
    d) one neuron fires on many targets

49. A skeletal muscle contraction in which a single Upper Motor Neuron recruits thousands of fibers is facilitated by
    a) diverging circuits   b) converging circuits
    c) oscillating circuits   d) parallel after-discharge circuits

50. Rhythmic movements such as arm/leg cross-crawling swing are facilitated by:
    a) diverging circuits   b) converging circuits
    c) oscillating circuits   d) parallel after-discharge circuits

1. Which is the correct sequence from the outermost to the innermost layer:
    a) dura mater, subarachnoid space, epidural space, arachnoid mater, pia mater
    b) arachnoid mater, subarachnoid space, pia mater, epidural space, dura mater
    c) epidural space, dura mater, arachnoid mater, subarachnoid space, pia mater
    d) pia mater, subarachnoid space, arachnoid mater, epidural space, dura mater

2. How does the Dura Mater of the brain differ from that of the spinal cord:
    a) the dura of the drain is a double layer and the spinal cord is single
    b) the dura of the brain has separations called sinuses
    c) the dura of spinal cord is separated from the periosteum of the vertebra
    d) a and b
    e) a, b and c

3. The Denticulate Ligaments:
    a) anchors the dura and pia to the coccyx
    b) fuse the periosteal and meningeal layers of the dura together
    c) attach the spinal pia to the dura
    d) anchors the dura to the cranium

4. Anesthetics can be administered for childbirth and abdominal surgery by injection into the:
    a) dural sinuses   b) subdural space
    c) subarachnoid space   d) epidural space

5. The Tentorium Cerebelli would be found within the:
    a) longitudinal fissure   b) fissure of Rolando
    c) fissure of Sylvius   d) transverse fissure

6. Which of the following regarding CSF is false:
    a) it is produced by the choroid plexus
    b) it circulates through the subarachnoid space
    c) it is cleansed and recycled like blood
    d) it collects in in the lumbar cistern
    e) all are true statements

7. Which statement regarding the Choroid Plexus is true:
    a) it separates the hypothalamus from arterial blood
    b) it is formed from the pseudopodia of astrocytes
    c) it is formed by separations between the layers of the dura mater
    d) it is formed by capillaries, epithelium and Ependymal Cells

8. The Filum Terminale is the:
    a) fused anchoring of the meninges to the coccyx
    b) swollen receptacle for CSF within the sacral canal
    c) tapered end of the spinal cord at the level of L2
    d) "horse's tail" extension of spinal nerves L3 through 1st Coccygeal

9. The Conus Medularis is the:
   a) fused anchoring of the meninges to the coccyx
   b) "horse's tail" extension of spinal nerves L3 through 1st Coccygeal
   c) tapered end of the spinal cord at the level of L2
   d) swollen receptacle for CSF within the sacral canal

10. The Cauda Equina is the:
    a) fused anchoring of the meninges to the coccyx
    b) "horse's tail" extension of spinal nerves L3 through 1st Coccygeal
    c) tapered end of the spinal cord at the level of L2
    d) swollen receptacle for CSF within the sacral canal

11. The gray matter of the spinal cord:
    a) consists of multipolar cell bodies and non-myelinated processes
    b) consists of ascending and descending tracts
    c) has lateral horns at all levels
    d) a and b
    e) a, b and c

12. Which is true of the Gray Commissure:
    a) Site of ascending tract decussation
    b) Site of Deep Tendon Reflex integration/synapse
    c) Connects the Left and Right Cerebellar Hemispheres
    d) a and b
    e) a, b and c

13. The nuclei/cell bodies of **Somatic Afferent** fibers are located in the:
    a) pre-central gyrus   b) post-central gyrus
    c) anterior horn   d) lateral horn   e) dorsal root ganglia

14. **Visceral-Efferent** fibers have their nuclei/cell bodies of origin in the:
    a) pre-central gyrus   b) post-central gyrus
    c) anterior horn   d) lateral horn   e) dorsal root ganglia

15. **Lower Motor Neurons** have their nuclei/cell bodies of origin in the:
    a) pre-central gyrus   b) post-central gyrus
    c) anterior horn   d) lateral horn   e) dorsal root ganglia

16. The Columns of the spinal cord:
    a) consists of multipolar cell bodies and non-myelinated processes
    b) consists of ascending and descending tracts
    c) has lateral horns at all levels
    d) are found only between levels T1–L2
    e) a and b

17. Anesthesia, the loss of conscious pain and temperature sense would be due to injury to which tract:
    a) Spinocerebellar   b) Corticobulbar
    c) Corticospinal   d) Spinothalamic   e) Vestibulospinal

18. Which of the following tracts decussates in the pyramids of the medulla:
    a) Spinocerebellar   b) Corticobulbar
    c) Corticospinal   d) Spinothalamic   e) Vestibulospinal

19. Which tract carries afferent data of unconscious proprioception:
    a) Spinocerebellar   b) Corticobulbar
    c) Corticospinal   d) Spinothalamic   e) Vestibulospinal

20. Which Plexus contains motor nerves to the Upper Extremity:
    a) Cervical   b) Brachial
    c) Thoracic   d) Lumbar   e) Sacral

21. A skier is paralyzed from the shoulders down following a spinal cord injury at the level of C5 and has lost function of his arm and hand; what is the most likely explanation:
    a) its motor nerve exits above the lesion
    b) its motor nerve exits below the lesion
    c) it is controlled by cranial nerve innervation
    d) it is controlled by the Sympathetic NS
    e) it does not ascend to the sensory cortex for integration

22. With regard to above patient, his Biceps Brachii reflex is preserved; why:
    a) its motor nerve exits above the lesion
    b) its motor nerve exits below the lesion
    c) it is controlled by cranial nerve innervation
    d) it is controlled by the Sympathetic NS
    e) it does not ascend to the sensory cortex for integration

23. With regard to the C5 injury of #21, chewing, speech and some head movement is preserved because:
    a) its motor nerve exits above the lesion
    b) its motor nerve exits below the lesion
    c) it is controlled by cranial nerve innervation
    d) it is controlled by the Sympathetic NS
    e) it does not ascend to the sensory cortex for integration

24. With regard to the C5 injury of #21: the diaphragm continues to function because:
    a) its motor nerve exits above the lesion
    b) its motor nerve exits below the lesion
    c) it is controlled by cranial nerve innervation
    d) it is controlled by the Sympathetic NS
    e) it does not ascend to the sensory cortex for integration

25. This individual's condition would be classified as:
    a) paraplegic   b) quadriplegic
    c) hemiplegic   d) myoplegic

26. The Cerebrum consists of all of the following areas except:
    a) Basal Nuclei   b) Limbic System
    c) Reticular Activating System d) Association Areas   e) all are part

27. Which of the following is not considered to be a lobe of the cerebral cortex:
    a) Frontal   b) Parietal
    c) Temporal   d) Insula   e) all are lobes

28. The folds of Cerebral gray matter are called:
    a) arbor vitae   b) folia
    c) vermis   d) fornix   e) convolutions

29. The Right and Left Cerebral Hemispheres are separated by the:
    a) Central Sulcus/Sylvius b) Transverse Fissure
    c) Lateral Sulcus/Rolando d) Longitudinal Fissure

30. The motor and sensory cortexes are separated by the:
    a) Central Sulcus/Rolando b) Transverse Fissure
    c) Lateral Sulcus/Sylvius d) Longitudinal Fissure

31. Upper Motor Neurons originate in which area:
    a) Frontal lobe   b) Temporal lobe
    c) Occipital lobe   d) Parietal lobe   e) Insula

32. The visual cortex is located within the:
    a) Frontal lobe   b) Temporal lobe
    c) Occipital lobe   d) Parietal lobe   e) Insula

33. The General Sense/Somatosensory cortex is located in the:
    a) pre-central gyrus   b) post-central gyrus
    c) insula   d) limbic system   e) basal nuclei

34. Integration between the right and left Cerebral Hemispheres is mediated by the:
    a) Corpus callosum   b) Fornix
    c) Anterior Commissure   d) Internal Capsule   e) Arbor vitae

35. Integration between lobes of the same hemisphere is carried out by the:
    a) Corpus Callosum   b) Fornix
    c) Anterior Commissure   d) Internal Capsule   e) Arbor vitae

36. Upper Motor Neuron tracts travel within the:
    a) Corpus Callosum   b) Fornix
    c) Anterior Commissure   d) Internal Capsule   e) Arbor vitae

37. Tremors are associated with dysfunction of which area:
    a) Pineal
    b) Basal Nuclei
    c) Limbic System
    d) Thalamus
    e) Pituitary

38. Inborn drives such as detecting danger/fear and arousal are regulated by the:
    a) Pineal Gland
    b) Hypothalamus
    c) Thalamus
    d) Basal Nuclei
    e) Limbic System

39. Which tract integrates the Limbic System with the Hypothalamus:
    a) Corpus Callosum
    b) Fornix
    c) Anterior Commissure
    d) Internal Capsule
    e) Arbor vitae

40. The Diencephalon consists of all of the following except:
    a) Pineal
    b) Thalamus
    c) Third Ventricle
    d) Hypothalamus
    e) all are part

41. Which structure is responsible for Circadian Rhythms and inhibits premature puberty:
    a) Pineal Gland
    b) Hypothalamus
    c) Thalamus
    d) Basal Nuclei
    e) Limbic System

42. The Thalamus:
    a) is the primary autonomic and endocrine control region
    b) directs sensory afferents to the post-central gyrus
    c) secretes melatonin and is associated with sleep/wake cycles
    d) is connected to the pituitary by the infundibulum
    e) creates a blueprint for smooth, coordinated skeletal muscle contraction

43. All of the following are functions of the Hypothalamus except:
    a) coordinates ANS responses
    b) coordinates Endocrine responses
    c) regulates Temperature
    d) regulates Thirst and Hunger
    e) all are function

44. All are part of the Brainstem except:
    a) Midbrain
    b) Pons
    c) Medulla Oblongata
    d) Cerebellum
    e) all are part

45. The Corpora Quadrigemma are located in the:
    a) medulla
    b) midbrain
    c) pons
    d) cerebellum
    e) basal nuclei

46. Medulla Oblongata is noted for all of the following except:
    a) the decussation of corticospinal tracts
    b) the vasomotor center
    c) regulating the rate of breathing
    d) regulating Thirst and Hunger
    e) all of these apply

47. The Cerebellum:
    a) directs sensory afferents to the sensory cortex
    b) is responsible for creating smooth, coordinated skeletal muscle contraction
    c) secretes melatonin and is associated with sleep/wake cycles
    d) is connected to the pituitary by the infundibulum
    e) is the primary autonomic and endocrine control region

48. The central gray matter region of the Cerebellum is known as the:
    a) arbor vitae   b) folia
    c) vermis   d) fornix   e) peduncle

49. The white matter tracts of the Cerebellum are known as:
    a) arbor vitae   b) folia
    c) vermis   d) fornix   e) convolutions

50. The importance of the Inferior Peduncles is that they advise the cerebellum of:
    a) proprioception   and kinesthesia   b) pain
    c) temperature   d) all of these

51. Parasympathetic motor nuclei originate in:
    a) Lateral Horn levels T1–L2   b) CNs III, VII, IX, X and S2,S3 and S4
    c) Adrenal Medulla   d) Hypothalamus

52. Which would be expected if one was nervous before a job interview:
    a) runny nose   b) tearing eyes
    c) excessive salivation   d) dry mouth   e) a, b and c

53. Which of the following are functions of the parasympathetic nervous system:
    a) urination   b) defecation
    c) sexual arousal   d) a and b   e)all are

54. Which is not a function of the Vagus Nerve:
    a) reduce the resting heart rate to 75 beats per minute
    b) control peristalsis
    c) stimulate gastric secretions
    d) stimulate salivation
    e) all are functions of the Vagus Nerve

55. The Hypogastric Plexus is formed by:
    a) Sacral Nerves 2,3 and 4   b) CN III
    c) CN IX   d) CN X   e) CN VII

56. Salivation is controlled by:
    a) Facial Nerve   b) Glossopharyngeal Nerve
    c) Vagus Nerve   d) a and b   e) all three

57. Constriction of the pupils is controlled by:
   a) Sacral Nerves 2,3 and 4   b) CN III
   c) CN IX   d) CN X   e) CN VII

58. Which would best describe the overall goal of Sympathetic reactions:
   a) increase oxygen and glucose supply to skeletal muscle
   b) increase oxygen and glucose supply to smooth muscle
   c) prepare the body for digestion
   d) prepare the body for mitosis and tissue repair

59. Which is true regarding the Sympathetic Nervous System:
   a) pre-ganglionics synapse in ganglion close to their origin
   b) pre-ganglionics travel in white rami
   c) pre-ganglionics secrete NE
   d) a and b
   e) a, b and c

60. Pre-ganglionic Sympathetic fibers may synapse with all of the following except:
   a) Prevertebral Ganglia   b) Adrenal Medulla
   c) Paravertebral Ganglia   d) Dorsal Root Ganglia   e) Synapse with all

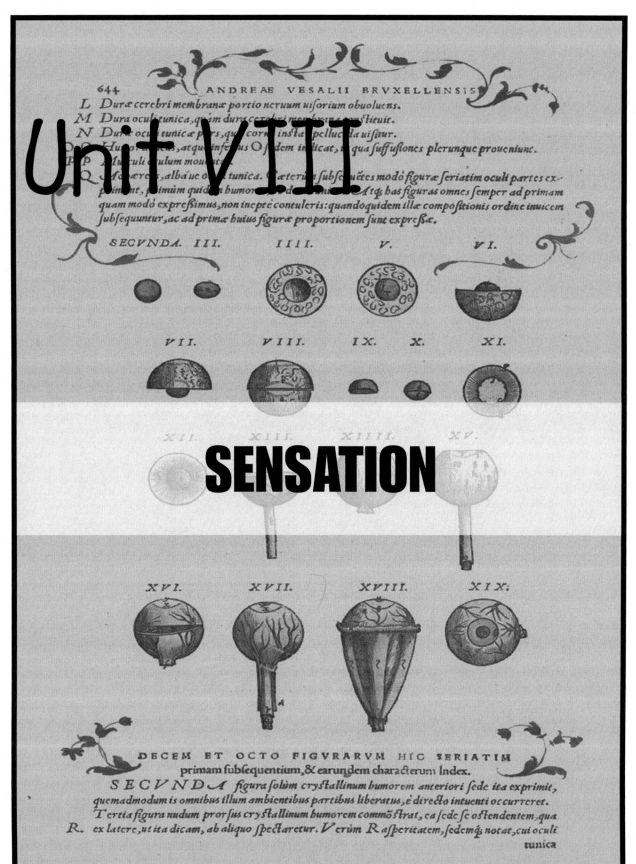

Unit VIII

SENSATION

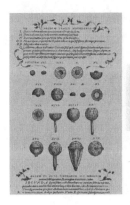

Part 1: **General Sense**

1. Sensory data is referred to as _____; motor responses are referred to as _____.

2. Sensory Afferent data is received by _____ _____ and reaches the CNS via _____ pathways; Motor Efferent data travel from the CNS via _____ pathways to reach their _____.

3. Sensory End organs conduct either _____ Senses or _____ Senses.

4. General Senses include: _____ _____, _____, _____, _____, and _____.

5. Special Senses include: _____, _____, _____ and _____. All Special Sense afferents are carried by _____ Nerves.

6. The process by which sensory end organs are stimulated is called _____; the process by which stimuli is converted into action potentials is called _____.

7. Reception is specialized based on the sensory end organ receptor's _____ _____ structure and surrounding _____ cells.

8. In Transduction, the stimulus to the receptor's cell membrane and supportive cells creates a _____ _____, which either depolarizes or hyperpolarizes.

9. The area covered by a specific receptor is called the _____ _____. Receptor Potentials, if adequate, create action potentials, which are called _____ Potentials.

10. Special Sense receptors synapse with a _____ _____, which propagates the generator potential. General Sense neurons conduct generator potentials to their cell bodies within the _____ _____ _____ before synapsing with ascending cell bodies, which are in the _____ _____ of the spinal cord.

11. Special Sense sensory neurons and ascending axons of Posterior Horn cells direct afferent data to the _____, which then directs impulses to the appropriate area of the _____ _____.

12. The neural link between a receptor and the sensory cortex is referred to as a _____ _____

13. The Labeled Line determines the specific type of sensory input whereas the characteristics or _____ _____ are determined by _____ and _____ of nerve impulses.

14. Patterns of Sensory Coding are created by _____ Receptors, which are always active and _____ Receptors, which are inactive until stimulated.

15. Tonic Receptors respond to changes in _____ of stimulation as in _____. Phasic Receptors respond to stimulus of _____ _____ as in _____.

16. The reduction in sensitivity to constant stimulus is called _____.

17. Adaptation occurs as _____ Adaptation and _____ Adaptation.

18. Peripheral Adaptation occurs when _____ sensitivity declines. Central Adaptation occurs when _____ _____ sensitivity declines.

19. Tonic Receptors are slow/fast adapting. How is this exemplified in pain perception?
    _____

    Phasic Receptors are slow/fast adapting. How is the exemplified in temperature perception?
    _____

20. How is Central (sensory neuron) Adaptation exemplified by olfaction? _____
    _____

21. List the fours classes of General Sense Receptors: _____ or _____, _____, _____, and _____.

22. Pain or Nociceptors are structurally described as _____ _____ endings and respond to four stimuli: extreme _____ changes, _____, _____ damage, and any _____ stimuli.

23. Stimulated free nerve endings secrete _____ and _____ _____ as neurotransmitters in the spinal cord; pain stimuli then ascends via the _____ _____ tract.

24. Sharp, focused pain is carried by Type _____ fibers; Diffuse, achy pain is carried by Type _____ fibers. Burning pain created by strong stimuli is called _____. Pain perception may be reduced by _____ Adaptation.

25. Like Nociceptors, Thermoreceptors structurally are _____ _____ _____ and are found in the _____, _____ _____, the _____ and the _____.

26. Mechanoreceptors have gated _____ _____, which open and close in response to changes in _____.

27. Mechanoreceptors fall into three groups: _____ or _____ Receptors, _____, and _____.

28. How does the structure of tactile receptor corpuscles differ from that of free nerve endings? _____ _____

29. Corpuscles composed of dendritic processes surrounded by specialized cells and matrix include _____, _____, and _____.

30. Meissner's Corpuscles receive _____ _____ and _____, and are located in the _____ layer of the dermis. Pacinian Corpuscles receive _____ _____ and are located in the _____ layer of the dermis. Ruffini Corpuscles perceive _____.

31. Other tactile receptors include _____ _____, which receive fine touch and pressure, and the _____ _____ _____ of the hair shaft.

32. Merkel's Discs have dendritic processes which reach into the _____ _____ of the epidermis.

33. Baroreceptors structurally are _____ _____ _____ located within _____.

34. Baroreceptors respond to changes in pressure via _____.

35. Propriceptors monitor _____ position, _____ and _____ tension, and _____ _____.

36. Joint positioning is monitored by _____ _____ _____ in the _____ _____. Tendon and ligament tension is monitored by the _____ _____ organ. Muscle contraction is monitored by the _____ _____.

37. Chemoreceptors monitor the concentration of _____ or _____, and _____.

38. H⁺ or pH and CO_2 concentration of the blood is monitored by the _____ and _____ Bodies; the CSF is monitored by the _____ center of the _____.

39. The Special Senses include _____, _____, _____ and _____. All Special Senses are received by _____ _____.

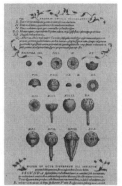

Part 2: The Cranial Nerves and Special Sense

40. The Twelve Cranial Nerves (CN) are:

    I   : _____   VII : _____
    II   : _____   VIII: _____
    III : _____   IX : _____
    IV   : _____   X   : _____
    V   : _____   XI : _____
    VI   : _____   XII : _____

41. Receptors of the Olfactory Nerve are located within the _____ _____ and pass through the perforations of the _____ _____ to synapse with sensory neurons within the _____ _____

42. The Olfactory Bulbs are on either side of the _____ _____ the axons of these sensory neurons form the _____ _____.

43. The receptors of CN II originate in the _____; these synapse with sensory neurons whose axons form the _____ _____.

44. Fibers of the medial/nasal fields of the Optic Nerves cross at the _____ _____, which overlies the _____ _____. The recombined axons continue to the visual cortex as the _____ _____.

45. The Oculomotor Nerve innervates the _____, _____, and _____ Rectus, and the _____ _____ muscles. CN III also supplies pre-ganglionic fibers to the _____ Ganglion, which control the muscles of the _____.

46. The CN IV, the Trochlear Nerve, innervates the _____ _____ muscle; CN VI, the Abducens Nerve, innervates the _____ _____

47. The Trigeminal Nerve is so named because _____.

48. The three nuclei of origin of CN V form the _____, the _____, and the _____ Branches.

49. In addition to sensory reception, the Mandibular Branch is also the motor output for muscles of _____. CN V also contributes Parasympathetic fibers (with CN III) to the _____ Ganglion, to the Sphenopalatine ganglia controlling _____, and Submandibular Ganglion controlling _____ glands.

50. The Facial Nerve receives both general sense from the _____ and _____ from the anterior _____, _____ of the tongue. CN VII also supplies both _____ and _____ motor output.

51. The Facial Nerve supplies pre-ganglionic parasympathetic motor fibers to the _____ Ganglion controlling the lacrimal glands, and the _____ Ganglion controlling salivary glands.

52. The somatic motor output of CN VII is divided into five branches: _____, _____, _____, _____, and _____.

53. Unilateral paralysis of the Facial Nerve is known as _____ _____. A chronic, pain-producing disorder of the Trigeminal nerve is _____ _____.

54. The Auditory Nerve is also referred to as the _____ Nerve.

55. The Vestibular Branch of CN VIII carries _____ sense, whereas the Cochlear Branch carries _____ sense.

56. The Glossopharyngeal Nerve carries the special sense _____ from the posterior _____ of the tongue, general sense from the _____, and BP and O_2 from the _____ _____.

57. CN IX supplies somatic motor output to the _____ and _____, and parasympathetic output to the _____ glands.

58. CN IX initiates the voluntary stage of _____ and mediates the _____ Reflex.

59. The Vagus Nerve supplies _____% of the parasympathetic output; it directly regulates the _____ rhythm and receives taste from the _____.

60. The Spinal Accessory Nerve is so named because _____. It innervates the _____ and _____ muscles. The Hypoglossal Nerve innervates the _____.

61. The Olfactory organs are composed of two layers: the _____ _____ and the _____ _____.

62. The Olfactory Epithelium contains the _____ _____, which has _____ cells and _____ cells.

63. Unlike other nerve cells, Olfactory receptors are _____ active and are replaced after _____ _____. The Lamina Propria contains Olfactory or _____ Glands, which produce _____.

64. Receptor neurons form _____, which embed in the mucus layer. Define Volatile: _____.

65. Substances diffuse through the mucus and interact with _____ _____ _____; this in turn opens _____ gates and _____ the receptor.

66. Receptor axons pass through the _____ _____ to synapse within _____ inside the _____ _____.

67. Receptor axons synapse within glomeruli with _____ cells whose axons form the _____ _____. These continue on to the Olfactory Cortex located below the _____ Lobe.

68. The ability to distinguish odors is called _____. One "gets used to" offensive odors via _____ adaptation. Emotional responses to odors are mediated by the _____ and the _____ System.

69. Aberrations in olfactory sense are called _____. Olfactory hallucinations are called _____ _____.

70. Ansosomias are due to _____ _____ and _____ _____; Unicinate Fits are associated with _____ and _____.

71. Taste is properly called _____.

72. Gustatory receptors and surrounding epithelium form _____ _____. The four classical tastes are: _____, _____, _____, and _____.

73. Sweet receptors respond to _____, _____ (Sweet and Low), _____ and some _____ _____ (Aspartame/Equal). Salt receptors respond to _____, which include _____.

74. Sour receptors respond to _____ and _____, which are associated with _____, or _____, food. Bitter receptors respond to _____, _____, and _____ as well as substances that are generally _____.

75. The newly discovered taste, _____, responds to _____. Sweet and salty receptors are located on the _____ of the tongue, sour on the _____, and bitter on the _____. Taste buds are located within _____ _____.

76. Lingual Papillae are _____, _____, and _____.

77. Unlike Fungiform and Circumvallate, Filiform papillae function by _____ _____.

How do Circumvallate and Fungiform papillae differ by location? _____ _____

78. Taste afferents are first directed to the _____ _____ of the medulla, then the _____, and finally the gustatory cortex within the _____ lobe. _____% of taste is smell.

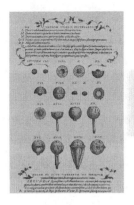

Part 3: The Eye and Vision

79. The eyebrows are depressed by the _____ _____ muscle and raised by the _____ muscle.

80. The eyelids are separated by the _____ _____ and meet at the Medial and Lateral _____.

81. The Medial Canthus is noted for the _____ _____. The underside of the palpebrae is supported by _____ _____.

82. The Lacrimal Caruncle houses _____ and _____ glands. Tarsal plates anchor the _____ _____ _____ muscle.

83. The Levator Palpebrae Superioris performs the reflex of _____, which spreads the secretions of Tarsal or _____ glands over the surface of the eye.

84. Infections of Tarsal/Meibomian glands are called _____; that of other eye glands are called _____. Eyelashes are separated by _____ glands.

85. The clear mucus membrane that covers the surface of the white portion of the eye is properly called the _____-_____ _____, and that covering the under side of the eyelid the _____ _____.

86. The Lacrimal Gland is located _____; tears collect at the _____ _____ and drain through the _____ _____ into the _____ _____.

87. Tears from the Lacrimal Canals collects in the _____ _____ then drains into the nasal cavity via the _____ _____.

88. Which four extrinsic muscles are innervated by CN III, the Oculomotor Nerve? _____ _____, _____ _____, _____ _____, and the _____ _____ Which is innervated by CN IV, the Trochlear Nerve? _____ _____ Which is innervated by CN VI, the Abducens Nerve? _____ _____

89. How does Diplopia differ from Strabismus? _____

_____

90. The lens divides the internal cavity of the eye into _____ and _____

segments.

91. The Anterior Segment is filled with _____ Humor and is divided into Anterior and

Posterior _____ by the _____ The Posterior Segment is filled with

_____ Humor.

92. How does the Aqueous Humor differ from the Vitreous with regard to formation? _____

_____

93. Production of Aqueous Humor is offset by drainage into the _____ _____

_____; blockage can lead to increased intraocular pressure, aka _____.

94. The wall of the eye is composed of three layers: the outer _____ _____,

the _____ _____, and the innermost _____

_____.

95. The Fibrous Tunic is composed of the white CT _____ and transparent

_____.

96. The junction of the Sclera and Cornea is called the _____. Transparency of the cornea is

maintained by specialized _____ _____.

97. The Vascular Tunic is also referred to as the _____ and forms three regions: the posterior

_____, the _____ _____, a thickened ring circling the

lens, and the pigmented _____.

98. The Choroid's melanocytes function by _____.

The Ciliary Body is composed of _____ _____, which control the shape

of the lens.

99. Extensions of the Ciliary Muscles, the _____ _____, are anchored to the

lens by the _____ _____.

100. The lens is composed of two specialized tissues, the lens _____ and the lens

_____. Clouding of the lens is called _____.

101. Lens fibers are noted for transparent proteins called _____. With age, lens fibers increase

in number. How does this affect the lens and vision? _____

_____

102. The size of the aperture of the iris is controlled by two bands of _____ muscle, an inner

_____ and outer _____.

103. In bright light the _____ NS stimulates the inner circular band to contract; this

_____ the iris. In dim light the _____ NS simulates the outer radial

band; this _____ the iris.

104. The Sensory Tunic is also known as the _____ and is composed of two layers, the _____ layer, which is in contact with the vitreous humor, and the underlying _____ layer.

105. The Pigmented layer of the Retina stores Vitamin _____; the Neural layer is noted for photoreceptors, _____ and _____, and forms the _____ _____ _____ at its junction with the ciliary body.

106. Cones function in _____ light and _____ vision; Rods function in _____ light and _____ vision.

107. Rods are noted for the photoreactive pigment _____; Cones, which react to colored light, are noted for the pigments _____ and 4 _____.

108. When stimulated by photons of white light, Rhodopsin, which is normally _____, is turned into an _____.

109. The isomer of Rhodopsin is _____ from purple to _____. This activates the enzyme _____.

110. Transducin opens/closes Na⁺ gates causing the Rod to depolarize/hyperpolarize and release _____.

111. Once stimulated, hyperpolarized Cones and Rods release glutamate depolarizing _____ neurons, which then depolarize _____ Cells, the axons of which form the _____.

112. The Optic nerve exits at the _____ _____, which creates a _____ _____ due to the lack of photoreceptors. The Posterior pole of the eye is marked by the _____ _____.

113. Unlike the blind spot created by the Optic Disc, the Macula lutea is noted for the _____ _____, the site of greatest _____ _____.

114. The shape of the lens is described as _____; this causes focused light rays to _____ on a central focal point. The process by which the lens changes shape to focus on near and far objects is called _____. The process by which the eyes turn inward to focus on near objects is called _____.

115. In near accommodation the lens _____ and the pupils _____ as the eyes converge; in far accommodation the lens _____ as the pupils _____ to increase visual acuity.

116. Normally shaped eyes are termed _____; elongate eyes are termed _____ and shorter eyes _____.

117. Myopic eyes create _____-sighted individuals whereas hyperoptic eyes create _____-sightedness. The loss of accommodation in normal aging Emmetroptic eyes requiring reading glasses is called _____.

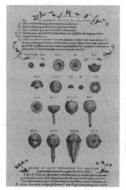

Part 4: The Ear, Hearing, and Equilibrium

118. The Outer Ear includes the _____ or Pinna and the _____ _____ Canal up to the _____ _____ or eardrum.

119. The outer border of the auricle is known as the _____. The Tympanic Membrane is noted for its characteristic light reflection, the _____.

120. The Middle Ear is also known as the _____ Cavity and is housed within the _____ _____ of the _____ bone.

121. The Tympanic Cavity extends from the Tympanic Membrane through the petrous portion of Temporal to the Oval or _____ Window and Round or _____ Window.

122. The Middle Ear is noted for its opening into the _____ or _____ Tube, which empties into the pharynx, and the smallest bones of the body, the _____ _____.

123. The three Auditory Ossicles are the _____, the _____, and the _____.

124. The Malleus transmits sound waves from the _____ Membrane to the Incus; the Stapes transmits sound from the Incus to the _____/_____ Window.

125. As a protective mechanism during loud noises, movement of the Stapes is restricted by the _____ muscle, and that of the eardrum by the _____ _____ muscle. Infection of the middle ear is called _____ _____.

126. The Inner Ear is also referred to as the _____.

127. The Labyrinth is subdivided into the _____ and _____ Labyrinth.

128. The Membranous Labyrinth is located within the Bony Labyrinth and is filled with _____. The Bony Labyrinth is filled with _____ and is noted for three structures: the _____, the _____ _____, and the _____.

129. The Vestibule is adjacent to the _____ and _____ Windows, and is noted for two structures the _____ and the _____.

130. The Utricle opens into the _____ _____, which lead into the Semicircular Canals. The Saccule opens into the _____ _____, which lead into the Cochlea.

131. The three Semicircular Canals lie at _____ angles to each other and are referred to as the _____, _____, and _____. Each canal ends at its swollen _____, which houses the equilibrium receptor, the _____ _____.

132. The center of the spiral-shaped Cochlea is the _____; the Cochlear Duct houses the auditory receptor, the _____ _____ _____. The Cochlea is divided into three chambers or _____: the _____ _____, the _____ _____, and the _____ _____.

133. The Scala Vestibuli abuts the _____ Window; the Scala Media or Cochlear Duct is noted for its roof, the _____ Membrane, and its floor, the _____ Membrane, which supports the Spiral Organ of Corti.

134. The Scala Tympani abuts the _____ Window and merges with the Scala Vestibuli to form the _____.

135. Sound waves can be likened to a sine wave. What determines the wavelength of sound? _____

What determines the frequency of the wavelength? _____

136. A single frequency is called a _____; different frequencies are perceived as _____.

137. How does pitch differ from Amplitude? _____
How is frequency expressed? _____ How is loudness expressed? _____

138. Sound waves directly vibrate the _____ _____, which transmits these vibrations to the _____ _____.

139. The movement of the ossicles vibrates the _____ Window, which sets the _____ within the _____ _____ to move towards the apex of the cochlea, the _____.

140. The perilymph of the scala vestibuli moves past the helicotrema through the _____ _____ and the _____ Window.

141. The movement of perilymph within the scala tympani causes the _____ Membrane to move up and down; this stimulates the _____ _____ Cells of the Organ of Corti.

142. The Cochlear Hair Cells are sandwiched in between the Basilar and _____ Membranes, and arranged in one row of _____ Hair Cells and three rows of _____ Hair Cells.

143. Hair Cells possess _____, which on movement open _____ channels. The depolarized Hair Cells now stimulate the afferent fibers of the _____ Nerve.

144. The afferent fibers of the Cochlear Nerve synapse with _____ neurons of the _____ _____ of the Cochlear Nerve. These then travel as part of the _____ Nerve.

145. The Vestibulocochlear Nerve travels first to the _____ _____ Nucleus, the _____ _____ (startle reflex), then on to the _____ to be directed to the Auditory Cortex of the _____ lobe.

146. How does Conduction Deafness differ from Sensorineural Deafness? _____
_____

What is Otosclerosis? _____

147. What is Tinnitis? _____
What is Meniere's Syndrome? _____

148. Vertigo is due to dysfunction of the _____ _____.

149. Equilibrium is monitored by the Vestibular Apparatus as both _____ equilibrium and _____ equilibrium.

150. Dynamic equilibrium is monitored by the _____ _____; Static equilibrium is monitored by the _____.

151. The maculae are located within the walls of the _____ and _____, and respond to _____ movement.

152. The Macula of the Saccule responds to _____ movement whereas that in the Utricle responds to _____ movement.

153. Vertical and horizontal movements stimulate receptor _____ Cells whose stereocilia are embedded within the _____ Membrane.

154. The Otolithic membrane is stabilized by CaCO$_3$ crystals called _____. Movement of the head causes the Hair Cells to stimulate the endings of the _____ Nerve which conduct impulses to sensory neurons within the _____ and _____ Ganglia.

155. Dynamic equilibrium monitors _____ motion by the movement of fluid within the _____ _____.

156. The Ampullae of the Semicircular Canals are noted for elevations called the _____ _____.

157. Receptor _____ Cells of the Crista Ampullaris extend into a gel-like mass called the
     _____.

158. During angular motion, the Hair cells within the Cupula respond to movement of the
     _____ within the canal by depolarizing on one side of the head and
     _____ on the opposite. These in turn stimulate dendrites of the
     _____ Nerve.

159. The Vestibular Nerve conducts impulses to either the _____ or the
     _____ _____ _____ of the brainstem.

160. The Vestibular Nuclear Complex also receives _____ and _____ sensory
     data and responds via eye movement and the _____ tract.

Unit VIII: Sensation

Part 1: **General Sense**

1. Afferent, Efferent
2. End Organs, Ascending; Descending, targets
3. General, Special
4. Pain, Temperature, Pressure, Touch, Vibration, Proprioception
5. Vision, Hearing, Taste, Smell; Cranial
6. Reception; Transduction
7. cell membrane, supportive
8. Receptor Potential
9. Receptive Field, Generator
10. Sensory Neuron; Dorsal Root Ganglion, Posterior Horn
11. Thalamus, Sensory Cortex
12. Labeled Line
13. Sensory Coding, frequency and pattern
14. Tonic, Phasic
15. frequency, pain; end receptors, temperature
16. Adaptation
17. Peripheral and Central
18. Receptor; Sensory Neuron
19. slow adapting: pain lingers after stimulus stops; fast adapting: one gets "used to" the change quickly
20. One gets "used to" offensive odors
21. Pain or Nociceptors, Thermoreceptors, Mechanoreceptors, Chemoreceptors
22. free nerve: temperature, chemicals, mechanical damage, strong stmuli
23. Glutamate and Substance P; Lateral Spinothalamic
24. A; C; Causalgia; Central
25. Free Nerve Endings; dermis, skeletal muscles, liver, and hypothalamus
26. ion channels; physical changes in the shape of the membrane
27. Tactile or touch, Baroreceptors, Proprioceptors
28. free nerve endings are bare dendrites; corpuscle endings are surrounded by supportive cells
29. Meissner's, Pacinian and Ruffini
30. light touch and pressure, papillary; deep pressure, reticular; skin stretch
31. Merkel's Discs, Root Hair Plexus
32. Stratum Germinatum
33. free nerve endings, walls of hollow organs and blood vessels
34. distention
35. joint position, tendon and ligament tension, muscle stretch
36. free nerve endings, joint capsule; Golgi Tendon, muscle spindle
37. H^+ or pH and CO_2
38. Aortic and Carotid; Respiratory center of medulla
39. vision, hearing, taste and smell; cranial nerves

Part 2: **Cranial Nerves and Special Sense**

40. Olfactory, Optic, Oculomotor
    Trochlear, Trigeminal, Abducens
    Facial, Acoustic/Vestibulocochlear, Glossopharyngeal,
    Vagus, Spinal Accessory, Hypoglossal
41. Olfactory mucosa, Cribiform plate, Olfactory Bulbs
42. Crista Galli; Olfactory Tract
43. Retina; Optic Nerves
44. Optic Chiasma; Optic Tracts
45. Superior, Inferior and Medial, Inferior Oblique. Ciliary, iris
46. Superior Oblique; Lateral Rectus
47. three nuclei of origin
48. Opthalmic, Maxillary, and Mandibular
49. mastication; Ciliary, Lacrimation, salivary
50. face, taste, two-thirds; visceral and somatic
51. Sphenopalatine, Submandibular
52. Temporal, Zygomatic, Buccal, Mandibular, Cervical
53. Bells' Palsy; Tic Douloureux
54. Vestibulocochlear
55. Equilibrium, Auditory
56. taste, third, pharynx, Carotid Sinus
57. tongue and pharynx, parotid
58. Swallowing, Gag
59. 90%; Cardiac, pharynx
60. receives contributions from gray matter C1–C5 and exists as a spinal nerve; Trapezius and SCM. Tongue
61. Olfactory Epithelium, Lamina Propria
62. Olfactory Receptors, Supporting and Basal
63. mitotically, 60 days; Bowman's, mucus

64. cilia; gas and water soluble
65. Odorant binding proteins; Na^+, depolarizes
66. Cribiform plate, Glomeruli, Olfactory Bulbs
67. Mitral, Olfactory Tracts, Temporal
68. Discrimination; Central; Hypothalamus and Limbic
69. Anosomias; Uncinate Fits
70. head trauma, nasal inflammation; epilepsy and migraines
71. Gustation
72. Taste Buds; salt, sweet, sour, bitter
73. sugar, saccharin, amino acids; metals, Na^+
74. H^+ and acids, spoiled or rancid; alkaloids, nicotine and caffeine, toxins
75. Umani, MSG; Tip, sides, back. Lingual Papillae
76. Filiform, Fungiform, Circumvallate
77. give the tongue a rough texture; Circumvallate located at posterior of tomgue, Fungiform are wide-spread
78. Solitary Nucleus, thalamus, Parietal. 80

Part 3: The Eye and Vision

79. Orbicularis oculi, Frontalis
80. Palpebral Fissure, Canthus
81. Lacrimal Caruncle; Tarsal Plates
82. sweat and sebaceous; Levator Palpebrae Superious
83. blikig, Meibomian
84. Chalazion; stys; Ciliary
85. Ocular-Bulbar Cojunctiva; Palpebral Cojunctiva
86. Superior-lateral eye; Medial Canthus, Lacrimal Puncta, Lacrimal Canal
87. Nasolacrimal Duct, Lacrimal Sac
88. Superior, Inferior and Medial Rectus and Inferior Oblique; Superior Oblique; Lateral Rectus
89. Diplopia: double vision; Strabismus: lazy eye
90. Anterior and Posterior
91. Aqueous, Chambers, Iris; Vitreous
92. Aqueous: constantly produced and drained; Vitreous: produced in embryo—constant volume
93. Canal of Sclemm; Glaucoma
94. Fibrous Tunic, Vascular Tunic, Sensory Tunic
95. Sclera, Cornea
96. Limbus; sodium pumps
97. Uvea; Choroid, Ciliary Body, Iris
98. absorb scattered light; Ciliary Muscles
99. Ciliary Processes, Suspensory Ligaments
100. Epithelium, Fibers; Cataracts
101. Crystallins; lens becomes denser and less elastic
102. Smooth; circular, radial
103. parasympathetic; constrict. Sympathetic; dilates

104. Retina, Pigmented, Neural Layer
105. A; Rods and Cones, Ora Serrata Retinae
106. Bright Light, color; dim, peripheral
107. Retinal, Opsins
108. purple, isomer
109. bleached, white; Transducin
110. Closes; hyperpolarize; glutamate
111. Bipolar, Ganglion Cell, Nerve
112. Optic Disc, Blind Spot; Macula Lutea
113. Fovea Centralis, Visual Acuity
114. Convex; converge; Accommodation, Convergence
115. bulges, constrict; flattens, dilates
116. Emmetropic; Myopic, Hyperoptic
117. Near, Far; Presbyopia

Part 4: The Ear, Hearing, and Equilibrium

118. Auricle, External Auditory, Tympanic Membrane
119. Helix; Umbo
120. Tympanic, Petrous Portion of temporal
121. Vestibular, Cochlear
122. Auditory/Eustachian; Auditory Ossicles
123. Malleus, Incus and Stapes
124. Tympanic; Oval/Vestibular
125. Stapedius, Tensor Tympani; Otitis Media
126. Labyrinth
127. Membranous and Bony
128. Endolymph; Perilymph, Vestibule, Semicircular Canals, Cochlea
129. Oval and Round, Utricle and Saccule
130. Semicircular Ducts; Cochlear Duct
131. Right, Anterior, Posterior and Lateral; Ampulla; Crista Ampullaris
132. Modiolis; Spiralorgan of Corti. Scala: Scala Vestibuli, Scala Media, Scala Tympani
133. Oval; Vestibular, Basilar
134. Round, Helicotrema
135. distance between two crests of the wave; number of cycles per unit of time
136. tone; pitch
137. Amplitude: intensity of sound; hertz; decibels
138. Tympanic membrane, Auditory Ossicles
139. Oval, Perilymph, Scala Vestibuli, Helicotrema
140. Scala Tympani, Round
141. Basilar; Cochlear Hair
142. Tectoral; Inner, Outer
143. Stereocilia, K^+; Cochlear
144. Bipolar, Spiral Ganglia; Vestibulocochlear

145. Superior Olivary, Inferior Colliculi, Thalamus, Temporal
146. Conduction: perforated ear drum or otosclerosis; Sensorineural: nerve damage
147. Ringing; ringing with vertigo
148. Vestibular Nerve/Apparatus
149. Dynamic and Static
150. Semicircular Canals; Maculae
151. Saccule and Utricle; linear
152. Verticle; Horizontal
153. Hair, Otolithic
154. Otoliths; Vestibular, Superior and Inferior Vestibular
155. Angular, Semicircular Canals
156. Cristae Ampullaris
157. Hair, Cupula
158. Endolymph; hyperpolarizing; Vestibular
159. Cerebellum, Vestibular Nuclear Complex
160. visual and somatic; Vestibulospinal

Unit VIII: Take a Test!

1. Olfaction is carried by which Cranial Nerve:
   a) I   b) II
   c) VII   d) IX   e) a and b

2. Gustation is carried by which Cranial Nerve:
   a) I   b) II
   c) VII   d) IX   e) a and b

3. Which taste buds are located in the back of the tongue and are most sensitive to alkaloids such and toxins:
   a) Salt   b) Sweet
   c) Bitter   d) Sour   e) Umami

4. Which Cranial Nerve initiates swallowing and the Gag Reflex:
   a) Facial   b) Vagus
   c) Hypoglossal   d) Glossopharyngeal   e) Spinal Accessory

5. Amino Acids will depolarize which type of taste receptor:
   a) Salt   b) Sweet
   c) Sour   d) Bitter

6. The meeting of the upper and lower palpebrae are referred to as the:
   a) tarsal plate   b) canthus
   c) conjunctiva   d) cornea

7. Tears drain into puncta located within the:
   a) cornea   b) caruncle
   c) lateral-superior palepbra d) lateral canthus

8. The clear, vascular covering of the anterior portion of the eye is called:
   a) cornea   b) conjunctiva
   c) sclera   d) uvea   e) choroid

9. Which of the following is innervated by the Abducens Nerve (VI):
   a) Medial Rectus   b) Superior Rectus
   c) Inferior Rectus   d) Lateral Rectus   e) Superior Oblique

10. Which of the following is innervated by the Trochlear Nerve (IV):
    a) Medial Rectus   b) Superior Rectus
    c) Inferior Rectus   d) Lateral Rectus   e) Superior Oblique

11. Which of the following is noted for being composed of avascular, fibrous CT:
    a) Cornea   b) Sclera
    c) Sensory Tunic   d) Conjunctiva   e) a and b

12. The Pigmented Epithelial layer is the inner-most layer of the:
    a) Fibrous Tunic   b) Uvea
    c) Sensory Tunic   d) Conjunctiva   e) Sclera

13. Which of the following forms the vascular Choroid, Iris and Ciliary Body:
    a) Fibrous Tunic   b) Uvea
    c) Sensory Tunic   d) Conjunctiva   e) Sclera

14. The area of greatest visual acuity is known as the:
    a) optic disc   b) fovea centralis
    c) cornea   d) lens   e) sclera

15. The aqueous humor is secreted by:
    a) ciliary processes   b) Pigmented Epithelial layer
    c) choroid   d) ciliary glands

16. Excess Aqueous Humor drains into the:
    a) Lacrimal Puncta   b) Nasal Cavity
    c) Canal of Schlemm   d) Lacrimal Caruncle

17. Vitreous Humor is found in which area:
    a) Anterior Segment   b) Posterior Segment
    c) Anterior Chamber   d) Posterior Chamber   e) in all areas

18. Which pupillary response is sympathetic:
    a) constriction   b) dilation
    c) accommodation   d) convergence

19. Damage to the Medial Recti muscles would affect which response:
    a) constriction   b) dilation
    c) accommodation   d) convergence

20. Near Focus Accommodation includes which of the following:
    a) Pupilary constriction   b) Convergence
    c) Lens bulges   d) a and b   e) a, b and c

21. Which area considered the photosensitive receptors of the retina:
    a) Cones   b) Rods
    c) Bipolar Neurons   d) Ganglion Cells   e) a and b

22. Axons of which of the following form the optic nerve:
    a) photoreceptors   b) bipolar neurons
    c) pigmented epithelium   d) ganglia cells

23. Which is the correct order in white light stimulation:
    a) Pigmented Epithelium, Rods, Bipolar Neuron, Ganglion Cell, Optic Nerve
    b) Bipolar Neuron, Rods, Pigmented Epithelium, Ganglion Cell, Optic Nerve
    c) Rods, Bipolar Neuron, Pigmented Epithelium, Ganglion Cell, Optic Nerve
    d) Ganglion Cell, Rods, Bipolar Neuron, Pigmented Epithelium, Optic Nerve

24. Clouding of the cornea:
    a) glaucoma   b) presbyopia
    c) cataract   d) strabismus   e) anosomia

25. Increased aqueous humor and intraocular pressure:
    a) glaucoma   b) presbyopia
    c) cataract   d) strabismus   e) anosomia

26. "Lazy eye" in children:
    a) glaucoma   b) presbyopia
    c) cataract   d) strabismus   e) anosomia

27. Which is the Auditory Nerve:
    a) I   b) II
    c) VII   d) VIII   e) XI

28. The Auditory Ossicles are located within the:
    a) external ear   b) middle ear
    c) inner ear   d) labyrinth   e) vestibule

29. The depression creating the "cone of light" on the tympanic membrane is called the:
    a) umbo   b) cochlea
    c) sebum   d) helicotrema   e) scala

30. The Pharyngotympanic Tube drains fluid:
    a) from the external auditory canal into the middle ear
    b) from the middle ear into the inner ear
    c) from the middle ear into the Nasopharynx
    d) from the bony labyrinth into the membranous labyrinth
    e) from the scala tympani into the scala vestibule

31. The Stapes articulates with the:
    a) Oval window   b) Round window
    c) Tympanic Membrane d) Cochlea   e) Auricle

32. Which does not help form the Bony Labyrinth:
    a) Vestibule   b) Semicircular Canals
    c) Auricle   d) Cochlea   e) all form it

33. Which is true of the Membranous Labyrinth:
    a) it floats in perilymph   b) it is filled with endolymph
    c) it is air-filled   d) a and b   e) all are true

34. Which opens into the Semicircular Canals:
    a) Utricle   b) Saccule
    c) Cochlear Duct   d) Round Window   e) Modiolis

35. Which of the following form the Vestibule:
    a) Utricle   b) Saccule
    c) Macula   d) a and b   e) a, b and c

36. Otoliths are receptors located in the:
    a) Maculae   b) Cochlea
    c) Organ of Corti   d) Cristae Ampullaris   e) Ampulla

37. Which is the receptor organ for hearing:
    a) Utricle   b) Saccule
    c) Macula   d) Otoliths   e) Organ of Corti

38. The Crista Ampullaris is located in the:
    a) Semicircular canals b) Cochlea
    c) Middle ear   d) Vestibule   e) Auricle

39. The Crista Ampullaris is involved with:
    a) Hearing   b) Pressure equalization
    c) Cerumen production   d) Static equilibrium
    e) Dynamic equilibrium

40. Static and Linear Equilibrium are sensed by:
    a) Ampulla   b) Semicircular Canals
    c) Macula e   d) Tectoral Membrane
    e) Basilar Membrane

41. The bony core of the Cochlea is called the:
    a) Amplla   b) Macula
    c) Saccule   d) Modiolis   e) Utricle

42. The Scala Vestibuli and Scala Tympani "meet" at the:
    a) Oval window   b) Round window
    c) Helicotrema   d) Scala media   e) Ampulla

43. The Cochlear Duct is also known as the:
    a) Scala Vestibuli   b) Scala Media
    c) Scala Tympani   d) Semicircular Duct   e) Modiolis

44. Which does not form the Organ of Corti:
    a) Basilar Membrane   b) Tectoral Membrane
    c) Vestibular Membrane d) Hair Cells   e) all are part

45. The Basilar Membrane vibrates as sound waves are conducted through the:
    a) Scala Vestibuli
    b) Scala Tympani
    c) Semicircular Canals
    d) Scala Media
    e) Maculae

46. Sound waves cause hair cells to bend (and depolarize) against which membrane:
    a) Basilar
    b) Tympanic
    c) Tectoral
    d) Vestibular
    e) Cochlear

47. Which implies fluid retention in the middle ear:
    a) Otosclerosis
    b) Tinnitis
    c) Otitis Media
    d) Sensorineural Deafness

48. Conduction deafness is also known as:
    a) Otosclerosis
    b) Tinnitis
    c) Otitis Media
    d) Sensorineural Deafness

49. "Ringing" in the ears is known as:
    a) Otosclerosis
    b) Tinnitis
    c) Otitis Media
    d) Sensorineural Deafness

50. Which is the correct order of sound conduction:
    a) Stapes, oval window, scala tympani, scala vestibuli, round window
    b) Stapes, round window, scala vestibuli, scala tympani, oval window
    c) Stapes, oval window, scala vestibuli, scala tympani, round window
    d) Stapes, round window, scala vestibuli, scala tympani, oval window

1:a, 2:e, 3:c, 4:d, 5:b, 6:b, 7:b, 8:b, 9:d, 10:e, 11:e, 12:c, 13:b, 14:b, 15:a, 16:c, 17:b, 18:b, 19:d, 20:e, 21:e, 22:d, 23:a, 24:c, 25:a, 26:d, 27:d, 2b:b, 29:a, 30:c, 31:a, 32:c, 33:d, 34:a, 35:c, 36:a, 37:c, 38:a, 39:e, 40:c, 41: d, 42:c, 43:b, 44:c, 45:b, 46:c, 47:c, 48:c, 49:a, 50: c

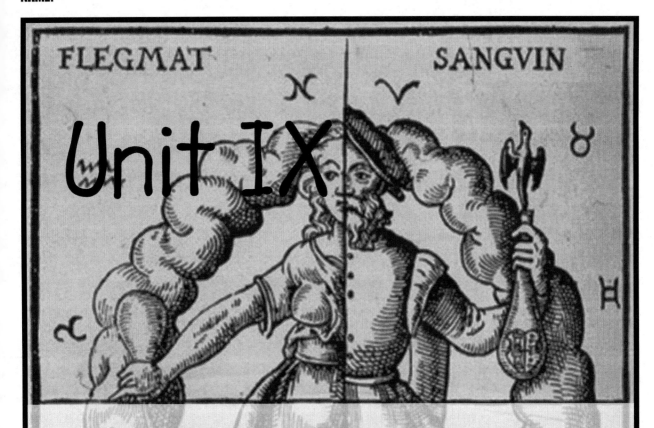

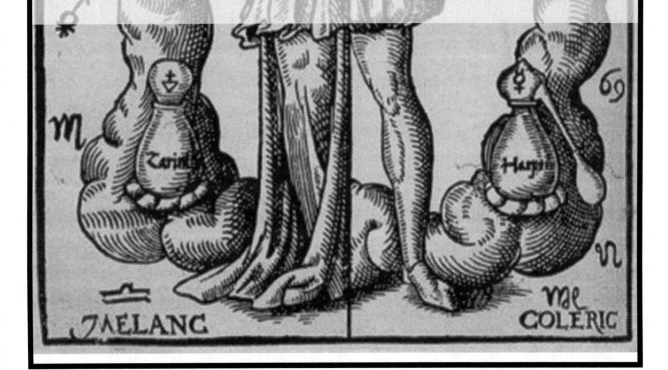

Unit IX

THE ENDOCRINE SYSTEM

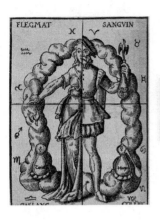

The Endocrine System

1. Endocrine glands function by secreting hormones into the _____ _____.

2. Exocrine glands function by secreting substances into _____ and onto _____. An example of an exocrine gland: _____.

3. Hormones function by only stimulating their _____ _____.

4. The five major regulatory effects of the endocrine system include:

   _____,

   _____,

   _____,

   _____, and

   _____.

5. The three classes of endocrine hormones include: _____,

   _____, and _____ _____ _____.

6. Due to their size, amino acid-based hormones must first _____,

   then use a _____ _____ to exert their effect on the nucleus.

7. Sources of amino acid-based hormones include the _____, the Anterior and Posterior

   _____, and the _____.

8. Steroids are based on _____ and exert their effect on the nucleus by _____

   _____.

9. Steroids are produced by the _____ _____ and by the

   _____. Steroids are grouped as _____, _____,

   and _____. Water soluble eicosanoids include _____ and local hormones.

10. Prostaglandins stimulate _____

    as well as _____ contractions.

    Local hormones include _____ which stimulate neighboring tissues such as _____

    and _____ such as _____ which stimulate the cell which released it.

11. The effects on the target cell by a hormone include:

_____,

_____,

_____,

_____, and

_____.

12. The magnitude of a hormone's effect is determined by _____,

_____, and _____.

13. A hormone's blood concentration is determined by its _____

and its _____.

14. The persistence of a hormone's blood concentration/period of activity is known as the

_____.

15. Receptor site availability may be affected by _____ and by

_____.

16. Define Affinity: _____.

17. The three modalities of hormonal secretion include _____, _____, and

_____ stimulation.

18. An example of hormonal stimulation is _____

_____.

19. An example of humeral stimulation is _____

_____.

20. An example of neural stimulation is _____

_____.

21. The Pineal is known to control _____ rhythms; its principal hormone,

_____, controls the _____.

22. Melatonin secretions peak at _____ and trough at _____.

23. The Pineal is also known to inhibit _____, which is also referred to

as _____ Puberty.

24. The Anterior Pituitary is also referred to as the _____. It is formed

from the embryonic invagination called _____ _____ and is composed of

_____ _____ tissue.

25. The Posterior Pituitary is also referred to as the _____. It is an

extension from the _____ and is composed of _____ tissue.

26. The Pituitary glands are connected to the hypothalamus by the _____ _____, also called the _____.

27. The hypothalamus communicates with the Adenohypophysis via the _____-_____ _____ System, and the Neurohypophysis via the _____-_____ _____.

28. The Hypothalamic-Hypophyseal Tract consists of _____ from cell bodies of the hypothalamus; the Neurohypophysis, therefore, consists of the _____ of these neurons.

29. The two principal hormones of the Posterior Pituitary are _____ and _____.

30. The _____ of the hypothalamus monitor blood water/solute concentration.

31. ADH is secreted by the _____ Nucleus and targets the _____; ADH functions by _____.

32. ADH secretion is inhibited by _____; a disease characterized by reduced ADH secretion causing increased urinary output is known as _____ _____.

33. Increased urinary output is also referred to as _____.

34. Oxytocin is secreted by the _____ Nucleus and in general it stimulate _____ _____ contraction. Its two principal functions include stimulating _____ and in conjunction with lactation, _____ _____.

35. The smooth muscle of the Lactiferous glands are known as _____.

36. The hypothalamus controls the Anterior Pituitary by sending releasing and inhibiting factors via the _____-_____ _____ _____; AP hormones are classified as _____ and fall into two functional categories: _____ and _____.

37. In general Tropic hormones function by: _____. The four include _____, _____, _____, and _____.

38. The two non-tropic hormones include _____ and _____.

39. Growth Hormone stimulates the _____ to release _____, which ultimately stimulate the target cells. Effects of GH include _____ and _____.

40. Growth Hormone inhibiting factor is also known as _____.

41. Prolactin releasing factor is stimulated by the _____; Prolactin levels also rise and fall with _____. Inappropriate lactation can be due to _____ _____.

42. FSH and LH/ICSH are classified as _____; FSH stimulates _____ and _____.

43. LH/ICSH in turn stimulate the secretion of hormones referred to as _____, which include _____, _____, and _____.

44. ACTH stimulates the _____ _____ to secrete the hormone group referred to as _____.

45. TSH is secreted by the _____ _____; Thyroid Hormone is properly referred to as _____ and _____.

46. TH is conjugated from the precursor _____, _____, and _____.

47. Dietary deficiency of iodine and L-Tyrosine can result in the accumulation of thyroglobulin causing the clinical finding called _____; when found regionally/geographically it is described as being _____.

48. Goiter is also a clinical finding in hypothyroidism, aka _____. Symptoms include _____, _____, _____, and _____.

49. Myxedema is treated by _____ and is/is not life threatening.

50. Hyperthyroidism is also known as _____ _____ and is/is not life threatening. It is most easily noted by the clinical finding _____ due to swelling of the fat pads behind the eye. Symptoms include _____, _____, _____, and _____.

51. Grave's Disease is treated surgically by _____ or by ingestion of _____ _____; both procedures usually result in _____ as a side effect.

52. TH production is stimulated by _____ response. The hierarchy of hormonal release when TH levels drop is: (1) _____, (2) _____, and (3) _____.

53. The thyroid also secretes _____, which stimulates osteoblast activity; this occurs when _____, which is a _____ response.

54. PTH is released in response to _____; this is considered _____ stimulation. PTH stimulates _____ activity.

55. Hyperparathyroidism therefore results in _____ serum calcium, causing _____ and _____.

56. Hypoparathyroidism results in _____ serum calcium and is characterized by _____ and _____.

57. The adrenal gland is divided into the outer _____ and inner _____. The adrenals are also referred to as the _____ glands.

58. The adrenal medulla is derived from _____ tissue and is a part of the _____ Nervous System. Its principal secretions are _____ (80%) and _____. These hormones are also part of the neurotransmitter group of _____, which are based on the amino acid _____.

59. Epinephrine brings about increased _____, _____, and _____ rate; it also dilates the _____ and stimulates _____.

60. The adrenal cortex is divided into three regions: outermost, the Zona _____, the Zona _____, and innermost, the Zona _____. The cortex produces hormones classified as _____, which are based on _____.

61. Corticosteroids are soluble/insoluble in lipids; they stimulate their target cells by _____ _____.

62. The Zona Glomerulosa secretes hormones referred to as _____, which control _____ and _____ balance. _____ is such a hormone.

63. The mineralcorticoid Aldosterone functions by stimulating the _____ _____ to increase _____ and _____ resorption, and increase _____ excretion.

64. Aldosterone release can be stimulated by reduced _____ and increased _____ levels; this is considered a _____ response. It may also be released in response to stress. This involves first the _____, which stimulates the _____ _____, which secretes _____ which stimulates the _____ _____, which in turn releases Aldosterone.

65. The Zona Fasiculata secretes hormones referred to as _____, which control _____ and _____ responses.

66. Glucocorticoids include the hormones _____ and _____; the release of these hormones is stimulated by _____, making this a _____ response.

67. Cortisol/Hydrocortisone functions by stimulating _____; at higher levels it acts as an _____ by preventing _____ . Excessive use of steroids can result in depressed _____ _____, pathology of the _____ and _____ systems.

68. The Zona Reticularis produces hormones referred to as _____, also known as _____, which include _____, _____ and its principal secretion, _____.

69. Adrenal insufficiency is also referred to as _____ Disease and is characterized by _____, _____, _____, and _____ discoloration.

70. Hyperadrenalism or _____ Disease can be due to _____ or induced by excessive use of _____. It is characterized by _____, _____, and distortion of the head or "_____."

71. The pancreas is referred to as dual gland, i.e., it has both _____ (ductless) and _____ (duct) functions.

72. The exocrine cells of the pancreas are known as _____ Cells; these cells secrete _____ _____, which leave the pancreas via the _____ Duct and enter the duodenum via the _____ _____ Duct.

73. The endocrine portion of the pancreas is known as the _____ of _____; these include _____ and _____ cells.

74. α Islet Cells secrete _____; β Islet secrete _____. Both cells are stimulated by _____ response.

75. Glucagon is known as the _____ hormone. It is released in response to _____ and functions by stimulating _____ and _____.

76. Insulin is known as the _____ hormone. It is released in response to _____ and functions by _____ and by inhibiting _____ and _____.

77. Hypoinsulinsim is better known as _____ _____; its three clinical cardinal signs include _____, _____, and _____.

78. Polyphagia is due to _____; polydypsia is due to _____, which results in _____.

79. Diabetes Melitus literally means _____ _____ whereas Diabetes Insipidus means _____ _____.

80. Type I Diabetes is also known as _____ _____; it is believed to be an _____ disease affecting the _____ resulting in _____ _____. These patients are classified as _____ _____.

81. Type II Diabetes is also known as _____ _____; it is considered _____ and generally affects _____.

82. Reduced insulin yielding elevated glucose results in the chemical state called _____; it also is noted by _____ in the urine.

83. Chronic complications of diabetes can lead to _____, most often of the lower extremities as well as _____ leading to blindness.

84. Diabetic neuropathy of the lower extremities predisposes the patient to developing _____ _____; these in turn can lead to _____ requiring _____.

85. The thymus produces _____ and _____, which are responsible for _____.

Unit IX: The Endocrine System

1. the circulatory system
2. ducts, surfaces. Salivary, Digestive
3. target cells
4. Homeostasis and Electrolyte Balance, BMR, Growth and Development, Immune and Stress Responses, Reproduction
5. Amino Acid-based, Steroids, water soluble Eicosanoids
6. Bind with Receptor Sites, Secondary Messenger
7. Hypothalamus, Pituitary, Thyroid
8. Cholesterol, Direct Gene Activation
9. Adrenal Cortex, Gonads. Mineralcorticoids, Glucocorticoids, Androgens, Prostaglandins
10. localized inflammation and pain, smooth muscle and uterine; paracrines, NO, autocrines, leukotrienes
11. change membrane permeability, stimulate synthesis, activate enzymes, secretion, mitosis and meiosis
12. Concentration, Available Receptor Sites, Hormone-Receptor Affinity
13. Rate of Release, Speed of inactivation
14. Half-life
15. Number of Sites, Competitive Inhibition
16. Strength of the Hormone-Receptor union
17. Hormonal, Humeral, Neural
18. Hypothalamus on the Anterior Pituitary
19. Glucose levels on the Pancreas
20. Hypothalamus on the Posterior Pituitary
21. Circadian; Melatonin, Sleep/Wake
22. Noon, Midnight
23. Premature puberty, Precocious
24. Adenohypophysis, Rathke's Pouch, Glandular Epithelial
25. Neurohypophysis; Hypothalamus, Neural
26. Pituitary Stalk, Infundibulum
27. Hypothalamic-Hypophyseal Portal, Hypothalamic-Hypophyseal Tract
28. Axons, Telodendria
29. ADH, Oxytocin
30. Osmoreceptors
31. Supraoptic, Kidney Tubules; stimulates tubules to resorb more water increaseing blood volume
32. Alcohol; Diabetes Insipidus
33. Polyuria
34. Paraventricular; Smooth Muscle, Uterine contractions of labor, milk let-down
35. Myoepithelia
36. Hypothalamic-Hypophyseal Portal System; Amino Acid Based, Tropic, Non-Tropic
37. Stimulating other endocrine glands to secrete. Thyroid Stimulating H, Follicle Stimulating H, Leutinizing/Interstitial Cell Stimulating H, Adrenocortico-tropic H
38. Growth H, Prolactin
39. Liver, Somatomedins. Synthesis, Mitosis
40. Somatostatin
41. Hypothalamus; Estrogen. Anterior Pituitary Tumor
42. Gonadotropins; Ovulation, Spermatogenesis
43. Androgens, Estrogen, Testosteone, Progesterone
44. Adrenal Cortex, Corticosteroids
45. Anterior Pituitary; Thyroxine, Triiodothyronine
46. Thyroglobulin, L-Tyrosine, Iodine
47. Goiter; Pandemic
48. Myxedema; reduced BMR, sluggish, weight gain, dry skin
49. Thyroid Hormone supplementation, not life threatening
50. Grave's Disease, life threatening. Exopthamos. Increased BMR, sweating, nervousness, irregular heart rate, weight loss
51. Thyroidectomy, Radioactive Iodine; Hypothyroidism
52. Hormonal; (1) Hypothalamus secretes TSH Releasing Factor (2) Anterior Pituitary secretes TSH (3) Thryoid secretes TH
53. Calcitonin; calcium levels rise above 11 mg/100ml, Humeral
54. Calcium drop below 9 mg/100ml; Humeral. Osteoclast
55. Elevated, depressed nervous system, weak muscles
56. reduced, convulsions, tetany
57. Cortex, Medulla; Suprarenal
58. Neural, Sympathetic. Epinephrine and Norepinephrine; Catecholamines, L-Tyrosine
59. BMR, Heart and Respiratory; Bronchioles, Glycogenolysis

60. Glomerulosa, Fasiculata, Reticularis; Corticosteroids, Cholesterol
61. Soluble; Direct Gene Activation
62. Mineralcorticoids, water, electrolyte. Aldosterone
63. Kidney Tubule, Sodium, Water, Potassium
64. Sodium, Potassium, Humeral. Hypothalamus, Anterior Pituitary, ACTH, Adrenal Cortex
65. Glucocorticoids, Immune, Metabolic
66. Cortisol, Cortisone; stress reduced cortisol, Hormonal
67. Gluconeogensis; anti-inflammatory, lysosomal membranes from bursting. Immune response, Cardiovascular, Nervous
68. Gonadocorticoids, Androgens, Estrogen, Progesterone, Testosterone
69. Addison's, weight loss, sodium imbalance, dehydration, skin
70. Cushing's, Tumors, Steroids. Hyperglycemia, loss of muscle tone, "moonface"
71. Exocrine, Endocrine
72. Acini; digestive enzymes, Pancreatic, Common Bile

73. Islets of Langerhan; a and b;
74. Glucagon; Insulin; Humeral
75. Hyperglycemic; reduced blood glucose, Glycogenolysis, Gluconeogenesis
76. Hypoglycemic; increased blood glucose, increasing glucose trans-membrane transport, Glycogenolysis, Gluconeogenesis
77. Diabetes Mellitus; Polyphagia, Polydypsia, Polyuria
78. Increased hunger due to insufficient glucose transport, increased glucose/water imbalance, increased urinary output
79. sweet urine, tasteless urine
80. Juvenile onset; autoimmune, Islet, Reduced insulin. Insulin dependent
81. Adult Onset; familial, middle age, overweight, sedentary
82. Ketosis; glucose
83. Neuropathy, Retinopathy
84. Non-healing ulcers; gangrene, ampuation
85. Thymosin, Thymopoietin, T-Lymphocyte production

Time allowed: 45 minutes

1. A hormone is best defined as any substance which is:
   a) secreted by glandular tissue
   b) delivered to its target cell by the vascular system
   c) secreted onto a surface
   d) secreted into a duct

2. Which of the following hormones produces its effects by direct-gene activation:
   a) lipid soluble   b) amino acid-based
   c) prostaglandins   d) neuroendocrine

3. Which would be classified as a local hormone producing smooth muscle contraction:
   a) steroid-based   b) amino acid-based
   c) prostaglandins   d) cholesterol-based

4. Steroids are produced by:
   a) Hypothalamus   b) Adrenal Cortex
   c) Pancreas   d) Parathyroid

5. Which affects the magnitude of Thyroid Hormone's effect on the body:
   a) Rate of release   b) availability of Receptor Sites
   c) Affinity   d) Half-life   e) all do

6. What determine the "Half-life" of a hormone:
   a) rate of passing through urine   b) rate of inactivation by the liver
   c) rate of release   d) a and b   e) a, b and c

7. How is hormone secretion regulated?
   a) by the nervous system   b) by other hormones
   c) by changes in blood composition   d) a and b   e) a, b and c

8. Which of the following glands inhibits early onset of puberty:
   a) Anterior Pituitary   b) Posterior Pituitary
   c) Hypothalamus   d) Pineal   e) Adrenal Medulla

9. The Hypothalamus exerts its influence over the Anterior Pituitary via the:
   a) Pineal   b) Hypophyseal portal
   c) Hypophyseal tract   d) Cranial Nerve X

10. The Hypothalamus exerts its influence over the Posterior Pituitary via the:
    a) Pineal   b) Hypophyseal portal
    c) Hypophyseal tract   d) Cranial Nerve X

11. Which are secreted by the Posterior Pituitary:
    a) ADH   b) oxytocin
    c) ACTH   d) a and b   e) a, b and c

12. Which of the following is secreted by the anterior pituitary:
    a) ADH   b) calcitonin
    c) ACTH   d) PTH   e) cortisol

13. Which of the following is not considered to be a 'tropic' hormone:
    a) FSH   b) LH   c) ACTH   d) GHe) TSH

14. Somatomedins of the liver are released in response to which of the following:
    a) FSH   b) LH   c) ACTH   d) GHe) TSH

15. Aldosterone would be released in response to which of the following:
    a) ADH   b) calcitonin   c) ACTH   d) PTHe) cortisol

16. Aldosterone functions by:
    a) increasing Na+ resorption   b) increasing K+ excretion
    c) increasing Na+ excretion   d) a and b   e) a and c

17. Eating a bag of salty pretzels will make one thirsty; this is due to the release of:
    a) ADH   b) calcitonin   c) ACTH
    d) PTH   e) cortisol

18. Which of the following reduces urinary output:
    a) ADH   b) calcitonin   c) ACTH
    d) PTH   e) cortisol

19. Which of the following stimulates testosterone production:
    a) FSH   b) TSH   c) ICSH   d) ADH

20. Which stimulates spermatogenesis:
    a) FSH   b) TSH   c) ICSH   d) ADH

21. The "suckling reflex" results in the release of which hormone/s:
    a) Prolactin   b) Oxytocin
    c) Estrogen   d) a and b   e) a, b and c

22. Which stimulates 'milk-letdown':
    a) prolactin   b) estrogen
    c) oxytocin   d) ADH   e) FSH

23. Which produces uterine and smooth muscle contractions:
    a) prolactin   b) estrogen
    c) oxytocin   d) ADH   e) FSH

24. Which stimulates milk production:
    a) prolactin   b) estrogen
    c) oxytocin   d) ADH   e) FSH

25. Goiter is associated with which of the following:
    a) myxedema   b) dietary I2 deficiency
    c) hypothyroidism   d) all of these

26. Which is released by the adrenal medulla in response to sympathetic stimulation:
    a) aldosterone   b) testosterone
    c) cortisol   d) Norepinephrine   e) glucagon

27. Aldosterone is considered a:
    a) mineralcorticoid b) glucocorticoid
    c) gonadocorticoid   d) neurotransmitter

28. Androgens are secreted by the:
    a) zona glomerulosa b) adrenal medulla
    c) zona fasiculata   d) zona reticularis   e) sertoli cells

29. Which is secreted by the Adrenal Cortex in females during sexual arousal:
    a) Testosterone   b) Estrogen
    c) Progesterone   d) Aldosterone   e) Epinephrine

30. Which of the following inhibits inflammation by strengthening lysosomal membranes from bursting:
    a) aldosterone   b) cortisol
    c) testosterone   d) epinephrine   e) norepinephrine

31. Insulin is secreted by:
    a) alpha cells   b) beta cells
    c) acini cells   d) sertoli cells   e) adrenal medulla

32. Which of the following is considered to have an exocrine function:
    a) alpha cells   b) beta cells
    c) acini cells   d) sertoli cells   e) adrenal medulla

33. Which increases blood glucose levels:
    a) insulin   b) glucagon
    c) thyroglobulin   d) thyroxine

34. The endocrine secretions of the pancreas are in response to which type of stimulation:
    a) neural   b) hormonal   c) humoral   d) all of these

35. Which increases glucose permeability and membrane transport:
    a) Insulin   b) Glucagon
    c) Thyroglobulin   d) Thyroxine   e) Somatostatin

36. Which of the following increases blood calcium levels:
    a) calcitonin   b) parathyroid hormone
    c) estrogen   d) prolactin   e) thyroxine

37. Which of the following is classified as a Tropic hormone:
    a) ADH   b) Oxytocin
    c) ACTH   d) GH   e) Prolactin

38. The adrenal cortex is the target of which hormone:
    a) ADH   b) Calcitonin
    c) Aldosterone   d) PTH   e) ACTH

39. Which stimulates oögenesis:
    a) FSH   b) TSH   c) ICSH   d) ADH   e) LH

40. Ovulation is in response to release of which hormone::
    a) FSH   b) TSH   c) ICSH   d) ADH   e) LH

41. Hyperadrenalism is also known as:
    a) Addison's   b) Grave's
    c) Cushing's   d) Diabetes Insipidus   e) Myxedema

42. Exophthalmos is associated with:
    a) Addison's   b) Hyperthyroidism
    c) Cushing's   d) Diabetes Insipidus   e) Myxedema

43. Glucagon is secreted by:
    a) alpha cells   b) beta cells
    c) acini cells   d) sertoli cells   e) adrenal medulla

44. A patient with Diabetes Mellitus complains they are always thirsty; this is known as:
    a) polydipsia   b) polyuria
    c) polyphagia   d) polygamy

45. The increased thirst associated with Diabetes Mellitus is due to increased secretion of:
    a) ACTH   b) ADH
    c) Insulin   d) Glucagon   e) none of these

46. How is Diabetes Mellitus related to Glycosuria:
    a) reduced insulin causes glomerular dysfunction
    b) reduced insulin increases normal glucose excretion
    c) increased glucose exceeds transport maximum
    d) increased glucose inhibits ADH
    e) increased glucose inhibits Aldosterone

47. A patient with Diabetes Insipidus complains of polyuria; this would be due to reduced secretion of:
    a) ACTH   b) ADH
    c) Insulin   d) Glucagon   e) none of these

48. Estrogen and progesterone are secreted by:
    a) anterior pituitary   b) posterior pituitary
    c) graafian follicle   d) corpus luteum   e) corpus albicans

49. Rising levels of which hormone signals the hypothalamus to signal the release of LH:
    a) FSH
    b) estrogen
    c) prolactin
    d) oxytocin
    e) TSH

50. Secretion of which hormone will lead to the development of the breasts during puberty:
    a) GH
    b) estrogen
    c) oxytocin
    d) prolactin
    e) FSH

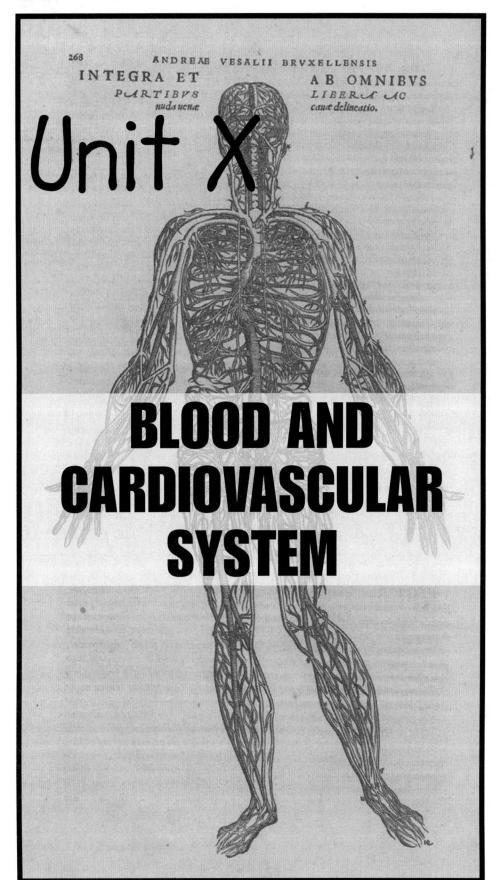

Unit X

BLOOD AND CARDIOVASCULAR SYSTEM

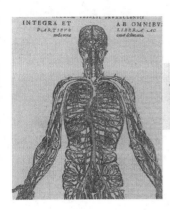

Part 1: **Blood**

1. Blood is classified as a connective tissue because:

   a. _____ ,

   b. _____ , and

   c. _____ .

2. The composition of blood includes cells or _____ _____ suspended in a semi-fluid matrix called _____ with fibers or _____ _____ , which come out of solution in response to injury/clotting.

3. By volume, blood is composed of _____% plasma and soluble proteins and _____ % formed elements. Formed elements include _____ , _____ , and _____ .

4. Erythrocytes form _____% of the total blood volume. The RBC concentration is called the _____ ; the normal range for adults include _____ for males and _____ for females.

5. The consistency of blood is described as _____ . The normal pH range is _____ . Normal total blood volume for adults is _____ for males and _____ for females.

6. General functions of blood include:

   a. _____ ,

   b. _____ ,

   c. _____ , and

   d. _____ .

7. Plasma is _____% water, _____% plasma proteins, and _____% _____ .

8. Plasma proteins are 60% _____ , 36% _____ , and only 4% _____ _____ .

9. Albumin functions by _____.
    Globulins include _____, _____, and _____. Clotting
    proteins include _____ and _____. All plasma proteins are
    synthesized in the _____.

10. Alpha and Beta globulins function as _____ _____, whereas Gamma
    globulins are _____.

11. The shape of an erythrocyte is _____. This is due to what event during formation?
    _____

12. The biconcave shape of the anucleate erythrocyte is supported by the compound _____.
    The RBC's oxygen binding compound is _____.

13. Free hemoglobin (Hb) without O_2 bound to it is called _____. When
    bound to O_2, it is called _____ and when bound to CO_2, it is called
    _____.

14. Hemoglobin is composed of four _____ _____, each wrapped around a
    central _____ group.

15. The heme group is bound to _____. The average adult has approximately
    _____ RBCs.

16. The general term for blood formation is _____; stem cells that give rise to all
    formed elements are called _____. The term for red blood cell production is
    _____.

17. Erythropoeisis occurs in the _____ _____ in red marrow. It is stimulated
    by the hormone _____, which is secreted by the _____ in response
    to _____.

18. Other factors stimulating hypoxia and therefore stimulating erythropoeisis include:
    a. _____,
    b. _____, and
    c. _____.

19. RBCs require the element _____, Vitamin _____, and _____
    _____.

20. Iron is transported bound to _____, but is stored as _____ and
    _____.

21. The average RBC lives for _____ days and is broken down in the _____.

22. Once degraded by the spleen, the RBC's iron is stored in the _____; the balance of the
    heme group is degraded to the pigment _____.

23. Bilirubin is used by the liver to produce _____, and is later metabolized into
    _____.

24. By definition, anemia is due to reduced _____, causing symptoms such as _____, _____, and _____.

25. Anemia due to reduced numbers of RBCs may be caused by blood loss/_____, infection/_____, or inhibition of hemopoeisis/_____.

26. Anemia due to reduced Hb may be due to deficiency syndromes as in _____ anemia due to insufficient iron and _____ anemia due to _____ deficiency.

27. Anemia due to abnormal Hb is _____ _____; these include _____ affecting individuals of Mediterranean descent, and _____ _____ anemia, affecting individuals of African descent.

28. Increased RBCs is referred to as _____; in this state the Hct rises above _____%. It affects the blood by increasing its _____.

29. Define:
    a. Diapedesis: _____
    b. Chemotaxis: _____
    c. Leukocytosis: _____

30. Leukocytes comprise _____% of the blood volume and are classified into two groups: _____ and _____.

31. Granulocytes include _____, _____, and _____.
    Agranulocytes include _____ and _____.

32. Neutrophils comprise _____% of leukocytes and _____ nuclei. Their granules contain _____ and _____, and they are involved in _____.

33. Eosinophils comprise _____% of leukocytes and possess _____ nuclei. Their granules contain _____ _____ and they are involved in _____ reactions and attack _____.

34. Basophils comprise _____% of leukocytes and possess _____ nuclei; their granules contain _____, which functions as a _____. Basophils are similar to _____ cells.

35. The two types of lymphocytes include:
    a. _____-Lymphocytes, involved in _____, and
    b. _____-Lymphocytes, involved in _____. These give rise to _____ cells, which produce antibodies.

36. Monocytes function as _____.

37. The formation of WBCs is known as _____. The hemocytoblast differentiates into two stem cell lines, the _____ and the _____.

38. The Lymphoid line gives rise to _____. The myeloid line differentiates into two stem lines, the _____ and the _____.

39. The monoblast will mature into _____; whereas the myeloblast will differentiate into _____, _____, and _____.

40. Reduced WBCs is known as _____ and is associated with use of _____; increased WBCs is referred to as _____ and is associated with _____.

41. The two forms of leukemia are _____ and _____.

42. Platelets are fragments of _____; their formation is stimulated by the hormone _____. Platelets function by _____.

43. Define:
    a. Hemorrhage: _____
    b. Hemostasis: _____

44. The four steps in hemostasis are:
    a. _____ _____
    b. _____ _____ _____
    c. _____, and
    d. _____ _____.

45. Vascular spasm principally functions by _____ and is brought about by _____. The purpose of platelet plug formation is to _____. Platelets secrete the hormone _____ which attracts more platelets to the plug.

46. Coagulation is divided into three phases:
    a. Phase I: _____ _____
    b. Phase II: _____, and
    c. Phase III: _____.

47. Prothrombin activation takes two pathways. The longer process with more steps takes place in the _____ is called the _____ pathway. The faster _____ pathway takes place in the tissues and is sped by the presence of _____ or tissue factor.

48. In Phase II Prothrombin is activated into the enzyme _____.

49. Thrombin catalyzes the polymerization of the plasma protein _____ into insoluble _____ strands, which form the temporary _____.

50. The purpose of clot retraction is to _____ and to prepare the area for the formation of _____.

51. After tissue is replaced, the clot is removed by the process of _____; this involves the activation of the plasma protein _____ into the enzyme _____, which dissolves fibrin.

52. Unwarranted clotting disorders are referred to as _____. A clot that persists in a closed blood vessel is a _____; one that breaks free and migrates is an _____. The blockage of a blood vessel is called an _____.

53. Occlusions due to emboli result in loss of blood flow or _____; this leads to cellular death or _____, creating an area of dead tissue referred to as an _____.

54. Bleeding disorders due to reduced platelets are known as _____. The sex-linked genetic disorder resulting poor/no clotting is _____.

55. Transfusions are required when blood loss exceeds _____%. Heparin is added to stored blood as an _____. The term to describe an individual's storing of their own blood for future surgery is _____.

56. Transfusion reactions of mismatched blood results in _____ and _____ of RBCs. Their released Hb accumulates in the _____ _____.

57. The four blood groups are _____, _____, _____, and _____.

58. Type A possesses _____ antigens, produces _____ antibodies, and can accept _____.
Type B possesses _____ antigens, produces _____ antibodies, and can accept _____.
Type AB possesses _____ antigens, produces _____ antibodies, and can accept _____.
Type O possesses _____ antigens, produces _____ antibodies, and can accept _____.

59. The Rh factor becomes a concern only when the mother is Rh _____, the father is Rh _____, and specifically with regard to the _____ pregnancy.

60. After an Rh⁻ woman's immune system is sensitized from the first pregnancy by an Rh⁺ man, her antibodies may cause _____ _____ in subsequent pregnancies, unless she is treated with _____.

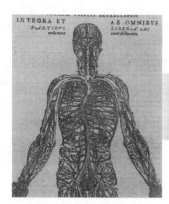

Part 2: The Heart

61. The heart is located within the _____ and is enclosed within the _____ _____ or _____.

62. The Pericardial Sac is divided into two layers, the outer _____ pericardium and the inner _____ pericardium.

63. The serous pericardium folds over forming two layers separated by the _____ _____. The _____ layer underlies the fibrous pericardium and the _____ layer becomes the outer layer of the heart or _____. Inflammation of the sac is called _____.

64. The three layers of the heart are the outer visceral pericardium or _____, the middle _____, and the innermost lining, _____, which is composed of _____ _____.

65. The heart chambers that receive blood from veins are called _____; their volumes are increased by small appendages called _____. Chambers that eject blood into arteries are called _____.

66. The atria are separated by the _____ _____; the ventricles are separated by the _____ _____. During fetal life the atria are connected by the _____ _____, which seals at/around birth.

67. The atria are divided into anterior and posterior portions by the _____ _____; the anterior wall is noted for its ridged _____ Muscles.

68. The right atria receives de-/oxygenated blood from the _____ _____ _____, the _____ _____ _____, and the _____ _____.

69. Deoxygenated blood travels from the right atrium to the right ventricle by passing through the _____ valve, one of the two _____ valves.

70. The ridged muscles of the ventricle's myocardium are known as the _____ _____; those that support the Tricuspid valve are called _____ muscles and are attached to the cusps by _____ _____.

71. Externally the atria and ventricles are demarcated by the _____ groove or _____ sulcus; the right and left ventricles are demarcated by the _____ sulci.

72. Blood travels from the right ventricle through the _____ valve and into the _____ _____ to the lungs. Blood that flows from the capillaries to the heart and then to the lungs is known as the _____ circulation.

73. All arteries carry oxygenated blood from the heart except the _____; all veins carry deoxygenated blood to the heart except the _____ _____.

74. Semilunar valves prevent backsplash of blood into the _____; the Bicuspid and Tricuspid valves prevent backsplash into the _____.

75. De-/oxygenated blood travels from the capillaries of the lungs to the left atrium via the _____ _____; it then passes through the _____/ _____ valve into the left ventricle, through the _____ valve and into the _____ , and on to the capillaries. This is referred to as the _____ circulation.

76. The Coronary circulation supplies blood to the _____; symptoms of cardiac ischemia are called _____ _____.

77. Cardiac fibers are interconnected by _____ _____, which are comprised of _____ for attachment and _____ junctions, which act as electrical connections. These facilitate all the fibers in a single chamber to act as a functional _____.

78. One percent of cardiac fibers are self-excitable and exhibit _____, initiating their own _____.

79. Unlike skeletal muscles, 20% of calcium for contraction diffuses in from the _____, creating a calcium _____; this creates the _____ contraction needed to propel blood.

80. The auto-rhythmic cells of the Cardiac Conduction System include the:
    a. _____ _____,
    b. _____ _____,
    c. _____ _____,
    d. Right and Left _____ _____, and the
    e. _____ _____.

81. The Sinoatrial (SA) node self-depolarizes at a rate of _____ beats/min without extrinsic control. The _____ nervous system reduces the rate to _____ beats/min. This establishes the normal _____ _____.

82. The Action Potential (AP) initiated by the SA node depolarizes both _____ for their simultaneous contraction; the AP then depolarizes the _____ _____.

83. The Atrioventricular node conducts the AP to the Bundle of His, but it is ultimately the
_____ _____ that depolarize the myocardium of the ventricles.

84. Systole implies Atrial and Ventricular _____; Diastole implies _____.

85. Describe the following arrhythmias:
   a. fibrillation: _____
   b. ectopic focus: _____
   c. heart block: _____

86. What is indicated by the following EKG segments?
   a. P wave: _____
   b. QRS complex: _____
   c. T wave: _____

87. Label the P, QRS and T waves
    Label the PQ, ST and QT intervals

| 0.0 | 0.2 | 0.4 | 0.6 | 0.8 |

88. Extended intervals result from delayed conduction, This is most likely due to _____ or
_____.

89. The cardiac cycle is divided into three phases: _____ _____,
_____ _____, and _____ _____.

90. Ventricular filling is noted as _____-_____ _____; 70% of
ventricular filling occurs _____. Ventricular filling is noted by the _____
on the EKG.

91. During ventricular systole, the ventricles _____ forcing the _____ valves
open at a pressure of _____ mm Hg.

92. Isovolumetric relaxation occurs during _____ _____ and is indicated by
the _____ on the EKG. Ventricular _____ also occurs during this period.

93. The first heart sound is created by the closing of the _____ valves and is associated with ventricular _____, which is indicated by the _____ on the EKG.

94. The second heart sound is created by the closing of the _____ valves and associated with ventricular _____, which is indicated by the _____ on the EKG.

95. The cardiac output is determined by the _____ _____ and the _____ _____.

96. The stroke volume is the _____ and is determined by the total volume after filling (_____ _____ Volume) minus the residual _____ _____ Volume. The average SV = _____ ml.

97. Factors affecting stroke volume include: ventricular stretch or _____, _____ of cardiac muscle, and _____ or arterial resistance.

98. Pressure receptors or _____ stimulate the ANS to influence heart rate. Hormones that influence heart rate include _____ and _____.

99. Increased calcium is known as _____ and can lead to _____ _____. Increased sodium is known as _____ and inhibits _____ _____. Increased potassium or _____ can lead to heart block and _____ _____.

100. Tachycardia is diagnosed when the heart rate exceeds _____ beats/min; bradycardia is diagnosed when the heart rate falls below _____ beats/min.

101. Left-sided Ccongestive heart failure leads to _____ _____; right-sided failure leads to _____ _____.

102. During fetal development, the sinus venosus will differentiate into the _____ _____, the _____ _____, and the _____ _____.

103. The Bulbus cordis will differentiate into the _____ _____, the _____ _____, and the _____.

104. In addition to the foramen ovale, the _____ _____ connects the fetal pulmonary trunk to the _____.

105. At birth the ductus arteriousus closes and remains as the _____ _____; when left open the defect is called _____ _____.

106. Patent ductus results in mixed arterial and venous blood; the most common clinical finding is _____.

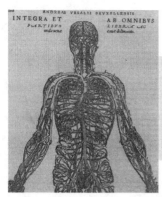

Part 3: Blood Vessels and Blood Pressure

107. All major blood vessels are composed of three layers. Facing the lumen is the _____ _____, the muscular _____ _____, and outermost, the _____ _____, also known as the _____. The tissues of the blood vessel walls are nourished by the _____ _____.

108. The tunica interna is lined by _____ _____. The tunica media, under autonomic influence, performs _____ and _____.

109. Vasoconstriction increases/decreases the diameter of the lumen, resulting in increased/decreased blood flow and pressure; vasodilation increases/decreases the diameter of the lumen, resulting in increased/decreased blood flow and pressure.

110. The two principal types of arteries are _____ or conducting arteries, and _____ or distributing arteries.

111. Elastic arteries have high amounts of the protein _____ allowing them to expand and _____, maintaining even blood flow.

112. With less elastin making them less distensible, muscular arteries are better suited for _____, enabling them to distribute blood to _____ and _____.

113. The three types of capillaries are _____, _____, and _____. Some capillary walls are supported externally by smooth muscle-like cells called _____.

114. Continuous capillaries are so named because _____. These capillaries generally supply the _____ and _____.

115. Fenestrated capillaries possess _____, which make them better suited for _____ in the intestine and _____ in the kidney.

116. Sinusoidal capillaries are described as _____; this allows for the passage of large molecules and _____. Sinusoids are found in the _____, _____, and _____ _____.

117. The flow of blood through the capillary bed is called the _____. The vessel supplying oxygenated blood to the capillary bed is called the _____; the vessel conveying deoxygenated blood from the capillaries is called the _____ _____.

118. Blood flow from the metarteriole to the true capillaries is controlled by the _____ _____. When constricted they divert blood directly to the thoroughfare channel through the _____ _____. Blood then enters the _____ _____.

119. Veins are also referred to as _____ vessels as they house up to 65% of the blood. Unlike arteries they possess _____ to prevent backflow.

120. Incompetent valves can lead to distended or _____ veins. Those commonly affected in the anal-rectal area are called _____. The merging of blood vessels is called an _____.

121. Define:
Blood flow _____
Blood pressure _____
Blood flows along a _____ _____.

122. What three factors affect peripheral resistance? _____, _____ _____, and _____ _____.

123. If viscosity is increased, peripheral resistance is increased/decreased and blood flow is increased/decreased. If the vessel diameter is increased, peripheral resistance is increased/decreased and blood flow is increased/decreased.

124. The magnitude of blood flow can be expressed as:

$$Blood\ Flow = \underline{\hspace{3cm}}$$

125. Blood pressure is highest in the _____ at _____ mm Hg, and lowest in the _____ _____ at _____ mm Hg.

126. Arterial blood pressure is a measure of the pressure in the _____. Systolic measures pressure during _____ _____ and averages _____ mm Hg. Diastolic is measured during _____ _____ and averages _____ mm Hg.

127. The pulse pressure is _____, and averages _____ mm Hg.

The MAP is determined by _____ + $\dfrac{\underline{\hspace{3cm}}}{3}$

128. On reaching the capillary beds, pressure drops to _____ mm Hg; pressure drops to _____ mm Hg on entering the venous system. Venous return is assisted by two mechanisms, the _____ and _____ _____.

129. The three factors affecting blood pressure are _____ _____, _____ _____, and _____ _____.

130. Cardiac output (CO) is determined by the _____ _____ (SV) and the _____ _____ (HR).

131. During rest conditions the heart rate is controlled by the _____ _____ and the stroke volume is simply a function of _____ _____. During stress both are stimulated by the _____ NS, increasing/decreasing CO and MAP.

132. Neural regulators adjust for blood pressure fluctuations by affecting _____ _____. These changes are controlled by the medulla's _____ _____. Within the walls of the carotid artery and the aorta are _____, which react to stretch due to pressure.

133. Baroreceptors stimulate the vasomotor center to induce _____, reducing peripheral resistance and increasing/decreasing blood pressure.

134. Close to the baroreceptors, chemoreceptors are sensitive to _____ _____ and _____, and _____ _____.

135. Epinephrine increases/decreases CO by inducing _____. NE causes _____. Nicotine causes _____.

136. How does increased ADH output affect blood pressure? _____

137. How does increased Atrial Natriuretic Peptide (ANP) affect blood pressure? _____

138. Angiotensin II functions as a _____. Nitric Oxide (NO) functions as a _____.

139. Long term pressure regulation involves changes in the _____ _____; this mechanism is controlled by the _____.

140. When pressure is increased, the kidneys increase/decrease urinary output to increase/decrease blood volume and restore correct pressure. When pressure drops, urinary output increases/decreases to increase/decrease blood volume.

141. When pressure drops, Renin from the kidney stimulates the production of the vasoconstrictor _____, as well as _____ and _____.

142. Hypotension is diagnosed when systolic BP falls below _____ mm Hg. Hypertension is considered sustained BP above _____/_____ mm Hg. 90% of these cases are labeled _____ or _____.

143. Secondary Hypertension is due to _____ or _____ and _____ disorders.

144. Blood flow through the tissues is called _____.

145. Tissue perfusion is determined by _____ and _____.

146. Blood velocity is determined by the _____ of the particular blood vessels. Autoregulation has _____ and _____ controls.

147. Metabolic controls respond to _____ and stimulate the release of the vasodilator _____. Myogenic controls affect _____ _____. When BP is elevated arterioles will dilate/constrict to control to the microcirculation; when it is low arterioles will _____.

148. Syncope occurs when BP falls below _____ mm Hg; cerebral edema occurs when BP exceeds _____ mm Hg.

149. The movement of fluid to and from the capillary is determined by Capillary _____ Pressure and the _____ _____ Pressure.

150. The Capillary Hydrostatic pressure measures _____ _____ and generally results with a net movement of fluid in/out. The Colloid Osmotic Pressure is created by _____ _____ and results with net movement of fluid in/out.

151. Define Circulatory Shock: _____ _____.

152. Define Hyperemia: _____.

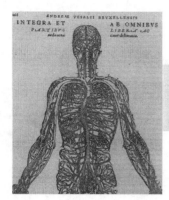

Part 4: Vascular Tree

153. Which chambers receive blood? _____ Which chambers propel blood?
     _____

154. What is meant by Pulmonary Circulation? _____
     _____ Which side of the heart is involved? _____

155. What is meant by Systemic Circulation? _____
     _____ Which side of the heart is involved? _____

156. What is meant by Coronary Circulation? _____
     _____

157. The right atrium receives blood from which three vessels? _____ _____
     _____, _____ _____ _____, and the
     _____ _____

158. Deoxygenated blood passes from the right atrium through the _____ Valve to reach
     the right Ventricle; it then passes through the _____ Valve to enter the enter the
     _____ Trunk.

159. The Pulmonary Trunk then divides into right and left _____ _____ to
     reach the microcirculation of the lung.

160. Oxygenated blood from the Pulmonary microcirculation enters the left atrium via the four
     _____ _____; blood then passes through the _____ or
     _____ Valve to enter the left ventricle.

161. Blood from the left ventricle passes through the _____ or _____ Valve to
     enter the _____.

162. The Aorta is classified as which type of blood vessel? _____. The Aorta ascends and
     curves into the _____ _____.

163. The three branches of the Aortic Arch, from right to left, are: _____,
     _____ _____, and _____
     _____ Arteries.

164. The Brachiocephalic Artery branches into the Right _____ _____ and Right _____ Arteries.

165. The Right and Left Subclavian Arteries branch into the _____ Artery to the neck and head and the _____ Artery, which services the upper extremities.

166. The Vertebral Artery is located within the _____ foramen of the cervical vertebra and will merge in the cranium to form the single _____ Artery.

167. The Basilar Artery services the rear of the brain by branching into the _____ _____ Artery.

168. The Posterior Cerebral Arteries then merge with the centrally located _____ of _____.

169. The Right and Left Common Carotid Arteries split into _____ and _____ branches.

170. The branches of the External Carotid service the _____; the Internal Carotid branches into the _____ and _____ _____ arteries and helps form the _____ of _____.

171. The Circle of Willis is completed by the Anterior and Posterior _____ Arteries.

172. Unlike arteries that split into smaller "branches," smaller veins merge forming larger veins. This is known as an _____.

173. The superficial veins of the occipital region and inner mandible anastomose into the _____ _____ vein. Blood and used CSF drain into the _____ _____ Vein.

174. The External Jugular and Vertebral Veins merge with the _____ Vein to form the _____ Vein.

175. The Internal Jugular merges with the Subclavian Vein to form the _____ Vein.

176. The Right and Left Brachiocephalic Vein merge into the _____ _____ _____.

177. After sending off branches to service the shoulder girdle, the Axillary Artery becomes the _____ Artery upon entering the arm.

178. The Brachial Artery branches at the elbow into the _____ and _____.

179. The Radial and Ulnar arteries merge in the hand to form the deep and superficial _____ before forming the _____ Artery for the microcirculation of the fingers.

180. The Digital Veins anastomose into the _____ and _____ Venous _____.

181. The Superficial Palmar Venous Arch forms the _____ (lateral) and _____ (medial) Veins. The Deep Palmar Venous Arch forms the _____ (lateral) and _____ (medial) Veins.

182. The Radial and Ulnar Veins anastomose into the _____ Vein. Which vein originates between them and merges with the Basilic Vein in the medial arm? _____ _____ Vein.

183. What vessel crosses from the lateral arm to connect the Cephalic Vein to the Basilic Vein?
_____

184. The Brachial and Basilic Veins merge forming the _____ Vein.

185. The Axillary Vein merges with the Cephalic Vein forming the _____ Vein.

186. The Subclavian Vein merges with the Internal and External _____ Veins from the head and neck to form the _____ Vein.

187. The Right and Left Brachiocephalic Veins merge into the _____ _____ _____.

188. Which vein drains blood from the intercostals muscles into the Superior Vena Cava? _____ Vein

189. What term describes the Aorta as it progresses inferiorly from the Arch? _____

190. Branches of the Descending Aorta that run between the ribs are known as _____ Arteries. Below the diaphragm, the Aorta is called the _____.

191. The first major branch of the Abdominal Aorta inferior to the diaphragm servicing the organs of the upper quadrants is called the _____ Artery.

192. The Celiac Artery splits into three branches: Left _____ Artery to the stomach, _____ Artery to the spleen, and the _____ _____ Artery.

193. The Common Hepatic Artery splits into the Right _____ Artery, the _____ _____ artery to the liver, and the _____ Artery.

194. Inferior to the Celiac Artery is the largest branch of the Abdominal Aorta, the _____ _____ Artery.

195. The Superior Mesenteric Artery services the _____. The branches to the kidneys are called the Right and Left _____ Artery.

196. Below the Renal Artery, the branches to the testes and ovaries exit the _____ Artery.

197. Below the Gonadal Artery is the last major branch of the Aorta, the _____ _____ Artery.

198. Below the Inferior Mesenteric Artery are four paired _____ Arteries to the posterior lumbar region. The Aorta then bifurcates into the Left and Right _____ _____ Artery.

199. The Common Iliac Arteries bifurcate into _____ and _____ branches.

200. The Internal Iliac Artery forms branches to the buttocks, the Inferior and Superior _____ Artery, and the medial thigh, the _____ Artery.

201. As it enters the thigh the External Iliac becomes the _____ Artery.

202. The Femoral Artery gives off a _____ _____ branch to the posterior thigh.

203. Branches of the Deep Femoral Artery that circle the femur head are called the _____ and _____ _____ Femoral Artery.

204. The Femoral Artery continues inferiorly behind the knee as the _____ Artery.

205. The Popliteal Artery splits into _____ _____ Artery, supplying muscles of dorsiflexion and the _____ _____ Artery, supplying those of plantarflexion.

206. The Anterior Tibial Artery becomes the _____ _____ on the dorsum of the foot.

207. The Dorsalis Pedis ends as the _____ Artery with its branches, the _____ Artery.

208. The Posterior Tibial's main branch, the _____ Artery, splits into Lateral and Medial _____ Artery.

209. The Metatarsal Veins merge forming the _____ _____ _____.

210. The Dorsal Venous Arch gives rise to the _____ Vein (lateral), the _____ _____ on the superior surface of the foot, and the _____ and _____ _____ Veins (medial).

211. What is the Great Saphenous Vein's claim to fame? _____

212. The Dorsalis Pedis becomes the _____ _____ Vein.

213. The Digital Veins merge forming the _____ _____.

214. The Plantar Arch forms the paired _____ Veins.

215. The Plantar Veins merge forming the _____ _____.

216. The Posterior Tibial merges with the Anterior Tibial and Fibular Veins to form the _____ Veins.

217. The Popliteal vein becomes the _____ and joins with the Great Saphenous to form the _____ _____ Vein.

218. The External and Internal Iliac Veins merge forming the _____ _____ Vein.

219. Right and Left Common Iliac Veins merge to form the _____ _____ _____.

220. Blood from the posterior abdominal wall drains into the Inferior Vena Cava via the paired _____ Veins.

221. The _____ Gonadal merges directly with the IFC, whereas the _____ Gonadal merges with the Renal Vein on that side.

222. In addition to the Proper Hepatic Artery, the liver receives nutrient rich blood from the digestive organs, spleen, and pancreas via the _____ _____ Vein.

223. The Hepatic Portal Vein receives blood from four main vessels: _____ and _____ _____ Veins, _____ Vein, and the Left _____ Vein.

224. The Inferior Mesenteric brings blood from the _____ _____; the Superior Mesenteric from the _____ _____. The Splenic brings blood from the spleen and _____; the Left Gastric Vein from the _____.

225. Processed blood leaves the liver and enters the Inferior Vena Cava via the Right and Left _____ Veins.

226. The Inferior Vena Cava drains into the _____ _____.

Unit X: Blood and Cardiovascular System

Part 1: Blood

1. Derived from Mesenchyme, Cells in a Non-living Matrix, Exhibits Vascularity
2. Formed Elements, Plasma, Soluble Proteins
3. 55%, 45%; Erythrocytes, Leukocytes, Platelets
4. 45%. Hematocrit; ♂45%, ♀42%
5. Viscous. 7.35–7.45, ♂5–6L, ♀4–5L
6. Oxygen delivery; Nutrient and waste transport; Temperature, pH and fluid volume maintenance; Protection against blood loss and infection
7. 90%, 8%, 2% electrolytes and gases
8. Albumin, Globulins, clotting factors
9. Creating Osmotic Pressure Gradient. Alpha, Beta, and Gamma. Prothrombin and Fibrinogen. Liver
10. Transport Proteins, Antibodies
11. Biconcave; Expulsing of organelles
12. Spectrin, Hemoglobin
13. Deoxyhemoglobin, Oxyhemoglobin, Carbaminohemoglobin
14. Polypeptide chains, Heme
15. Iron; 2.5 Trillion
16. Hemopoeisis; Hemocytoblasts; Erythropoeisis
17. Blood Sinusoids. Erythropoietin, Kidney, Hypoxia/Reduced O_2
18. Hemorrhage, Increased O_2 demand, Reduced O_2 availability
19. Iron, B_{12}, Folic Acid
20. Transferrin, Ferritin and Hemosiderin
21. 120, Spleen
22. Liver; Bilirubin
23. Bile, Urobilinogen
24. O_2, weakness, palor, shortness of breath
25. Hemorrhagic, Hemolytic, Aplastic
26. Microcytic, Pernicious, B_{12}
27. Genetically linked; Thallasemias, Sickle Cell
28. Polycemia; 80%; Viscosity
29. Movement of WBCs through capillary wall; Chemical attraction for WBCs; Normal WBC elevation to 11k with infection
30. 1%, Granulocyte, Agranulocyte
31. Neutrophils, Eosinophils, Basophils, Lymphocytes, Monocytes
32. 40–70%, Polymorph. Peroxidase and Defensin; bacterial and fungal infection
33. 1–4%, Bilobed. Digestive enzymes, allergic, parasites
34. 0.5%, U-shaped; Histamine, Vasodilator. Mast
35. T-: immune Rx to viral and cancer cells; B-: immune Rx, Plasma
36. Macrophages
37. Leukopoeisis. Lymphoid, Myeloid
38. Lymphocytes. Monoblast, Myeloblast
39. Monocytes, Neutrophils, Eosinophils and Basophils
40. Leukopenia, Anticancer/Steroids Drugs; Leukemia, Cancer
41. Myelocytic, Lymphocytic
42. Megakaryocytes; Thrombopoeitin. adhering to breaches in BV walls
43. RBCs outside the vascular tree. Halting of hemorrhage by sealing of breach
44. Vascular Spasm, Platelet Plug formation, Coagulation, Clot Retraction
45. Reduce flow to injured area. Prostaglandins. Seal Breach. Thromboxane
46. Prothrombin, Thrombin, Fibrin
47. Blood, Intrinsic. Extrinsic, Thromboplastin
48. Thrombin
49. Fibrinogen, Fibrin, Clot
50. Pull edges of breach together, new tissue growth
51. Fibrinolysis; Plasminogen
52. Thromboembolytic. Thrombus; Embolus. Occlusions
53. Ischemia; Necrosis, Infarct
54. Thrombocytopenias. Hemophilia
55. 30%. Anticoagulant. Autologous
56. Agglutination, Lysing; Kidney Tubules
57. A, B, AB, O
58. A, B, A, and O; B, A, B, and O; A and B, None, A,B,AB, and O; None, A and B, O only
59. Rh$^-$, Rh$^+$, 2nd
60. Erythroblastosis Fetalis, RhoGAM

Part 2: The Heart

61. Mediastinum, Pericardial Sac, Pericardium
62. Fibrous, Serous
63. Pericardial Cavity, Parietal, Visceral. Pericarditis
64. Epicardium, Myocardium, Endocardium, Squamous

Epithelium
65. Atria; Auricles. Ventricles
66. Interatrial Septum; Interventricular Septum. Foramen Ovale
67. Crista Terminalis; Pectinate
68. Superior Vena Cava, Inferior Vena Cava, Coronary Sinus
69. Tricuspid, Atrio-Ventricular
70. Trabeculae Carne, Papillary, Chordae Tendinae
71. Atrioventricular, Coronary. Interventricular
72. Semilunar, Pulmonary Artery; Pulmonary
73. Pulmonary; Pulmonary Vein
74. Ventricles; Atria
75. Oxygenated, Pulmonary Vein; Bicuspid/Mitral Seminlunar, Aorta. Systemic
76. Myocardium; Angina Pectoris
77. Intercalated Discs, Desmosomes, Gap. Syncytium
78. Autorhythmicity, Depolarizations
79. ECF, Surge, Sustained
80. Sinoartial Node, Atrioventricular Node, Bundle of His, Bundle Branches, Purkinje Fibers
81. 100; Parsympathetic, 75; Sinus Rhythm
82. Atria; Atriventricular Node
83. Purkinje Fibers
84. Contraction; Relaxation
85. Rapid, irregular contractions; Abnormal Pacemaker sets rhythm; No impulses from AV Node, ventricles beat at 30/m
86. Atrial Depolarization; Ventricular Depolarization; Ventricular Repolarization
87.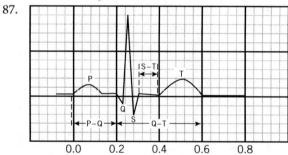
88. Ischemia, infarct
89. Ventricular Filling, Ventricular Systole, Isovolumetric Relaxation
90. Mid-late Diastole; Passive, P Wave
91. Contract, Semilunar, 120 mm Hg
92. Early Diastole, T wave. Repolarization
93. Atrioventricular, Contraction, QRS
94. Semilunar, Diastole, T Wave

95. Stroke Volume, Heart Rate
96. Volume of blood ejected, End Diastolic, End Systolic. 70 ml
97. Preload, Contractility, Afterload
98. Baroreceptors; Epinephrine, Thyroxine
99. Hypercalcemia, spastic contractions. Hpernatremia, calcium transport. Hyperkalemia, cardiac arrest
100. 100; 60
101. Pulmonary Edema; Peripheral Edema
102. Right Atrium, Coronary Sinus, SA Node
103. Pulmonary Trunk, Right Ventricle and Aorta
104. Ductus Arteriousus, Aorta
105. Ligamentus Arteriousum; Patent Ductus
106. Cyanosis

Part 3: Blood Vessels and Blood Pressure

107. Tunica Interna, Tunica Media, Tunica Externa, Adventitia. Vasa Vasorum
108. Squamous Epithelium. Vasoconstriction and Vasodilation
109. Decreased, increased; Increased, decreased
110. Elastic, Muscular
111. Elastin, recoil
112. Vasoconstriction, organs, capillaries
113. Continuous, Fenestrated, Sinusoidal. Pericytes
114. no breaks between cells. Skin, muscles
115. Pores, Absorption, Filtration
116. Leaky; cells; Liver, Lymph Bone Marrow
117. Microcirculation. Metarteriole; Postcapillary Venule
118. Precapillary Sphincter; Vascular Shunt. Postcapillary Venule
119. Capacitance. Valves
120. Varicose. Hemorrhoids. Anastomoses
121. Volume of Blood through a specific area over a specific time; Force per unit area on the BV wall. Pressure gradient
122. Viscosity, Vessel Length and Vessel Diameter
123. Increased, Decreased. Decreased, Increased
124. Difference in BP/Peripheral Resistance
125. Aorta, 120, Right Atrium, 0
126. Aorta, Ventricular Contraction, 120. Ventricular Relaxation, 80
127. The difference between Systolic and Diastolic pressure. 40, Diastolic + Pulse Pressure/3
128. 40, 20. Respiratory, Muscular Pump
129. Cardiac Output, Peripheral Resistance, Blood Volume

130. Stroke Volume, Heart Rate
131. Vagus Nerve, Venous Return. Sympathetic, Increasing
132. Peripheral Resistance. Vasomotor Center. Baroreceptors
133. Vasodilation, decreasing
134. Reduced O_2, pH, increased CO_2
135. Increases, Vasodilation. Vasoconstriction.
136. Increases water resorption and BV and BP
137. Increases sodium and water excretion, reducing BV and BP
138. Vasoconstrictor; Vasodilator
139. Blood Volume; Kidney
140. Increase, decrease. Decreases, increase
141. Angiotensin II, ADH, Aldosterone
142. 100. 140/90. Primary, Essential
143. Atherosclerosis, Endocrine, Kidney
144. Perfusion
145. Velocity, Autoregulation
146. Cross Sectional area. Metabolic and Myogenic
147. Reduced O_2, NO. Smooth muscle; constrict, dilate
148. 60; 160
149. Hydrostatic, Colloid Osmotic
150. Force exerted on capillary wall, out. Soluble Proteins, in
151. Reduced BV due to hemorrhage, dehydration, and burns
152. Redness due to increased/restored blood flow

Part 4: The Vascular Tree

153. Atria; Ventricles
154. Transport of deoxygenated blood from the tissues to the lungs; Right
155. Transport of oxygenated blood from the lungs to the tissues; Left
156. Transport of blood to and from the Myocardium
157. Superior and Inferior Vena Cava, Coronary Sinus
158. Tricuspid; Semilunar; Pulmonary
159. Pulmonary Arteries
160. Pulmonary Veins, Mitral or Bicuspid
161. Semilunar or Aortic, Aorta
162. Elastic; Aortic Arch
163. Brachiocephalic, Left Common Carotid, Left Subclavian
164. Common Carotid, Subclavian
165. Vertebral, Axillary
166. Transverse, Basilar
167. Posterior Cerebral

168. Circle of Willis
169. External and Internal
170. Superficial face and head; Anterior and Middle Cerebral, Circle of Willis
171. Communicating
172. Anastomosis
173. External Jugular; Internal Jugular
174. Axillary, Subclavian
175. Brachiocephalic
176. Superior Vena Cava
177. Brachial
178. Radial and Ulnar
179. Palmar Arch, Digital Artery
180. Deep and Superficial Palmar Venous Arch
181. Radial and Ulnar; Cephalic and Basilic
182. Brachial; Median Antebrachial
183. Median Cubital
184. Axillary
185. Subclavian
186. Jugular, Brachiocephalic
187. Superior Vena Cava
188. Azygous
189. Descending
190. Intercostal; Abdominal
191. Celia
192. Gastric, Splenic, Common Hepatic
193. Gastric, Proper Hepatic, Gastroduodenal
194. Superior Mesenteric
195. Small and Large Intestines; Renal
196. Gonadal
197. Inferior Mesenteric
198. Lumbar; Common Iliac
199. Internal and External
200. Gluteal; Obturator
201. Femoral
202. Deep Femoral
203. Medial and Lateral Circumflex
204. Popliteal
205. Anterior Tibial, Posterior Tibial
206. Dorsalis Pedis
207. Arcuate, Metatarsal
208. Fibular, Plantar
209. Dorsal Venous Arch
210. Fibular, Dorsalis Pedis, Small and Great Saphenous
211. Longest vein in the body
212. Anterior Tibial
213. Plantar Arch
214. Plantar

215. Posterior Tibial
216. Popliteal
217. Femoral, External Iliac
218. Common Iliac
219. Inferior Vena Cava
220. Lumbar

221. Right, Left
222. Hepatic Portal
223. Inferior and Superior Mesenteric, Splenic, Left Gastric
224. Large Intestine, Small Intestine, Pancreas, Stomach
225. Hepatic
226. Right Atrium

Unit X: Take a Test!

1. Which of the following is NOT function of blood?
    a) transports nutrients, wastes and gases   b) regulates pH
    c) prevents blood loss   d) protection against infection
    e) all are functions

2. Formed Elements comprise what portion of blood:
    a) 1%   b) 8%
    c) 45%   d) 55%   e) 90%

3. Which is not considered to be a formed element:
    a) erythrocyte   b) thrombocyte
    c) leukocyte   d) immunoglobulin   e) all are formed elements

4. Plasma proteins such as albumin and globulin form what portion of plasma:
    a) 1%   b) 8%
    c) 45%   d) 55%   e) 90%

5. Which plasma protein functions by creating an osmotic gradient:
    a) albumin   b) gamma globulin
    c) fibrinogen   d) plasmin   e) thrombin

6. Which cell exudes its nucleus and organelles prior to maturing:
    a) erythrocyte   b) thrombocyte
    c) leukocyte   d) platelet   e) megakaryocyte

7. Which compound supports the biconcave shape of erythrocytes:
    a) heparin   b) spectrin
    c) hemoglobin   d) histamine   e) erythropoeitin

8. Which compound is classified as an anticoagulant:
    a) heparin   b) spectrin
    c) hemoglobin   d) histamine   e) erythropoeitin

9. Which compound is classified as a vasodilator:
    a) heparin   b) spectrin
    c) hemoglobin   d) histamine   e) erythropoeitin

10. Which compound is secreted by the kidney is response to O2 demand:
    a) heparin   b) spectrin
    c) hemoglobin   d) gamma globulin   e) erythropoeitin

11. De-oxyhemoglobin is also referred to as:
    a) reduced hemoglobin   b) HHb
    c) carbaminohemoglobin   d) Hb   e) a and b

12. Hemoglobin bound to CO2 is referred to as:
    a) reduced hemoglobin   b) carbaminohemoglobin
    c) HHb   d) Hb   e) a and c

13. Anemia is characterized by:
    a) reduced blood volume   b) reduced O2
    c) reduced leukocytes   d) reduced platelets   e) a and c

14. Which of the following disorders increases blood viscosity:
    a) aplastic anemia   b) polycemia vera
    c) sickle cell anemia   d) pernicious anemia   e) microcytic anemia

15. Which disease implies reduced or no erythrocyte production:
    a) aplastic anemia   b) polycemia vera
    c) sickle cell anemia   d) pernicious anemia   e) microcytic anemia

16. Which of the following is due to B12 deficiency:
    a) aplastic anemia   b) polycemia vera
    c) sickle cell anemia   d) pernicious anemia   e) microcytic anemia

17. Polycemia vera affects blood flow by:
    a) increasing peripheral resistance
    b) increasing blood pressure
    c) decreasing peripheral resistance
    d) decreasing blood pressure

18. B12 deficiency can cause anemia by which modality:
    a) reduced RBC production   b) improperly formed hemoglobin
    c) reduced hemoglobin production d) RBC lysis

19. In which condition is anemia due to bacterial or viral infection:
    a) aplastic   b) hemorrhagic
    c) hemolytic   d) hemophilia   e) sickle cell

20. In the spleen, hemoglobin is degraded to:
    a) stercobilin   b) bilirubin
    c) urobilinogen   d) erythropoeitin   e) deoxyhemoglobin

21. The movement of leukocytes from capillaries into the interstitial tissues is referred to as:
    a) diapedesis
    b) hemorrhage
    c) chemotaxis
    d) leukocytosis
    e) thrombus

22. The process by leukocytes are attracted to the by-products of cellular injury is called:
    a) diapedesis
    b) hemorrhage
    c) chemotaxis
    d) leukocytosis
    e) thrombus

23. Which of the following is normally the most abundant leukocyte:
    a) basophils
    b) eosinophils
    c) monocytes
    d) lymphocytes
    e) neutrophils

24. Which leukocyte secretes histamine:
    a) basophils
    b) eosinophils
    c) monocytes
    d) lymphocytes
    e) neutrophils

25. Which leukocyte is associated with allergic reactions:
    a) basophils
    b) eosinophils
    c) monocytes
    d) lymphocytes
    e) neutrophils

26. Which leukocyte is considered a phagocyte:
    a) basophils
    b) eosinophils
    c) monocytes
    d) lymphocytes
    e) neutrophils

27. Which leukocyte produces antibodies:
    a) basophils
    b) eosinophils
    c) monocytes
    d) lymphocytes
    e) neutrophils

28. Platelets secrete which substance to attract more platelets to the area:
    a) thromboxane
    b) heparin
    c) histamine
    d) defensins
    e) plasmin

29. Which of the following is derived from a megakaryocyte:
    a) erythrocyte
    b) leukocyte
    c) thrombocyte
    d) macrophage
    e) all are

30. Which is the correct sequence of the following events:
    1: fibrinogen fibrin
    2: clot retraction
    3: formation of thromboplastin
    4: prothrombinthrombin
    a) 3,4,1,2   b) 1,2,3,4   c) 4,3,1,2   d) 3,2,1,4   e) 4,2,3,1

31. Coagulation occurs faster within the interstitial spaces than within the blood due to the presence of:
    a) heparin
    b) histamine
    c) thromboplastin
    d) spectrin
    e) plasmin

32. Fibrin functions by:
   a) stimulating thrombocyte formation
   b) activating the prothrombin activator
   c) attracting more platelets to the area
   d) stimulating vascular spasm
   e) drawing the broken ends of blood vessels together

33. Prostaglandins are involved in which process of Hemostasis:
   a) Vascular Spasm   b) Coagulation
   c) Platelet Plug formation d) Clot Retraction

34. Which must occur for a clot to be dissolved:
   a) prothrombin is activated into thrombin
   b) fibrinogen is activated into fibrin
   c) thromboplastin is activated into thromboxane
   d) plasminogen is activated into plasmin
   e) erythropoeitin is activated into thrombopoeitin

35. Fibrin is involved in which process of Hemostasis:
   a) Vascular Spasm   b) Coagulation
   c) Platelet Plug formation d) Clot Retraction

36. A blood clot that has broken free and migrates is known as a:
   a) thrombus   b) embolus
   c) hemorrhage   d) infarct   e) macrophage

37. Of the blood groups, which does not possess any antigens making it the universal donor:
   a) A   b) B   c) AB   d) O

38. Of the blood groups, which does not produce any antibodies making it the universal recipient:
   a) A   b) B   c) AB   d) O

39. In a cross between an Rh- man and an Rh+ woman, who is at greatest risk of hazardous antigen-antibody reactions:
   a) mother   b) father
   c) first child   d) second child   e) no one

40. Which is a sex-linked genetic disorder resulting in defective clotting factors:
   a) polycemia vera   b) sickle cell anemia
   c) hemophilia   d) thallasemia minor

1: e; 2: c; 3: d; 4: b; 5: a; 6: a; 7: b; 8: a; 9: d; 10: e; 11: e; 12: b; 13: b; 14: b; 15: a; 16: d; 17: a; 18: c; 19: c; 20: b; 21: a; 22: c; 23: c; 24: a; 25: b; 26: c; 27: d; 28: a; 29: c; 30: a; 31: c; 32: e; 33: a; 34: d; 35: b; 36: b; 37: d; 38: c; 39: d; 40: c

Part 2: Time allowed:30 minutes

1. Cardiac fibers are similar to skeletal fibers in that both types are:
    a) uninucleate   b) involuntary
    c) striated   d) botha and b   e) a, b and c

2. Which insures simultaneous contraction of all cardiac fibers in the same chamber:
    a) purkinje fibers   b) endocardium
    c) CT skeleton   d) intercalated disc   e) ECF calcium

3. The epicardium is also known as the:
    a) Fibrous pericardium   b) Serous Visceral Layer
    c) Serous Parietal Layer d) Serous Pleura   e) Serous Peritoneum

4. Which of the following layers is described as a functional syncytium:
    a) Endocardium   b) Myocardium
    c) Epicardium   d) Pericardium

5. Which of the following explain why the atria contract before the ventricles:
    a) the CT skeleton insulates the atria from the ventricles
    b) the action potential to the ventricles is delayed by the cardiac conduction system
    c) ventricular depolarization takes much longer than atrial
    d) a and b
    e) a, b and c

6. Which is the correct sequence in the propagation of a cardiac action potential
    1. Purkinje fibers
    2. SA node
    3. right and left bundle branches
    4. AV bundle
    5. AV node
    a) 2, 4, 5, 3, 1   b) 5, 2, 4, 1, 3
    c) 5, 2, 4, 3, 1   d) 2, 4, 3, 1, 4   e) 2, 5, 4, 3, 1

7. Which is the correct sequence in the flow of blood through the valves of the heart:
    1. Mitral Valve
    2. Pulmonary Valve
    3. Aortic Valve
    4. Tricuspid Valve
    a) 2, 4, 3, 1   b) 4, 2, 1, 3
    c) 2, 4, 3, 1   d) 4, 1, 2, 3   e) 2, 4, 3, 1

8. Which delivers de-oxygenated blood to the right atrium from the myocardium:
    a) Superior Vena Cava   b) Inferior Vena Cava
    c) Coronary Sinus   d) Pulmonary Vein   e) Pulmonary Artery

9. Which delivers oxygenated blood to the left atrium:
   a) Superior Vena Cava   b) Inferior Vena Cava
   c) Coronary Sinus   d) Pulmonary Vein   e) Pulmonary Artery

10. Which delivers deoxygenated blood to the lungs:
   a) Pulmonary Vein   b) Inferior Vena Cava
   c) Pulmonary Artery   d) Superior Vena Cava   e) Pulmonary Artery

11. Which make-up the ridged muscles of the ventricles:
   a) papillary muscles   b) trabeculae carnea
   c) Pectinate muscles   d) crista terminalis   e) fossa ovalis

12. Which make-up the ridged muscles of the atria:
   a) papillary muscles   b) trabeculae carnea
   c) Pectinate muscles   d) crista terminalis   e) fossa ovalis

13. The chordae tendinae anchor the valve cusps to the:
   a) papillary muscles   b) trabeculae carnea
   c) Pectinate muscles   d) interventricular septum e) fossa ovalis

14. Mitral Valve Prolapse could be due to poor function of the:
   a) Pectinate muscles   b) Trabeculae Carne
   c) Myocardium   d) Papillary muscles   e) crista terminalis

15. Which is the closed remnant of the fetal inter-atrial septal shunt:
   a) crista terminalis   b) trabeculae carnea
   c) coronary sulcus   d) coronary Sinus   e) fossa ovalis

16. Which prevents backsplash of blood into the left atrium:
   a) Tricuspid Valve   b) Bicuspid Valve
   c) Semilunar Valves   d) Pulmonary Valve   e) Aortic Valve

17. Which prevents backsplash of blood into the right atrium:
   a) Tricuspid Valve   b) Bicuspid Valve
   c) Semilunar Valves   d) Pulmonary Valve   e) Aortic Valve

18. The first heart sound is created by:
   a) the closing of the aortic valve   b) the closing of the pulmonary valve
   c) the closing of the bicuspid valve   d) the contraction of the ventricles
   e) the flow of blood through the AV valves

19. The second heart sound associated with ventricular diastole is created by the closing of which valve:
   a) Tricuspid Valve   b) Bicuspid Valve
   c) Semilunar Valves   d) Atrioventricular Valve e) Mitral Valve

20. Without autonomic influences the Sinoatrial node depolarizes at what rate/min:
   a) 30   b) 40
   c) 60   d) 75   e) 100

21. Which would be the resting sinus rhythm:
    a) 100   b) 75
    c) 60   d) 40   e) 30

22. The myocardium of the ventricles is depolarized directly by:
    a) Sinoatrial node   b) Right and Left Bundle branches
    c) Purkinje Fibers   d) Atrioventricular node   e) Bundle of His

23. Which is located in the interventricular septum:
    a) Sinoatrial node   b) Right and Left Bundle branches
    c) Purkinje Fibers   d) Atrioventricular node   e) Bundle of His

24. In which cardiac disorder do the ventricles depolarize and contract at their own rate of 30 beats/min:
    a) Fibrillation   b) Ectopic focus
    c) Infarct   d) Heart Block   e) Ischemia

25. In which cardiac disorder does an abnormal pacemaker depolarize the myocardium at an abnormal rate:
    a) Fibrillation   b) Ectopic focus
    c) Infarct   d) Heart Block   e) Ischemia

26. Which indicates an area of dead tissue:
    a) Fibrillation   b) Ectopic focus
    c) Infarct   d) Heart Block   e) Ischemia

27. Reduced blood flow to an area of myocardium is known as:
    a) Fibrillation   b) Ectopic focus
    c) Infarct   d) Heart Block   e) Ischemia

28. Which portion of the ECG indicates ventricular systole:
    a) P wave   b) QRS complex
    c) T wave   d) P-Q interval   e) S-T segment

29. Which indicates ventricular diastole:
    a) P wave   b) QRS complex
    c) T wave   d) P-Q interval   e) S-T segment

30. Which portion of the ECG indicates atrial depolarization:
    a) P wave   b) QRS complex
    c) T wave   d) P-Q interval   e) S-T segment

31. A heart rate of 60 beats/min or less is considered:
    a) Right-sided Heart Failure   b) Bradycardia
    c) Tachycardia   d) Left-sided Heart Failure   e) Angina Pectoris

32. A patient's P wave is missing from the ECG, but they still have a positive net cardiac output. Why:
    a) 70% of ventricular filling is passive
    b) AV node is now the pacemaker
    c) the Bundle Branches are still depolarizing the Purkinje fibers
    d) a and b
    e) a, b and c

33. The Stroke Volume is best described as:
    a) the volume of blood ejected from the ventricle per minute
    b) the volume of the left ventricle
    c) the total volume of all four cardiac chambers
    d) the volume of blood ejected from the ventricle per cardiac cycle
    e) the total blood volume of the body

34. Which of the following do not influence the Stroke Volume:
    a) contractility   b) sinus rhythm
    c) afterload   d) preload
    e) all of these factors affect stroke volume

35. Norepinephrine will directly affect which of the following:
    a) preload   b) contractility
    c) afterload   d) heart rate   e) venous return

36. Epinephrine will directly affect which of the following:
    a) preload   b) contractility
    c) afterload   d) heart rate   e) venous return

37. Increased ventricular stretch affects which of the following factors:
    a) afterload   b) contractility
    c) preload   d) sinus rhythm   e) venous return

38. A heart rate of 100 beats/min or more is considered:
    a) Right-sided Heart Failure   b) Bradycardia
    c) Tachycardia   d) Left-sided Heart Failure   e) Angina Pectoris

39. Pulmonary edema is associated with:
    a) Right-sided Heart Failure   b) Bradycardia
    c) Tachycardia   d) Left-sided Heart Failure   e) Angina Pectoris

40. The pallor and pale-blue discoloration of the lips and nail-beds associated with poor oxygenation is termed:
    a) ischemia   b) angina pectoris
    c) cyanosis   d) anastomoses

23: c, 24: d, 25: b, 26: c, 27: c, 28: b, 29: c, 30: a, 31: b, 32: e, 33: d, 34: b, 35: d, 36: b, 37: c, 38: c, 39: d, 40: c

1: c, 2: d, 3: b, 4: b, 5: d, 6: e, 7: b, 8: c, 9: d, 10: c, 11: b, 12: c, 13: a, 14: d, 15: e, 16: b, 17: a, 18: c, 19: c, 20: e, 21: b, 22: c,

Part 3: Time allowed: 30 minutes

1. Which of the following is correct:
   a) All arteries carry blood from the heart
   b) Elastic arteries are also known as Conducting arteries
   c) Muscular arteries have larger tunica medias
   d) a and b
   e) a, b and c

2. Vasoconstriction is accomplished by the:
   a) Tunica Interna   b) Tunica Media
   c) Tunica Externa   d) Adventitia   e) Vasa Vasorum

3. Blood is supplied to the layers of the vessel wall by the:
   a) Tunica Interna   b) Tunica Media
   c) Tunica Externa   d) Adventitia   e) Vasa Vasorum

4. How do veins differ from arteries:
   a) They do not possess a Tunica Interna
   b) They do not possess Tunica Media
   c) They do not possess Tunica Externa
   d) They have valves
   e) They do not possess a Vasa Vasorum

5. The movement of fluids from the microcirculation into the tissues is called:
   a) anastomoses   b) perfusion
   c) varicosities   d) vascular shunting   e) coarctation

6. Which vessels deliver blood to organs and are referred to as distributing vessels:
   a) Elastic Arteries   b) Muscular Arteries
   c) Arterioles   d) Capillaries   e) Venules

7. Conducting vessels such as the Aorta are referred to as:
   a) Elastic Arteries   b) Muscular Arteries
   c) Arterioles   d) Capillaries   e) Venules

8. Which of the following is found principally in the kidney's glomerulus for filtration:
   a) Continuous capillaries b) intercellular clefts
   c) Fenestrated capillaries d) Sinusoidal capillaries   e) anastomoses

9. Which of the following is found principally in Red Marrow:
   a) Continuous capillaries b) intercellular clefts
   c) Fenestrated capillaries d) Sinusoidal capillaries   e) anastomoses

10. Blood exits the capillary bed via the:
    a) terminal arteriole   b) post-capillary arteriole
    c) thoroughfare channel   d) post-capillary venule   e) metarteriole

11. Vascular shunts bypass the microcirculation directing blood through the:
   a) terminal arteriole
   b) post-capillary arteriole
   c) thoroughfare channel
   d) post-capillary venule
   e) metarteriole

12. The merging of veins to form larger vessels is called:
   a) anastomoses
   b) perfusion
   c) varicosities
   d) vascular shunts
   e) coarctation

13. The "ballooning" and thinning of a blood vessel wall is called:
   a) anastomoses
   b) perfusion
   c) varicosities
   d) aneurysm
   e) coarctation

14. Separation of the tunicas of a major vessel such as the aorta is called:
   a) anastomoses
   b) perfusion
   c) varicosities
   d) aneurysm
   e) coarctation

15. Faulty venous valves of the lower extremities can lead to the formation of:
   a) varicosities
   b) swollen hemorrhoids
   c) pulmonary edema
   d) a and b
   e) a, b and c

16. Baroreceptors:
   a) are located in the aorta and carotid arteries
   b) stimulate the vasomotor center of the medulla
   c) stimulate vasodilation
   d) reduce peripheral resistance
   e) all of these

17. An elevated BP above 120/80 will most likely result in which response:
   a) vasoconstriction of the muscular arteries and vasoconstriction of the metarteriole
   b) vasoconstriction of the muscular arteries and vasodilation of the metarteriole
   c) vasodilation of the muscular arteries and vasoconstriction of the metarteriole
   d) vasodilation of the muscular arteries and vasodilation of the metarteriole

18. Which of the following concerning peripheral resistance (PR) is true:
   a) PR increases as vessel length decreases
   b) PR decreases as vessel diameter increases
   c) PR decreases as viscosity increases
   d) PR increases as vessel diameter increases

19. All of the following assist venous return except:
   a) skeletal muscle activity
   b) respiration
   c) venous valves
   d) increased urinary output

20. What would be the most likely response to elevated CO2:
    a) increasing urinary output to reduce blood volume
    b) vasodilation to reduce peripheral resistance
    c) vasoconstriction to reduce blood flow
    d) increasing the cardiac output to increase pulmonary venous return
    e) forming an anastomoses

21. Which of the following factors affecting BP is directly controlled by the kidneys:
    a) stroke volume   b) blood volume
    c) peripheralresistance d) heart rate

22. Which factor is affected by venous return and arterial afterload:
    a) stroke volume   b) blood volume
    c) peripheralresistance d) heart rate

23. Which factor is directly affected by Vasomotor center of the medulla:
    a) stroke volume   b) blood volume
    c) peripheralresistance d) heart rate

24. Which represents blood pressure on exiting the microcirculation and entering the venous system:
    a) 0 mm Hg   b) 20 mm Hg
    c) 40 mm Hg   d) 80 mm Hg   e) 120 mm Hg

25. Which is the average blood pressure on entering the microcirculation:
    a) 0 mm Hg   b) 20 mm Hg
    c) 40 mm Hg   d) 80 mm Hg   e) 120 mm Hg

26. Which represents the average pressure in the aorta during ventricular Diastole:
    a) 0 mm Hg   b) 20 mm Hg
    c) 40 mm Hg   d) 80 mm Hg   e) 120 mm Hg

27. Which represents the average pressure in the aorta during ventricular Systole:
    a) 0 mm Hg   b) 20 mm Hg
    c) 40 mm Hg   d) 80 mm Hg   e) 120 mm Hg

28. Which represents the average pressure in the right atrium during atrial diastole:
    a) 0 mm Hg   b) 20 mm Hg
    c) 40 mm Hg   d) 80 mm Hg   e) 120 mm Hg

29. Which of the following acts as a vasodilator:
    a) ADH   b) Atrial Natriuretic Polypeptide
    c) Aldosterone   d) Nitric Oxide   e) Angiotensin II

30. Which of the following decreases blood volume by increasing sodium and water excretion:
    a) ADH   b) Atrial Natriuretic Polypeptide
    c) Aldosterone   d) Nitric Oxide   e) Angiotensin II

31. ADH functions by:
    a) increasing water resorption to increase blood volume and BP
    b) increasing water excretion to decrease blood volume and BP
    c) increasing sodium and water excretion to increase blood volume and BP
    d) increase sodium and water resorption to decrease blood volume and BP
    e) increase sodium and water excretion to decrease blood volume and BP

32. Which does the kidney secrete in response to BP below 80 mmHg:
    a) spectrin   b) ADH
    c) erythropoietin   d) Renin   e) ANP

33. Which of the following is responsible for the movement of interstitial fluid into the capillaries:
    a) hydrostatic pressure   b) arterial pressure
    c) colloid osmotic pressure d) velocity   e) viscosity

34. Which of the following is responsible for the movement of interstitial fluid into the capillaries:
    a) hydrostatic pressure   b) arterial pressure
    c) colloid osmotic pressure d) velocity   e) viscosity

35. Which vessel is preferred measuring a patient's pulse rate:
    a) brachial artery   b) radial artery
    c) jugular vein   d) axillary   e) coronary

36. Which vessel is preferred measuring a patient's blood pressure:
    a) brachial artery   b) radial artery
    c) jugular vein   d) axillary   e) coronary

37. Which does not branch from the aortic arch:
    a) brachiocephalic artery   b) right common carotid artery
    c) left common carotid artery d) left subclavian   e) all are branches

38. Which does not contribute to the hepatic portal vein:
    a) splenic vein   b) superior mesenteric vein
    c) inferior mesenteric vein d) hepatic vein   e) all contribute

39. Which is a midline branch off the abdominal aorta:
    a) superior mesenteric artery b) celiac artery
    c) inferior mesenteric artery d) a and b   e) a, b and c

40. Which is not a branch off the Celiac Artery:
    a) phrenic artery   b) left gastric artery
    c) common hepatic artery   d) splenic   e) all are branches

1: e; 2: b; 3: e; 4: d; 5: b, 6: b, 7: a, 8: c; 9: d, 10: d, 11: c; 12: a, 13: d, 14: e, 15: e, 16: e, 17: c, 18: b, 19: d, 20: d, 21: b, 22: a, 23: c, 24: b 25: c, 26: d, 27: e, 28: a, 29: d, 30: d, 31: a, 32: d, 33: a, 34: c; 35: b, 36: a, 37: b, 38: d; 39: c, 40: a

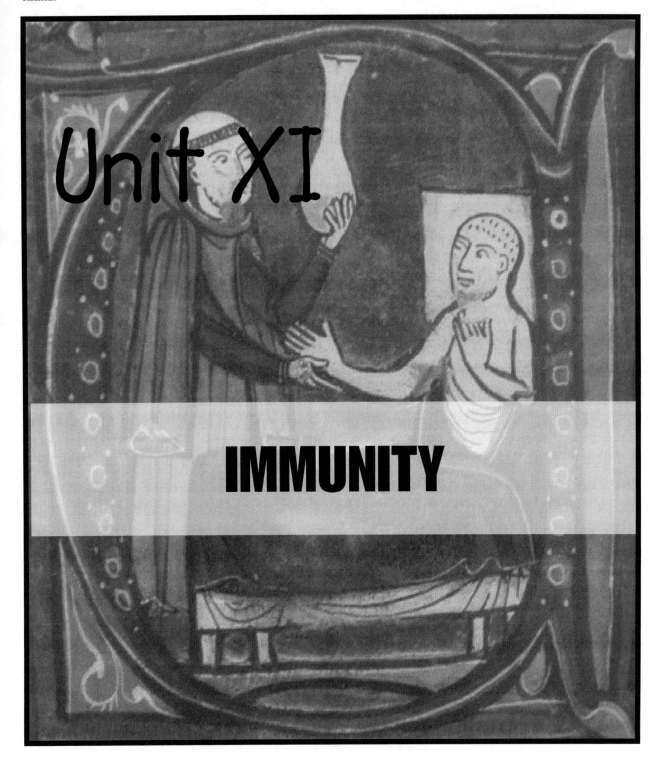

Unit XI

IMMUNITY

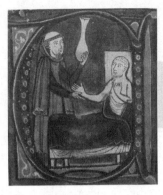

Part 1: Lymphatic System

1. The two principal functions of the lymphatic system include _____ _____ and _____.

2. Lymphatic capillaries collect up to _____ liters of interstitial fluid per day; phagocytes and lymphocytes are housed within _____ _____ and organs.

3. Lymphoid tissue is composed primarily of _____ connective tissue. The lymphatic capillary is described as having a _____ end.

4. Specialized lymphatic capillaries of the small intestine villi are called _____; intestinal lymph is known as _____.

5. Lymphatic capillaries drain into _____ and then into either the _____ _____ _____, collecting fluid from the head and arms, or the _____ _____, collecting fluid from the lower body.

6. Both the Right Lymphatic Duct and Thoracic Duct empty into the junctions of the _____ _____ and _____ veins.

7. Lymphatic drainage into the internal jugular and subclavian veins is assisted, as in veins, by the presence of _____, as well as _____ and _____ pumps.

8. The inflammation of lymphatic tissue is called _____; the accumulation of lymphatic fluid is called _____.

9. The four types of lymphoid cells include immunocompetent _____, phagocytizing _____, _____ cells, which activate T cells and the _____ cells, which form a network of anchoring fibers.

10. Lymphocytes are either _____- Lymphocytes or _____- Lymphocytes; both types of cells originate in the _____ _____.

11. T-Lymphocytes are named as they acquire immunocompetency in the _____; these cells function by _____.
    B- Lymphocytes give rise to _____ cells.

12. Plasma Cells function by producing _____.

13. Define antigen: _____
_____.

14. How do antibodies function? _____
_____

15. Antigen-antibody complexes on foreign cells make them more recognizable to _____,
which engulf them, and to _____, which attack and destroy them.

16. Lymphoid tissue is a fibrous network composed of _____ connective tissue on which
_____ and _____ cells cling.

17. Macrophages are also called _____. Dendritic Cells function by _____
_____.

18. Slightly more organized than diffuse lymphatic tissue are non-capsulated lymphatic _____;
these are noted for their central concentration of cells called the _____
_____.

19. The cells found within the lymphatic follicles' germinal centers are _____ cells and
_____.

20. Both Dendritc cells and B-Lymphocytes both function similarly by _____
_____.

21. The specialized lymphatic follicles of the small intestine wall are called _____
_____.

22. Peyer's Patches increase/decrease in number progressing towards the caecum.

23. Unlike follicles, lymph nodes are enclosed within a _____ _____;
like other solid organs, the lymph node is divided into an outer _____ and inner
_____.

24. The cortex is subdivided into compartments by extensions of the fibrous capsule called
_____. The cortex is noted for _____ _____ as
seen in follicles. The medulla is formed by extensions of cortical tissue called _____
_____.

25. The cortical Germinal Centers are noted for concentrations of _____ cells and
_____, both of which activate in-transit _____. The medullary cords
also contain _____, as well as antibody producing _____ cells.

26. Lymph enters the capsule on the convex side of the node via _____ _____
_____, which drain into the _____ _____.

27. Lymph from the subcapsular sinus filters into the _____ sinus, then exits the
node at its concave _____ through _____ _____
_____.

28. There are more/fewer efferent lymphatic vessels than afferent causing lymph to accumulate within the sinuses; this allows for _____

_____

29. The spleen is located in the _____ _____ _____ and is composed of _____ CT. Like lymph nodes, it is surrounded by a _____ _____, which form subdividing _____.

30. The reticular tissue of the spleen is subdivided as _____ _____ and _____ _____.

31. White pulp has an _____ function and is noted for _____; red pulp provides the spleen's _____ _____ function and is noted for its fibrous _____ _____.

32. As part of its blood cleansing function, _____ cling to the splenic cords to engulf the remains of old and defective _____ and _____.

33. After destroying old RBCs and platelets, the spleen stores _____ and sends _____ to the liver for use in bile synthesis.

34. The spleen also stores _____ and is a site of _____ in the fetus.

35. The thymus is located _____. Its hormones _____ and _____ make naïve lymphocytes immunocompetent.

36. Structurally, the thymus appears _____; its tissue is subdivided into _____ and is referred to as the _____.

37. The purpose of the Blood-Thymus Barrier is to _____

_____

38. The tonsils are incomplete lymphatic organs that _____; they are noted for invaginations called _____, which trap foreign cells.

39. The appendix is an extension off the _____ and is noted for its concentration of _____.

40. Define Lymphadenopathy: _____.

41. Define Lymphoma: _____.

42. How does Hodgkin's Disease differ from lymphoma? _____

_____

43. What is Non-Hodgkin's Lymphoma? _____

_____

44. The concern over acute appendicitis requiring removal is _____

_____

45. What is splenomegaly? _____

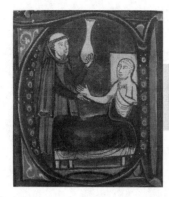

Part 2: Immune System

46. The immune system is composed of two defense systems: the _____, or non-specific defenses, and the _____, or specific defenses.

47. Innate or non-specific defenses include _____ _____ and automated responses to tissue injury or _____.

48. Surface barriers include the _____ and _____, as well as anti-microbial _____.

49. The secretions of skin have a pH of _____; tears and saliva contain the enzyme _____.

50. Non-specific internal defenses include the action of _____, _____ _____ cells, and anti-microbial _____.

51. Anti-microbial proteins are released in response to _____ and _____ markers recognized on foreign particles. These cells and proteins release chemicals which signal/stimulate the _____ response.

52. Anti-microbial proteins include _____ and _____.

53. Interferon functions by _____
_____,
whereas the Complement system functions by _____
_____

54. The complement system enhances inflammation and opsonization by fixation, which involves _____, _____ _____ and the alternate pathway, which involves _____.

55. By definition a phagocyte is any cell that _____
_____.

56. Migrating phagocytes include macrophages, which develop from _____ and _____ cells of the epidermis.

57. Stationary phagocytes include _____ cells of the liver and _____ of the CNS. Other phagocytes include _____, the most abundant of WBCs, and _____ cells, which are generally associated with allergic reactions.

58. Phagocytosis requires recognition of the invading cell's _____; this is enhanced by the attaching of complement and antibodies, also known as _____.

59. Non-phagocytic Natural Killer cells function by secreting _____, which cause the invader cell to _____.

60. The four cardinal/clinical signs of inflammation are _____, _____, _____, and _____.

61. The redness and swelling associated with injury is called _____ and is due to _____.

62. In addition to causing vasodilation creating hyperemia, chemicals released in injury also cause RBCs to congregate or _____; those that attract WBCs are described as being _____.

63. Chemotaxic signals attract _____ and _____ cells that adhere to vessel walls; this is called _____.

64. Following margination, neutrophils squeeze through the capillary wall into the interstitial spaces via _____; when RBCs accompany them, it is called a _____. When plasma escapes with them it creates _____.

65. Mast cells secrete _____ and _____.

66. Histamine functions as a _____; Heparin functions as an _____ and also _____ _____.

67. After heparin is exhausted, WBCs congregate forming _____, more commonly called _____.

68. Inflammatory exudates composed of dead WBCs are referred to as being _____; the exudates of chronic inflammation are tissue based due to organization or degeneration, and are called _____.

69. Histogenous exudates are either _____ if the stimulus is strong or _____ if the stimulus is constant but weak.

70. Degenerative changes are described as _____ if protein based due to bacteria, or _____ if due to toxicity or anoxia.

71. Proliferative changes are the organization of tissue forming _____ externally and _____ internally.

72. Anti-microbial proteins include _____ and the _____.

73. Interferon functions by _____
_____.

74. The Complement System is composed of some 20 _____ _____, which work in two pathways: _____ _____ and the _____ _____.

75. In Complement fixation, plasma proteins attach to _____-_____ _____; in the alternate pathway, they attach directly to _____. Both enhance _____ or recognition.

76. Fever is caused by the release of _____.

77. Adaptive defenses include the production of _____ and are described as being _____ _____.

78. An antigen is any substance that _____.
Antigens are large molecules, generally _____ and _____.

79. Complete antigens possess two characteristics. Define:
Immunogenicity: _____
Reactivity: _____

80. What is a hapten? _____
Haptens combine with body proteins initiating _____ _____.

81. What are antigen determinants? _____
What are MHCs? _____

82. The process by which lymphocytes acquire the ability to recognize foreign antigens is called _____. This occurs in primary lymphoid organs, either in the _____ _____ or the _____.

83. T-Lymphocytes acquire immunocompetence in the thymus; this constitutes _____-_____ immunity. B-Lymphocytes become immunocompetent in the _____ _____; this constitutes _____-_____ immunity.

84. T-Lymphocytes of cell-mediated immunity develop immunocompetency due to the influence of the hormones _____ and _____; these cells must then develop recognition of a specific _____ while developing _____-_____, or self-recognition.

85. B-Lymphocytes from the bone marrow form the humoral-mediated immunity by developing _____ _____ to a specific antigen.

86. Antigen Presenting Cells are those cells which _____
_____.

87.   APCs include _____, _____ cells, and _____.

88.   An immature B-Lymphocyte completes differentiation by _____
_____.

89.   The antigen-receptor site complex enters the B-Lymphocyte by _____; this triggers a
series of rapid divisions producing an army of _____.

90.   Most of the clones produced will further differentiate into _____ _____.

91.   These plasma cells then produce _____ over the next 4–5 days before
_____. Clones that do not become plasma cells will become long-lived
_____ _____.

92.   Memory cells function by _____
_____.

93.   The initial exposure to an antigen and the ensuing clonal selection and production of antibodies is known
as the _____ _____ _____.

94.   During the primary immune response antibody levels peak after _____ days after exposure. Memory
cells are responsible for the _____ _____ _____.

95.   During the secondary immune response antibody levels peak after _____ days.

96.   Active immunity implies that B-cells _____
_____. Active immunity is either _____ or
_____ acquired.

97.   Active immunity is naturally acquired by _____; artificially acquired active immunity is
accomplished by use of _____.

98.   Vaccines produce an immune response by _____
_____.

99.   Passive immunity implies that _____
_____.

100. In naturally acquired passive immunity, antibodies are _____
_____.

In artificially acquired passive immunity, antibodies are _____
_____.

101. Antibodies are also referred to as _____ and comprise the _____
_____ portion of blood.

102. The general structure of antibodies is composed of _____ _____ chains. Antibodies
are noted for two functional regions: the _____, which is identical in all antibodies of the
same class, and the _____ region.

103. The constant region of an antibody determines _____; the variable region possesses the _____ _____ _____.

104. Antibodies are grouped based on their constant region as _____, _____, _____, _____, and _____.

105. Upon binding to an antigen, antibodies expose their _____-_____ site on its constant region.

106. The exposing of the antibody's complement-binding site triggers _____ _____.

107. Complement fixation then triggers _____ of viruses and bacterial toxins; these complexes are then _____.

108. Antibodies also cause the clumping or _____ of multiple antigens. Antibodies complex with chemical toxins causing _____.

109. Precipitation causes toxins to _____ to be phagocytized.

110. Monoclonal antibodies are produced by _____ _____; they are significant in _____ _____.

111. In cell-mediated immunity, T-cells recognize both _____ _____ and self _____ proteins.

112. In addition to recognition, T-cells require _____ by _____ before clonal proliferation can occur.

113. The costimulation of T cells is accomplished by the cytokines _____ and _____.

114. The three types of T-cells include _____ or T4 cell, presenting the _____ protein, the _____ or T8 cell, presenting the _____ protein, and _____ cells.

115. T_H Helper/T4 cells secrete cytokines and therefore function as a _____; T_C Cytotoxic/T8 kill their target cells by secreting _____ and _____. Memory cells function in _____ _____ _____.

116. T-Cells must exhibit double recognition; this means _____ _____.

117. Self MHC proteins are divided into two groups based on their foreign particle Interaction: _____ MHC proteins, which are displayed by all body cells and recognized by _____ cells, and _____ MHC proteins, which are associated with _____.

118. Class I MHC proteins complex with _____ antigens; Class II MHC proteins complex with _____ antigens.

119. Endogenous antigens are formed by MHC I proteins binding with _____

    _____.

    Exogenous antigens are formed by MHC II proteins binding with _____

    _____.

120. Endogenous antigens are recognized by _____ T-cells; exogenous antigens are recognized

    by _____ T-cells.

121. Once Cytotoxic T_C CD8 T-cell receptors bind to MHC I endogenous antigens and Helper T_H CD4
    T-cell receptors bind to MHC II exogenous antigens, they still require _____ before
    proliferation.

122. Costimulation factors include _____, _____, and _____.

123. Cytokines are secreted by _____ and _____-cells; Interleukin 1 is secreted by
    _____ and Interleukin 2 is secreted by _____.

124. The cytokines secreted by macrophages and T-cells actually stimulates _____

    _____.

125. Interleukin 1, which is also secreted by macrophages, stimulates _____
    _____ as well as _____ and _____.

126. The Interleukin 2 secretions of T_H Helper T-Cells stimulate _____

    _____.

127. Define Anergy: _____

128. After activation, T cells enlarge and form _____; activity peaks _____ days after initial
    exposure. After 30 days, those remaining will become _____ cells.

129. In addition to Perforin and Lymphotoxin, T_C Cytotoxic T-cells also secrete _____
    _____ _____ and _____ _____.

130. Tumor Necrosis Factor causes apoptosis of its target cell. Describe Apoptosis: _____

    _____.

131. Gamma Interferon functions by _____.

132. Suppressor T-cells function by _____

    _____.

133. Define:
    Autograft: _____
    Isograft: _____

134. Define:
    Allograft: _____
    Xenograft: _____

135. Immunosuppression can be caused by _____, _____, and _____.

136. Congenital immunodeficiency diseases include _____ _____ _____. Examples of acquired immunodeficiency include _____ and _____ Disease.

137. The HIV virus infects which cell? _____

138. In autoimmune diseases, antibodies cause _____ cells to attack body cells. These include _____ _____, _____ _____, _____ Disease, and _____ _____ _____.

139. Allergic reactions are also known as _____ reactions.

140. In allergic hypersensitivity reactions, tissue is damaged due to _____ _____. Allergens or incomplete antigens are also known as _____.

141. Allergic hypersensitivity reactions are grouped in three categories: _____ or _____, _____, and _____.

142. Acute or Immediate reactions are also known as Type ____; these include _____ and _____. The antibody _____ is involved.

143. Describe Atopy: _____

144. Describe Anaphylaxis: _____
_____

145. What is Anaphylactic shock? _____
_____

146. Subacute Reactions begin _____ hours after exposure; the antibodies _____ and _____ are involved. These include Types ____ and ____.

147. Type II reactions are also known as _____; Type III reactions are noted for the formation of an _____ _____.

148. In Cytotoxic Type II reactions, antibodies are directed against _____ _____; in Immune Complex Type III reactions, tissue is damaged _____.

149. Delayed Hypersensitivity reactions are also known as Type ____ reactions; these can take between _____ hours after exposure before symptoms appear.

150. Type IV reactions, also known as _____ _____, include _____ _____.

Unit XI: Immunity

Part 1: Lymphatic System

1. Drain interstitial fluid, House phagocytes/lymphocytes
2. 3, Lymph nodes
3. Reticular, Blind
4. Lacteals, Chyle
5. Trunks, Right Lymphatic Duct, Thoracic Duct
6. Internal Jugular, Subclavian
7. Valves, Muscular, Respiratory
8. Lymphangitis; Lymphedema
9. Lymphocytes, Macrophages, Dendritic, Reticular
10. B, T, Red marrow
11. Thymus; Attacking and destroying foreign cells/particles; Plasma
12. Antibodies
13. Any substance that initiates/generates an antibody/immune response
14. By forming complexes with antigens making them more recognizable as foreign
15. Macrophages, Lymphocytes
16. Reticular, Macrophages, Dendritic
17. Phagocytes, Activating T-cells
18. Follicles, Germinal Centers
19. Dendritic, B-Lymphocytes
20. Activating T-lymphocytes
21. Peyer's Patches
22. Increase
23. Fibrous Capsule; Cortex Medulla
24. Trabeculae, Germinal Centers, Medullary Cords
25. Dendritic B-Lymphocytes, T-Lymphocytes; Macrophages, Plasma
26. Afferent Lymphatic Vessels, Subcapsular Sinus
27. Medullary, Hilus, Efferent Lymphatic Vessels
28. Fewer, Immune complexing, Recognition and Engulfing
29. Left upper quadrant, reticular. Fibrous Capsule, Trabeculae
30. White Pulp, Red Pulp
31. Immune, Lymphocytes; Blood cleansing, Splenic Cords
32. Macrophages, RBCs, Platelets
33. Iron, Bilirubin
34. Platelets, Erythropoeisis
35. Anterior spine/posterior to the sternum in the mediastinum; Thymosin, Thymopoeitin
36. Bilobed; Lobules, Stroma
37. Prevent immature lymphocytes from being prematurely activated
38. Ring the pharynx; Crypts
39. Caecum, Lymphocytes
40. Any disease of the lymph nodes
41. Benign or malignant tumor of any lymph tissue
42. Malignancy of lymph nodes
43. All other cancers of lymphoid tissue besides that of the lymph nodes
44. Rupture leading to peritonitis/infection
45. Enlargement of spleen due to accumulation of infectious material

Part 2: Immune System

46. Innate, Adaptive
47. Surface barriers, Inflammation
48. Skin, Mucosa, Secretions
49. 3–5, lysozyme
50. Phagocytes, Natural Killer, Proteins
51. Polysaccharide, Protein, Inflammatory
52. Interferon, Complement
53. Interfering with the protein synthesis of viral infected cells preventing their synthesis of new viral particles; Complexing and enhancing recognition/Opsonization
54. Antigen-antibody complexes; Direct attachment to microbes
55. Engulfs foreign bodies
56. Monocytes, Dendritic
57. Kuppfer, Microglia. Neutrophils, Mast
58. Antigens, Opsonization
59. Perforins, Lyse
60. Redness, Swelling, Heat, Pain
61. Hyperemia, Vasodilation
62. Sludge, Chemotaxic
63. Neutrophils, Mast, Margination
64. Diapedesis, Hemorrhage. Edema
65. Heparin, Histamine
66. Vasodilator, Anticoagulant, Repels WBCs
67. Exudates, Pus

68. Hematagenous, Histogenous
69. Degenerative, Proliferative
70. Cloudy, Fatty
71. Scars, Adhesions
72. Interferon, Complement System
73. Interfering with the protein synthesis of viral infected cells preventing their synthesis of new viral particles
74. PlasmaProteins, Complement Fixation, Alternate Pathway
75. Antigen-Antibody Complex; Microbes. Opsonization
76. Pyrogens
77. Antibodies, Antigen specific
78. Generates an immune response; Glycoproteins, Proteins
79. Stimulate an immune reaction; React to antibodies and immune cells
80. Foreign particle too small to trigger immune response. Allergic reactions
81. Regions on antigen that trigger response; Self-proteins
82. Immunocompetence; Red Marrow, Thymus
83. Cell-Mediated. Red Marrow; Humeral-Mediated
84. Thymosin, Thymopoeitin; Antigen, Self- Tolerance
85. Receptor Sites
86. Engulf foreign particles and present their antigens on their own surface for T-cell recognition
87. Macrophages, Dendritic, B-Lymphocytes
88. Binding with its specific antigen
89. Endocytosis; Clones
90. Plasma Cells
91. Antibodies, Dying, Memory Cells
92. Producing Secondary Immune Response
93. Primary Immune Response
94. 10, Secondary Immune Response
95. 2–3
96. Form antibodies to foreign particles; Naturally, Artificially
97. Exposure; Vaccines
98. Use of dead or attenuated microbes
99. Antibodies are delivered from another source
100. Passed from mother to child via placenta or colostrum; Injected as in gamma globulin
101. Immunoglobulins, Gamma Globulin
102. 4 Peptide; Constant; Variable
103. General class and functions; Antigen Binding Site
104. IgM, IgA, IgD, IgG, IgE
105. Complement binding
106. Complement fixation
107. Neutralization, Phagocytized
108. Agglutination; Precipitation
109. Come out of solution

110. Fusing a B cell with a tumor cell; Diagnostic tests
111. Foreign antigens, MHC
112. Costimulation, Cytokines
113. Interleukin 1, Interleukin 2
114. Helper, CD4, Cytotoxic, CD8, Memory
115. Costimulator; Perforin, Lymphotoxin; Secondary Immune Response
116. Exhibiting self-tolerance and foreign recognition
117. Class I, CD8; Class II, B cells
118. Endogenous, Exogenous
119. Proteins produced by virus infected or tumor cells; Proteins of engulfed bacteria
120. Cytotoxic, Helper
121. Costimulation
122. Cytokines, Interleukin 1, Interleukin 2
123. Macrophages, T; Macrophages, Helper T_H
124. Macrophage and T-Cell Proliferation and activity
125. T- and B-Cell proliferation, inflammation and fever
126. T- and B-Cell Proliferation and Natural Killer Cells
127. T-Cell binding w/o costimulation yields intolerance to the antigen
128. Clones; 7. Memory
129. Tumor Necrosis Factor, Gamma Interferon
130. Gradual cellular death without lysis
131. Stimulates Macrophages
132. Inhibiting T- and B-Cell activity and autoimmune diseases
133. Tissue transplant from one area of the body to another (self graft); Tissue donated by Identical Twin
134. Tissue donated by member of same species; Tissue acquired from another species
135. Steroids, Cytotoxic Drugs, Radiation
136. Severe Combined Immuno-deficiency; AIDs, Hodgkin's
137. T_H-Helper
138. T_C-Cytotoxic; Multiple Sclerosis, Myasthenia Gravis, Grave's, Type I Diabetes
139. Hypersensitivity
140. Inappropriate Immune Cell activity; Haptens
141. Acute or Immediate, Subacute, Delayed
142. I; Anaphylaxis, Atopy; IgE
143. Immediate but mild Rx to environmental allergens
144. Histamine Rx: Watery eyes, runny nose; Asthma, GI symptoms
145. Allergen enters blood creating systemic Histamine Rx
146. 1–3 hours; IgM, IgG
147. Cytotoxic; Immune Complex
148. Body's Blood Cells and Tissues; By Antibodies and Complement
149. IV; 12–72
150. Cell Mediated, Contact Dermatitis

Time allowed: 45 minutes

1. Functions of the Lymphatic System include:
   a) reabsorbing fluid lost from the capillaries and returning it to the blood
   b) housing immune cells
   c) absorbing lipids form the small intestine
   d) a and b
   e) a, b and c

2. Lymphatic tissue is primarily composed of:
   a) glandular tissue   b) secretive tissue
   c) reticular tissue   d) smooth muscle   e) plasma

3. The Right Lymphatic Duct:
   a) drains fluid from the cisternae chili
   b) empties into the jugular and subclavian veins
   c) drains fluid from the right lower extremity
   d) a and b
   e) a, b and c

4. Which of the following structures actually filters lymph:
   a) Peyer's Patches   b) Spleen
   c) Lymph Node   d) Tonsils   e) Thymus

5. Which indicates interstitial accumulation of lymphatic fluid:
   a) Lymphadenopathy   b) Lymphoma
   c) Hodgkin's Disease   d) Lymphangitis   e) Lymphedema

6. Which of the following is noted as specifically malignancy of the lymph nodes:
   a) Lymphadenopathy   b) Lymphoma
   c) Hodgkin's Disease   d) Lymphangitis   e) Lymphedema

7. Intestinal lymph is absorbed through:
   a) Crypts   b) Germinal centers
   c) Lacteals   d) Trabeculae   e) Subcapsular Sinus

8. Which of the following considered an adaptive/specific defense:
   a) Integument   b) Antibodies
   c) Mucosa   d) Lysozyme   e) Interferon

9. The immune function of the spleen is performed in the:
    a) Trabeculae   b) Medullary Cords
    c) White Pulp   d) Stroma   e) Red Pulp

10. Lysis of the invader's cell and nuclear membranes is accomplished :
    a) Pyrogens   b) Perforins
    c) Interferon   d) Histamine   e) Heparin

11. Which cell secretes histamine and heparin:
    a) Mast cell   b) Dendritic Cell
    c) Natural Killer Cell   d) Neutrophil   e) Macrophage

12. Which of the following inhibits viral-infected cells from synthesizing new viral particles protecting other healthy cells:
    a) Pyrogens   b) Perforins
    c) Interferon   d) Histamine   e) Heparin

13. Which acts as an anti-coagulant and repels WBCs:
    a) Pyrogens   b) Perforins
    c) Interferon   d) Histamine   e) Heparin

14. Which functions as the phagocyte of the epidermis:
    a) B-Cells   b) T-Cells
    c) Dendritic Cells   d) Mast Cells   e) Kuppfer Cells

15. Inflammation is described as *"calor, rubor, tumor et dolor"*; what does *"tumor"* mean:
    a) redness   b) heat
    c) swelling   d) pain   e) fever

16. The adhering of leukocytes to blood vessel walls during an inflammatory response is called:
    a) Sludging   b) Margination
    c) Chemotaxis   d) Edema   e) Diapedesis

17. Erythema in inflammation would be the result of:
    a) Chemotaxis   b) Edema
    c) Sludging   d) Diapedesis   e) Margination

18. The migration of WBCs through the capillary walls and into the interstitial spaces is called:
    a) Sludging   b) Margination
    c) Chemotaxis   d) Diapedesis   e) Edema

19. Which is the correct sequence of events:
    1: margination
    2: diapedesis
    3: chemotaxis
    4: exudates formation
    5: phagocytosis

a) 2,1,3,4,5   b) 1,3,5,2,4

c) 5,3,2,1,4   d) 3,1,2,5,4   e) 3,5,4,1,2

20. Which indicates a proliferative inflammatory exudate:
   a) pus formation
   b) a raised red swelling
   c) adhesion and scar tissue formation
   d) fatty deposits
   e) vascular leakage

21. The Complement System functions by:
   a) attaching directly to microbes
   b) attaching to antigen-antibody complexes
   c) enhancing opsoniztion
   d) increasing inflammation
   e) all of these

22. Pyrogens function by:
   a) increasing body temperature
   b) preventing microbes from using zinc and iron
   c) fragmenting the nuclear membrane and DNA of microbes
   d) a and b
   e) a, b and c

23. Primary Lymphoid organs:
   a) are those where immunocompetence occurs
   b) include the bone marrow and thymus
   c) filter the lymphatic fluid
   d) a and b
   e) a, b and c

24. The term "Opsonization" is best defined as:
   a) Recognition
   b) Neutralization
   b) Precipitation
   d) Lysis
   e) Apoptosis

25. "Immunogenicity" is defined as:
   a) The development of immune cells from marrow
   b) The embryologic development of all lymphatic organs
   c) An irritant stimulating inflammation
   d) The engulfing of foreign particles by macrophages
   e) An antigen stimulating the formation of antibodies to it

26. The process by which an immune cell learns to recognize specific antigens is known as:
   a) Immunogenicity
   b) Opsonization
   c) Immunocompetence
   d) Reactitivty
   e) Anergy

27. The Humoral Immune Response is facilitated by:
   a) B-Cells
   b) T-Cells
   c) Dendritic Cells
   d) Mast Cells
   e) Kuppfer Cells

28. "Dual recognition" is best defined by:
   a) T-Cell recognition of both viruses and bacteria
   b) T-Cell recognition of foreign and MHC antigens
   c) T-Cell recognition of both B-cells and Macrophages
   d) B-Cell recognition of more than one non-self antigen
   e) B-cell recognition during Primary and Secondary Responses

29. Which of the following statements is true:
   a) Individual B-cells have receptors sites which bind with any foreign antigen
   b) B-cells mediate the cellular immune response
   c) Individual B-cells develop receptors sites for only one non-MHC antigen
   d) B-cells learn to recognize a foreign antigen by first binding with it
   e) B-cells must undergo costimulation to recognize an antigen

30. Haptens are responsible for stimulating which of the following:
   a) Immunogenesis   b) Reactivity
   c) Anaphylaxis   d) Anergy   e) all of these

31. Clonal selection results in the differentiation and proliferation of:
   a) Plasma Cells   b) T-Cells
   c) Dendritic Cells   d) Mast Cells   e) Kuppfer Cells

32. Which is the correct sequence of events:
   1: plasma cell differentiation
   2: exposure
   3: B-cell proliferation
   4: clonal selection
   5: incubation
   6: antibody formation
   a) 6,4,3,1,5,2   b) 4,6,5,3,1,2
   b) 5,3,1,6,2,4   d) 1,5,4,2,3,6   e) 2,5,4,3,1,6

33. The antigen-receptor site complex enters B-cells via:
   a) Phagocytosis   b) Endocytosis
   c) Diffusion   d) Osmosis   e) Lysis

34. Which occurs as a result of Secondary Immunity:
   a) Natural Killer Cells are the second line of defense
   b) Microbes are phagocytized within seconds on entering the body
   c) Microbes are repelled from the body at the surface level
   d) Clonal selection begins within hours of exposure rather than days
   e) Antibodies remain active for years and attach on exposure

35. Artificial Active Immunity is acquired by:
   a) exposure to the pathogen   b) placenta or colostrum in breast milk
   c) vaccines   d) gamma globulin injection   e) antibiotics

36. Natural Passive Immunity is acquired by:
    a) exposure to the pathogen b) placenta or colostrum in breast milk
    c) vaccines   d) gamma globulin injection   e) antibiotics

37. Which of the following is not a function of antibodies:
    a) Neutralization   b) Complement Fixation
    c) Phagocytosis   d) Agglutination   e) Precipitation

38. How does Passive Immunity differ from Active Immunity:
    a) Memory Cells are not produced   b) B-cell proliferation does not occur
    c) Antibodies are produced by T-cells   d) a and b
    e) a, b and c

39. Which antibody class is principally involved in agglutination:
    a) IgA   b) IgD   c) IgE
    d) IgG   e) IgM

40. Which antibody function is used in toxicology studies:
    a) Neutralization   b) Complement Fixation
    c) Phagocytosis   d) Agglutination   e) Precipitation

41. Immunosurveillance is performed by:
    a) T-Cells   b) B-Cells
    c) Reticular Cells   d) Dendritic Cells   e) any lymphoid cell

42. Which recognizes Endogenous Antigens:
    a) THelper   b) TCytotoxic
    c) B-Cell   d) Plasma Cell   e) Dendritic Cell

43. Endogenous Antigens are produced by:
    a) viral infected cells   b) cancer cells
    c) Dendritic cells   d) a and b   e) a, b and c

44. Which recognizes Exogenous Antigens:
    a) THelper   b) TCytotoxic
    c) B-Cell   d) Plasma Cell   e) Dendritic Cell

45. Which of the following functions in costimulation:
    a) THelper   b) TCytotoxic
    c) TSuppressor   d) TMemory

46. Which of the following actively attacks and kills invading foreign cells:
    a) THelper   b) TCytotoxic
    c) TSuppressor   d) TMemory

47. Which cell is the target of the HIV virus:
    a) THelper   b) TCytotoxic
    c) B-Cell   d) Plasma Cell   e) Dendritic Cell

48. What are the consequences if there is no costimulation:
    a) TCytotoxic will not proliferate and produce clones
    b) Anergy will develop
    c) The TCytotoxic will tolerate the non-MHC antigen it has attached to
    d) a and b
    e) a, b and c

49. Which describes the use of a pig's aortic valve in transplant/replacement surgery:
    a) Autograft   b) Allograft
    c) Isograft   d) Xenograft

50. Which is an immediate localized hypersensitivity reaction associated without pronounced histamine reaction:
    a) Atopy   b) Anaphylaxis
    c) Cytotoxic   d) Immune Complex   e) Anergy

1: e, 2: c, 3: b, 4: c, 5: e, 6: c, 7: c, 8: b, 9: c, 10: b, 11: a, 12: c, 13: e, 14: c, 15: c, 16: b, 17: c, 18: d, 19: d, 20: c, 21: e, 22: d, 23: d, 24: a, 25: e, 26: c, 27: a, 28: b, 29: c, 30: c, 31: a, 32: e, 33: b, 34: d, 35: c, 36: b, 37: c, 38: d, 39: e, 40: e, 41: a, 42: b, 43: d, 44: a, 45: a, 46: b, 47: a, 48: e, 49: d, 50: a

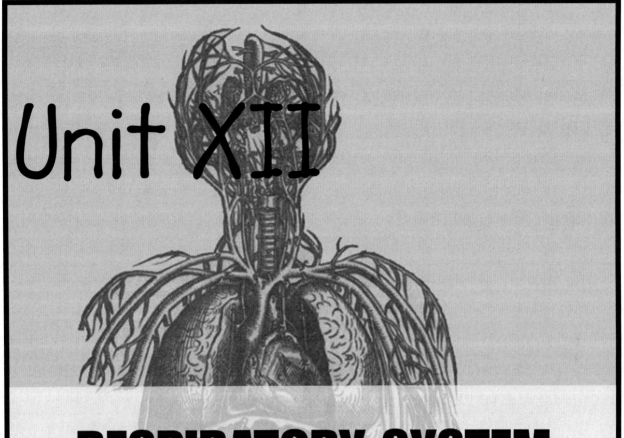

Unit XII

RESPIRATORY SYSTEM

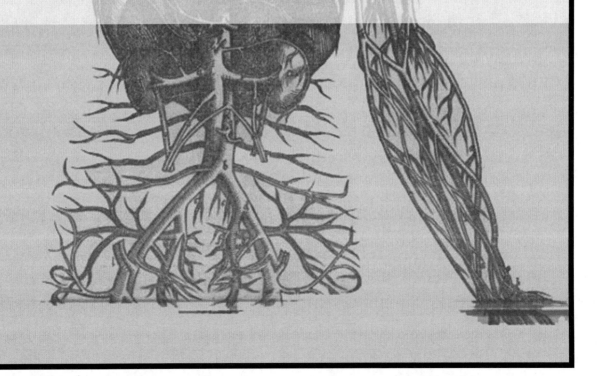

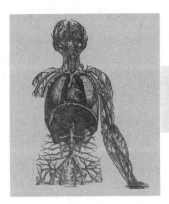

Respiratory System

1. The Respiratory Zone is defined as _____ and includes
   _____ _____, _____ _____, and
   _____.

2. The Conducting Zone is defined as _____ and
   includes the _____ and the rest of the _____ _____.
   The air in the conducting zone is also referred to as the _____ Air Space.

3. Functions of the nose include _____ and _____ air to match the air
   within the lung, _____ and _____ air of impurities, and housing the
   _____ receptors.

4. The Nasal bones make up the _____ of the nose; this slopes into the
   _____ _____. The tip of the nose is called the _____.

5. The external nares are separated at their vestibules by the _____; the nasal cavity is
   divided by the _____. Nasal hairs are also called _____.

6. The nasal cavity is lined by two types of membranes: the _____ mucosa,
   which is associated with smell, and the _____ mucosa, which is noted for its
   _____ _____ _____ epithelium and
   _____ cells.

7. The respiratory mucosa and its PSCCE also line the conchae of the _____ bone, which
   have a vascular underlining; these function to _____ and _____ inspired air.

8. The four paranasal sinuses are the _____, _____, _____,
   and _____.

9. How does Rhinitis differ from Sinusitis? _____
   _____

10. The three segments of the pharynx are the _____, _____, and
    _____.

11. The oral cavity opens into the oropharynx at the arch-like _____. The oropharynx is also noted for the _____ and _____ tonsils.

12. Food is blocked from entering the nasopharynx during swallowing by the upward movement of the _____; food is blocked from entering the trachea during swallowing by the _____, which is located in the _____.

13. The larynx is also known as the _____ _____. The larynx is also point where the common conduit for food and air separate into _____ and _____.

14. The bulk of the larynx is formed by two fused cartilage plates, the _____ cartilage.

15. The thyroid cartilage is anchored to the trachea by the _____ cartilage. The posterior and lateral walls of the larynx are formed by three paired cartilages: the _____, _____, and _____.

16. Of the three, the Arytenoid stands out because _____ _____.

17. The variable opening between the vocal cords is called the _____. The false vocal cords are also called the _____ _____.

18. What is Valsalva's Maneuver? _____

19. What are the three layers of the trachea? _____, _____, and outer _____

20. The Mucosa is lined by _____ _____ _____ Epithelium; the Submucosa is noted for _____ glands.

21. Patency of the trachea is maintained by C-shaped _____ _____ in the Adventitia.

22. The last of the tracheal cartilages is called the _____; it is split to accommodate the _____ of the trachea.

23. The trachea bifurcates into right and left _____ _____, which enter the lung at its _____.

24. Primary bronchi subdivide into Secondary or _____ _____, one going to each lobe. There are _____ right lobes and _____ left lobes.

25. The 5 Lobar Bronchi subdivided into 10 Tertiary or _____ Bronchi in each lung. Bronchi of 1 mm or less are now called _____.

26. The smallest of conducting vessels, the _____ bronchioles, are less than 0.5 mm; these lead into the _____ bronchioles.

27. How does the distribution of cartilage and smooth muscle change as one progresses from the primary bronchi to the alveoli? _____

_____

28. How does the epithelium change from trachea to alveoli? _____

_____

29. The Respiratory Membrane (aka _____-_____ Membrane) is composed of three elements: _____ _____ of the alveoli, _____ _____, and the capillary _____.

30. The alveoli wall is composed of _____ _____ epithelium or _____ _____ Cells.

31. Unlike squamous cells, Cuboidal Type II cells secrete _____.

32. The left lobe is noted for its depression, the _____ _____. Its two lobes are divided by _____ fissure.

33. The three lobes of the right lung are divided by _____ and _____ fissures.

34. Lobes are subdivided into _____ _____, 10 in each lung.

35. Each bronchopulmonary segment is serviced by a segmental or _____ bronchi. Lung tissue other than alveoli is serviced by the _____ Arteries.

36. Motor and Sensory innervation of the lung is supplied by the _____ _____. The double-layered serosa surrounding the lung is called the _____.

37. How does the Parietal Pleura differ from the Visceral Pleura? _____

_____

38. The space separating the two pleurae is called the _____ _____; this space contains _____ _____.

39. Define Pleurisy: _____.

40. Define Pleural Effusion: _____.

41. Define Pneumonia: _____.

42. What is Intrapulmonary pressure? _____

43. How does Intrapulmonary pressure compare to Atmospheric pressure during inspiration: _____? During expiration? _____

44. What is Intrapleural pressure? _____
    What is its significance to inspiration? _____

_____

45. Define Atelectasis: _____.
Define Pneumothorax: _____.

46. Boyle's Law states that when volume increases, _____ _____.

47. Intrapulmonary pressure rises/drops with inspiration; inspiration ends when intrapulmonary and atmospheric pressure reach _____.

48. During inspiration, the ribs move _____ and _____, and the diaphragm moves _____. Inspiration increases/decreases thoracic volume.

49. During inspiration, intrapulmonary pressure drops 1mm Hg below atmospheric, causing air to be _____.

50. During expiration the ribs move _____ and _____, and the diaphragm moves _____. Expiration increases/decreases thoracic volume.

51. Forced expiration is assisted by the _____ _____ muscles.

52. Surfactant functions by reducing _____ and preventing _____.

53. Lung Compliance is a measure of the _____ of lung tissue. Define Spirometry: _____.

54. Define:
Tidal Volume (TV):_____.
What is the average volume for both adult male and females: _____ ml

55. Define:
Inspiratory Reserve Volume (IRV): _____
What is the average volume for adult males: _____ml, adult females: _____ml.

56. Define:
Expiratory Reserve Volume (ERV): _____
What is the average volume for adult males: _____ml, adult females: _____ml.

57. Define Residual Volume (RV) _____
What is the average volume for adult males: _____ml, adult females: _____ml..

58. Define:
Inspiratory Capacity: _____
Which lung volumes contribute to it: _____
What is the average volume for adult males: _____ml, adult females: _____ml.

59. Functional Residual Capacity _____
Which lung volumes contribute to it: _____
What is the average volume for adult males: _____ml, adult females: _____ml.

60. Vital Capacity (_____ ml): _____
    Which lung volumes contribute to it: _____
    What is the average volume for adult males: _____ml, adult females: _____ml.

61. Total Lung Capacity: _____
    Which lung volumes contribute to it: _____
    What is the average volume for adult males: _____ml, adult females: _____ml.

62. On the following graph indicate the area/areas for the following values:
    Tidal Volume: _____
    Inspiratory Reserve: _____
    Inspiratory Capacity: _____
    Expiratory Reserve: _____
    Residual Volume: _____
    Functional Residual Capacity: _____
    Vital Capacity: _____
    Total Lung Capacity: _____

63. What is the normal breathing rate? _____ breaths/minute.
    How do you determine the Minute Ventilation Volume: _____ x _____ = _____ ml/min
    What is the value during aerobic exercise? _____ L/min

64. What is meant by the "Dead Air Space" _____.
    What is the average volume for both adult males and females: _____ ml.
    What is the Minute Alveolar Ventilation Volume _____ ml/min

65. How is the dead air space related to body weight: _____.
    How does this affect the alveolar ventilation volume: _____.

66. What characterizes Obstructive Respiratory Diseases: _____.
    What are examples: _____ and _____
    How do they affect lung volumes: _____

67. What characterizes Restrictive Respiratory Diseases: _____.
    _____
    What are examples: _____, _____ and _____
    How do they affect lung volumes: _____

68. Dalton's Law of Partial Pressures states: _____
    _____.

69. O_2 comprises approximately _____% of air. According to Dalton's Law, the PO_2 at sea level
    (760 mm Hg) is _____ mm Hg. The PO_2 increases/decreases with elevation.

70. Henry's Law states that the greater the concentration of a gas, the _____
    _____.

71. According to Henry's Law, the direction of gas flow is determined by _____
_____.

72. Which is more soluble in water: O_2 or CO_2?
What is oxygen toxicity? _____
_____

73. Describe the mechanism causing "The Bends": _____
_____.

74. In what three ways does alveolar gas differ from atmospheric? _____
_____, and _____

75. What is meant by "External Respiration"? _____
_____

76. Gases move from alveoli to capillary along a _____ _____
_____.

77. The partial pressure gradient for O_2 in external respiration is _____ mm Hg in the pulmonary
capillaries and _____ mm Hg in the alveoli. That for CO_2 is _____ mm Hg in the pulmonary
capillaries and _____ in the alveoli.

78. What is meant by "Internal Respiration"? _____
_____

79. The partial pressure gradient for O_2 in internal respiration is _____ mm Hg in the tissues and
_____ mm Hg in the blood. That for CO_2 is _____ mm Hg in the tissues and _____ in
the blood.

80. Define Perfusion: _____.

81. When ventilation is poor, PO_2 increases/decreases and terminal arterioles constrict /dilate.
When ventilation is enhanced, PO_2 increases/decreases and terminal arterioles constrict/dilate.

82. Constricting terminal arterioles during reduced PO_2 will _____
_____.

83. When PCO_2 is high, capillaries constrict/dilate and bronchioles constrict/dilate.

84. In Emphysema, alveoli enlarge and chambers break through. How does this affect gas exchange? _____
_____

85. How is O_2 transported in the blood? _____
_____

86. Each Hb molecule can bind with up to _____ O_2. When bound to O_2, Hb is referred to
as _____ (_____). Reduced Hb is also known as
_____ (_____). The binding of O_2 to Hb is called
_____.

87. An HbO_2 with 4 O_2 is described as being _____.

88. How does Hb's affinity for O_2 change as it approaches saturation? _____ _____ How is it affected by increasing temperature, pH, and PCO_2? _____

89. When the PO_2 is 40 mm Hg, as in the tissues, the Hb saturation is _____%. Hb saturation reaches 98% at _____ mm Hg, the same PO_2 in the alveoli.

90. The Bohr Effect states that rising PCO_2 levels cause the release of _____ ions. How does this affect the pH? _____

91. How does the acidic pH created by increased H^+ affect the Hb-O_2 bond? _____ _____ This will eventually result in _____ _____.

92. Define Hypoxia: _____, Hb = _____%.

93. Define Cyanosis: _____.

94. Briefly describe:
Anemic Hypoxia: _____.
Ischemic: _____.

95. Define Histotoxic: _____.
Hypoxemic: _____.

96. Describe the effect of carbon monoxide (CO) poisoning: _____ _____.

97. By what three mechanisms is CO_2 transported?
(_____%) _____,
(_____%) _____, and
(_____%) _____.

98. When Hb is bound to CO_2 (20%), it is referred to as _____.

99. 70% of CO_2 diffuses into the RBCs and combines with _____ to form _____ _____ (H_2CO_3).

$$CO_2 + H_2O \rightleftarrows H_2CO_3 \rightleftarrows H^+ + HCO_3^-$$

100. The formation of carbonic acid from CO_2 and water is catalyzed by the enzyme _____ _____. Carbonic acid then disassociates into _____ (HCO_3^-) and _____.

101. What is the affect of the released H^+? _____.
As bicarbonate diffuses out of the RBC, _____ diffuses in.

102. What happens to HCO_3^- on reaching the pulmonary capillaries? _____
_____

103. According to the Haldane Effect, what is the relationship between PO_2, Hb saturation, and CO_2
transport? _____
_____

104. As a function of the Carbonic Acid--Bicarbonate Buffer System, during alkaline conditions,
_____ _____ will disassociate releasing _____; this results in a
higher/lower pH.

105. The two Medullary Respiratory Centers are the _____ _____
_____ and the _____ _____ _____.

106. The Dorsal Respiratory Group is referred to as the _____ _____; the
DRG fires the _____ and _____ nerves.

107. What is Eupnea? _____

108. The Phrenic nerve stimulates the _____ to contract, whereas the Intercostal nerve
stimulates the _____ _____. The action of these muscles increases/
decreases thoracic volume and increases/decreases intra thoracic pressure.

109. The Ventral Respiratory Center stimulates the _____ _____.

110. The two respiratory centers of the pons are the _____ and the _____
Centers.

111. The Pneumotaxic Center shortens _____ and prevents _____-
_____ of the lung.

112. The Apneustic Center prolongs _____ and allows one to _____
_____.

113. Irritants stimulate _____ and _____.

114. In the Herring-Brewer Inflation Reflex, _____ send inhibitory signals via the
_____ Nerve to halt inspiration/expiration.

115. Central chemoreceptors are located in the _____; Peripheral chemoreceptors are located
within the _____ and _____ _____.

116. Define Hypercapnia: _____.

117. The resulting increased H^+ from elevated CO_2 is countered by _____ to increase O_2.

118. Hyperventilation can lead to reduced CO_2, a condition called _____; this can cause
cerebral ischemia and _____.

119. Hypocapnia is countered by a reduced breathing rate or _____. The cessation of
breathing is called _____.

120. How does Hyperpnea differ from hyperventilation? _____
_____

121. What is Acclimatization? _____
_____

122. Define Dyspnea: _____ .

123. How are the alveoli altered in Emphysema? _____
How does this affect respiratory function? _____

124. How does Bronchitis differ from Asthma? _____
_____

125. What are the three principal types of lung cancer? _____ _____
_____ (40%), _____ (35%), and _____
_____ _____ (25%).

126. What are the principal effects of Cystic Fibrosis? _____
_____

Unit XII: Respiratory System

1. Regions of gas exchange, Respiratory Bronchioles, Alveoli Ducts, Alveoli
2. All other rigid, non-exchange pathways, Nose, Respiratory Tree. Dead
3. Moisten, Warm, Filter, Clean, Olfactory
4. Bridge, Dorsum Nasi. Apex
5. Philtrum; Septum. Vibrissae
6. Olfactory, Respiratory, Pseuodostratified Ciliated Columnar, Goblet
7. Ethmoid, Warm, Humidify
8. Ethmoid, Sphenoid, Frontal, Maxillary
9. Rhinitis: inflammation of lining; Sinusitis: fluid within cavity
10. Nasopharynx, Oropharynx, Laryngopharynx
11. Fauces. Palatine, Lingual
12. Uvula; Epiglottis, Larynx
13. Voice Box. Esophagus, Trachea
14. Thyroid
15. Cricoid. Arytenoid, Corniculate, Cuneiform
16. Anchoring of the Vocal Cords
17. Glottis. Vestibular Folds
18. Closing off of larynx to build internal pressure forcing bowel movement, urination
19. Mucosa, Submucosa, Adventitia
20. PSCCE; Seromucus
21. Cartilage Rings
22. Carina; Bifurcation
23. Primary Bronchi, Hilus
24. Lobar Bronchi. 3, 2
25. Segmental. Bronchioles
26. Terminal; Respiratory
27. Cartilage decreases as smooth muscle increases
28. PSCCE in Trachea and Primary Bronchi, changing to Columnar, Simple Cuboidal in Terminal Bronchioles and Simple Squamous in Alveoli
29. Alveolar-Capillary: Simple Squamous, Basal Lamina, Endothelium
30. Simple Squamous, Type I
31. Surfactant
32. Cardiac Notch. Oblique
33. Oblique, Horizontal
34. Bronchopulmonary Segments
35. Tertiary. Bronchial
36. Pulmonary Plexus. Pleura
37. Parietal covers Thoracic wall; Visceral overlies external surface of lung
38. Pleural Cavity; Pleural Fluid
39. Inflammation of Pleura, produces friction rub
40. Accumulation of fluid in Pleural cavity
41. Fluid within the Alveoli
42. Pressure within the alveoli
43. Negative, less; Positive, exceeds
44. Pressure within the Pleural Cavity. Negative pressure gradient adheres lung tissue to thoracic wall, expanding lung and opening alveoli
45. Collapsed area of lung due to break in visceral pleura; Air in lung due to puncture
46. Pressure decreases
47. Drops; Equilibrium
48. Up and Out, Down. Increases
49. Inhaled
50. Down and In, Up; Decreases
51. Internal Intercostal
52. Surface tension of water, collapsing of alveoli walls
53. Extensibility. Measurement of Respiratory Volumes
54. TV: Volume of air exchanged during normal breathing cycles; 500 ml
55. IRV: Volume of air forcibly inspired after TV: male: 3100 ml, female 1900 ml
56. ERV: Volume forcibly expired after TV; male: 1200 ml, female 700 ml
57. TV: Volume of air remaining after ERV; male: 1200 ml, female 1100 ml
58. IC: Total volume of air that can be inspired after normal expiration; TV + IRV; male: 3600 ml, female 2400 ml
59. FRC: Total volume of air remaining in the lungs after a normal expiration; ERV + RV; male: 2400 ml, female 1800 ml
60. VC: Total volume of air that can be forcibly expired after a forced inspiration; TV + IRV + ERV; male: 4800 ml, female 3100 ml
61. TLC: Total volume of air in the lungs after a forced inspiration TV + IRV + ERV + RV; male: 6000 ml, female 4200 ml

62. TV: B; IRV: A; IC: E; ERV: C; RV: D; FRC: F; VC: G; TLC: H

63. 12; 12 x TV = 6000 ml/minute; 200L/min

64. Non-respiratory air in the conducting zone; 150 ml; 4800 ml/minute

65. Dead air space is equal to 1 ml per pound; it decreases 1 ml per pound.

66. Obstructive: increased airway resistance; Bronchitis and Asthma; Cause hyperinflation of the lung, increasing TLC, FRC, RV

67. Restrictive: Structural or Functional changes in Lung tissue; TB, Fibrosis, Emphysema Cause reductions in total lung capacities

68. The pressure exerted by a combination of gases is equal to the sum of the pressures exerted by each individual gas

69. 21%; 159 mm Hg; Decreases

70. The greater the volume and speed of dissolving in solution

71. Along the gradient created by the partial pressures of the gas vs. liquid phases

72. CO_2; When PO_2 exceeds 2.5 atm causing CNS disturbance

73. Deep water diving increases P_{N2}; with rapid ascent P_{N2} drops causing N_2 to bubble out of solution

74. Higher CO_2, lower O_2, and higher moisture

75. Pulmonary gas exchange, Alveoli-Capillary

76. Partial Pressure Gradient

77. 40, 104, 45, 40

78. Exchange of gases between Capillaries and Tissues

79. 40, 104, 45, 40

80. Blood flow into Pulmonary Capillaries

81. Decreases, Constrict. Increases, Dilate

82. Redirect blood to better ventilated areas

83. Capillaries Constrict, Bronchioles Dilate

84. Reduces surface area for gas exchange

85. 98.5% bound to Hb; 1.5% dissolved in plasma

86. 4. Oxyhemoglobin HbO_2. Deoxyhemoglobin HHb. Loading

87. Saturated

88. Affinity increases with saturation; Increasing all decreases O_2-Hb affinity

89. 75%. 70 mm Hg

90. H^+; decreased pH creating acidosis

91. Weakens the bond. Increased O_2 Unloading and increased acidity

92. Decreased O_2 to tissues when Hb saturation drops below 75%

93. Bluish discoloration of skin and membranes due to increased HHb

94. Reduced RBCs or Hb; Due to impaired or blocked blood flow

95. Cells unable to use O_2 due to poisons; Reduced PO_2 due to disease or CO toxicity

96. CO permanently binds to Hb, reducing and eliminating O_2 transport

97. 7–10% dissolved in plasma; 20% bound to Hb; 70% converted to HCO_3^-

98. $HBCO_2$: Carbaminohemoglobin

99. H_2O, Carbonic Acid

100. Carbonic Anhydrase. Bicarbonate, H^+

101. Decreases pH, triggering Bohr Effect, increasing O_2 unloading. Cl^-

102. Reenters RBC, forms Carbonic Acid and is then split into CO_2 and H_2O

103. The lower the PO_2 and Hb saturation the more CO_2 can be transported

104. Carbonic Acid, H^+; Lower

105. Dorsal Respiratory Group, Ventral Respiratory Center

106. Inspiratory Center; Phrenic and Intercostal

107. Regular Inspiratory Rhythm: 2 sec insp/3 sec exp

108. Diaphragm, External Intercostals. Increases, decreases

109. Internal Intercostals

110. Pneumotaxic, Apneustic

111. Inspiration, over-inflation

112. Inspiration, hold one's breath

113. Cough, Sneeze

114. Baroreceptors, Vagus, Inspiration

115. Medulla; Aorta Carotid Sinus

116. Increased PCO_2, increasing H^+

117. Hyperventilation

118. Hypocapnia, Fainting

119. Hypoventilation; Apnea

120. Deep, vigorous ventilation with exercise rather than rapid, shallow

121. The gradual physiologic accommodation to living at high altitudes with reduced PO_2

122. Difficult or labored breathing

123. Enlargement and Deterioration of walls; reduces surfaces for gas exchange

124. Bronchitis: swelling of Submucosa causing stenosis of airways; Asthma: constriction of respiratory bronchioles and alveoli

125. Squamous Cell Carcinoma; Adenocarcinoma; Small Cell Carcinoma

126. Thickened mucus leading to respiratory infection

Time allowed: 45 minutes

1. Which describes the exchange of intrapulmonary and atmospheric air:
   a) Ventilation
   b) External Respiration
   c) Internal Respiration
   d) Perfusion
   e) Cellular Respiration

2. The flow of gases across the respiratory membrane is called:
   a) Ventilation
   b) External Respiration
   c) Internal Respiration
   d) Perfusion
   e) Cellular Respiration

3. During Expiration:
   a) the diaphragm moves up, the ribs down and in
   b) the diaphragm moves up, the ribs up and out
   c) the diaphragm moves down, the ribs up and out
   d) the diaphragm moves down, the ribs down and in

4. During Inspiration:
   a) atmospheric pressure exceeds intrapulmonary pressure
   b) intrapleural pressure exceeds intrapulmonary pressure
   c) intrapleural pressure exceeds atmospheric pressure
   d) intrapulmonary pressure exceeds atmospheric pressure
   e) atmospheric pressure equals intrapulmonary pressure

5. Which of the following is not part of the Conducting Zone:
   a) Nasal Cavity
   b) Pharynx
   c) Larynx
   d) Alveoli
   e) All are part

6. Which describes the function of the Uvula:
   a) directs food into esophagus during swallowing
   b) covers the trachea during swallowing
   c) closes the fauces during swallowing
   d) directs air through the nasopharynx during sneezing
   e) blocks food from entering the nasopharyx during swallowing

7. Inflammation of the olfactory mucosa is properly called:
   a) Sinusitis
   b) Laryngitis
   c) Rhinitis
   d) Pharyngitis
   e) Uvulitis

8. The vocal cords attach to the:
   a) epiglottis
   b) cuneiform cartilage
   c) corniculate cartilage
   d) arytenoid cartilage
   e) cricoid cartilage

9. "Patency" of the trachea is maintained by:
   a) thyroid cartilage   b) serous glands in the Submucosa   c) smooth muscle in the Adventitia
   d) Trachealis muscle   e) cartilage rings in the Adventitia

10. The Carina:
    a) attaches the larynx to the trachea
    b) attaches the vocal cords to the larynx
    c) forms the split between the trachea and esophagus
    d) forms the bifurcation of primary bronchi
    e) covers the trachea during swallowing

11. Which is true of the bronchial tree progressing from the trachea to the alveoli:
    a) smooth muscle increases   b) cartilage decreases   c) smooth muscle decreases
    d) cartilage increases   e) a and b are true

12. Which is not part of the Respiratory Membrane:
    a) Basal Lamina   b) Cartilage Plates   c) Squamous Type I Cells
    d) Capillary Endothelium   e) All are part of the respiratory membrane

13. Surfactant is secreted by which of the following:
    a) Squamous Type I   b) Cuboidal Type II   c) Serous glands
    d) Mucus glands   e) Goblet Cells

14. Which is true regarding Surfactant:
    a) reduces surface tension of water   b) prevents alveoli from collapsing
    c) liquefies mucous in the bronchioles   d) a and b
    e) a, b and c

15. Inspiration normally ends when:
    a) lung compliance ends
    b) intrapulmonary and atmospheric pressure equalize
    c) intrapulmonary and intrapleural pressure equalize
    d) intrapleural exceeds intrapulmonary pressure
    e) intrapulmonary exceeds atmospheric pressure

16. Which lines the wall of the Thoracic Cavity:
    a) Visceral Peritoneum   b) Parietal Peritoneum   c) Visceral Pleura
    d) Parietal Pleura

17. What is meant by "lung compliance":
    a) the respiratory rate changes with altitude
    b) the surface area of the alveoli increase with exercise
    c) the lung expands and alveoli open during inspiration
    d) a and b
    e) a, b and c

18. Which of the following is responsible for the adhering of the lung to the expanding rib cage during inspiration:
    a) intrapleural pressure
    b) intrapulmonary pressure
    c) atmospheric pressure
    d) alveolar pressure
    e) partial pressure

19. Which of the following conditions will reduce Lung Compliance:
    a) Pleurisy
    b) Pleural Effusion
    c) Dyspnea
    d) Pneumonia
    e) Bronchitis

20. Pneumothorax will most likely result from:
    a) inflammation of the pleura
    b) increased intrapleural fluid
    b) fluid in the alveoli
    d) puncture of the parietal pleura
    e) deterioration of the alveoli

21. How could one determine if a patient has Pleurisy:
    a) "Bubbling" can be auscultated during expiration
    b) "Friction Rub" can be auscultated
    c) Fluid levels can be seen on x-rays
    d) a and b
    e) a, b and c

22. Which of the following conditions will reduce surface area for O_2 transport:
    a) Pleurisy
    b) Pleural Effusion
    c) Pneumothorax
    d) Pneumonia
    e) Bronchitis

23. How does alveolar air differ from atmospheric air:
    a) it has a lower PO_2
    b) it has a higher PCO_2
    c) it has less water vapor
    d) a and b
    e) a, b and c

24. The concentration of oxygen is always the same regardless of the altitude, but why can't one survive above 25,000 feet :
    a) the atmospheric pressure is too high for ventilation
    b) the PCO_2 is too high for external respiration
    c) the PO_2 is too low for external respiration
    d) a and b
    e) a, b and c

25. According to Henry's Law which of the following conditions must exist for External Respiration to occur:
    a) PO_2 capillaries 104 mm Hg/tissues 40 mm Hg
    b) PO_2 capillaries 40 mm Hg/tissues 104 mm Hg
    c) PCO_2 capillaries 104 mm Hg/tissues 40 mm Hg
    d) PCO_2 capillaries 40 mm Hg/alveoli 104 mm Hg
    e) PO_2 capillaries 40 mm Hg/alveoli 104 mm Hg

26. The Vital Capacity is the:
    a) Air within the Conducting Zone
    b) Air exchanged during Hyperpnea
    c) Air exchanged during a normal breathing cycle
    d) Minimum volume of air needed to survive
    e) The volume of air needed to prevent hypoxia

27. The Tidal Volume is the:
    a) Air within the Conducting Zone
    b) Air exchanged during Hyperpnea
    c) Air exchanged during a normal breathing cycle
    d) Minimum volume of air needed to survive
    e) The volume of air needed to prevent hypoxia

28. The Dead Air Space:
    a) the air within the Conducting Zone
    c) increases with excessive weight gain
    e) a, b and c

    b) the air in Non- Respiratory areas
    d) a and b

29. Which will occur when the PO_2 is high and is PCO_2 low:
    a) Pulmonary capillaries dilate and bronchioles dilate
    b) Pulmonary capillaries dilate and bronchioles constrict
    c) Pulmonary capillaries constrict and bronchioles constrict
    d) Pulmonary capillaries constrict and bronchioles dilate

30. Hemoglobin can bind with which of the following:
    a) O_2
    d) a and b

    b) CO_2
    e) a, b and c

    c) NO

31. Which best describes the mechanism behind CO poisoning:
    a) CO creates an acidic pH
    b) CO reduces O_2 solubility
    c) CO combines with O_2 increasing CO_2 levels and $HbCO_2$
    d) CO permanently binds to O_2 receptors reducing O_2 transport

32. According to the Bohr Effect which of the following will weaken Hb-O_2 affinity:
    a) increased CO_2
    d) a and b

    b) decreased pH
    e) a, b and c

    c) decreased temperature

33. At what point would a patient be diagnosed with hypoxia:
    a) the hematocrit is below normal
    c) the O_2 saturation is below 75%
    e) a, b and c

    b) they present cyanosis
    d) a and b

34. In which of the following do cells suffer from localized hypoxia due to lack of blood flow
    a) Anemic
    d) Hypoxemic

    b) Ischemic
    e) Apneustic

    c) Histotoxic

35. While climbing in the Adirondacks one may reach summits as high as 7,500 feet above sea level, but without experiencing altitude sickness; why:
    a) blood is directed to alveoli of higher PO_2
    b) the lower the oxygen saturation the higher the CO_2 transport
    c) O_2 is unloaded during high metabolic activity
    d) O_2^-Hb saturation is still above 75% when under 10,000 feet
    e) erythropöeitin is released in response to altitude sickness

36. Which of the following statements regarding CO_2 transport is false:
   a) 70% is transported as bicarbonate
   b) CO_2 combines with water to form carbonic acid
   c) bicarbonate travels in plasma rather than the RBC
   d) HCO_3^- creates an acidic pH
   e) all statements are true

37. According to Haldane which will occur as a result of reduced O2–Hb saturation
   a) decreases CO_2 transport as HCO_3^-
   b) increases CO_2 transport as HCO_3^-
   c) increases CO_2 transport as $HbCO_2$
   d) decreases CO_2 transport as $HbCO_2$

38. A rising CO_2 level leads to acidosis because it also increases:
   a) carbonic acid   b) bicarbonate   c) H^+
   d) carbonic anhydrase   e) Cl^-

39. Decreased CO_2 is also known as:
   a) Hyperpnea   b) Hypopnea   c) Hypocapnia
   d) Hypercapnia   e) Apnea

40. Hypoventilation will lead to:
   a) Respiratory Alkalosis   b) Respiratory Acidosis   c) Metabolic Alkalosis
   d) Metabolic Acidosis

41. Which of the following would be noted in Respiratory Acidosis:
   a) Increased CO_2 b) Increased HCO_3^- c) Decreased CO_2
   d) Decreased HCO_3^-

42. What will be the most likely respiratory response to Hypercapnia
   a) Apnea   b) Eupnea   c) Hyperpnea
   d) Hyperventilation   e) Hypoventilation

43. Hyperventilation will lead to:
   a) Respiratory Alkalosis   b) Respiratory Acidosis   c) Metabolic Alkalosis
   d) Metabolic Acidosis

44. Which describes the respiratory symptoms associated with COPD:
   a) Apnea   b) Dyspnea   c) Hyperventilation
   d) Hypoventilation   e) Hyperpnea

45. Which center allows us to hold our breath:
   a) Apneustic Center   b) Pneumotaxic Center   c) Ventral Respiratory Group
   d) Dorsal Respiratory Group

46. How does Hyperventilation differ from Hyperpnea:
    a) Hyperventilation is rapid shallow breathing
    b) Hyperventilation focuses on eliminating excess CO_2
    c) Hypernea is deep breathing
    d) a and b
    e) a, b and c

47. Which occurs in bronchioles in chronic allergic reactions:
    a) smooth muscle constricts
    b) the adventitia swells and expands
    c) the cartilage rings constrict
    d) the Submucosa swells inward
    e) surfactant production is reduced

48. Emphysema is noted for:
    a) stenosis of terminal bronchioles
    b) constriction of terminal bronchioles
    c) reduced surface area due to destruction of alveolar walls
    d) cavitating masses
    e) inflammation of the olfactory mucosa

49. Which of the following is characterized by constriction of smooth muscle:
    a) Bronchitis   b) Asthma   c) Emphysema
    d) Cystic Fibrosis   e) Adenocarcinoma

50. Which is a genetic defect in chloride transport resulting in excessive, thickened mucous production:
    a) Squamous Cell Carcinoma   b) Cystic Fibrosis   c) Adenocarcinoma
    d) Small Cell Carcinoma   e) Atelectasis

NAME:

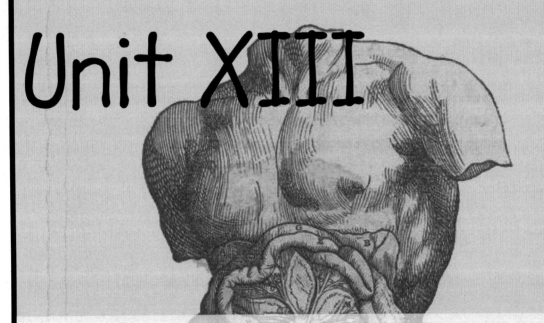

DE HVMANI CORPORIS FABRICA LIBER V.

DECIMA QVINTI LIBRI FIGVRA·

Unit XIII

THE DIGESTIVE SYSTEM

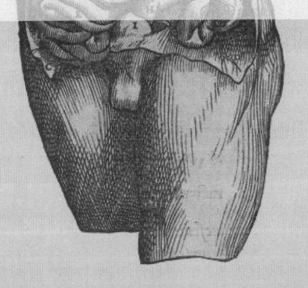

DECIMAE FIGVRAE EIVSDEMQVE CHA-

racterum Index.

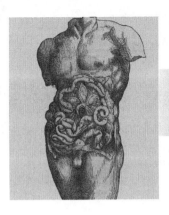

The Digestive System

1. Define Ingestion: _____
   _____.

2. Define Propulsion: _____
   _____.

3. How do the peristaltic contractions of propulsion differ from segmentation? _____
   _____.

4. Define Chemical Digestion: _____
   _____.

5. Define Absorption: _____
   _____.

6. Mechanoreceptors of the intestinal wall respond to _____; Chemoreceptors
   respond to changes in _____ and _____ _____ within the
   _____.

7. Neurologic receptors include both local _____ as well as _____ controls.

8. Local Intrinsic control is provided by the _____ _____; Extrinsic control
   is provided by the _____ and _____.

9. The serous membrane of the abdominal and pelvic cavities is known as the _____ and is
   divided into two layers, the _____ and _____ layers.

10. The Visceral Peritoneum covers _____,
    whereas the Parietal Peritoneum lines _____ _____. Both are separated
    by the fluid-filled _____ _____.

11. How does Peritonitis differ from Ascites? _____
    _____
    _____.

12. Define Mesentery: _____.
    Organs that do not face the peritoneal cavity do/do not possess a mesentery and are described as
    _____

13. The four principal layers of the Alimentary Canal from innermost to outermost are the
    _____, _____, _____ _____, and the
    _____.

14. Unlike intraperitoneal organs which have an outer serosa, retroperitoneal organs possess an outer
    _____.

15. The Mucosa is noted for three sublayers: innermost is the secretory _____
    _____, which is noted for its secretory _____ tissue.

16. The columnar epithelium of the mucous membrane is noted for _____ cells; underlying
    this membrane is the capillary-rich _____ _____.

17. Surrounding the lamina propria is the _____ _____, which underlies the
    submucosa.

18. Surrounding the submucosa is the _____ _____, which in turn is covered
    by the serosa. The serosa is covered by a layer of simple squamous epithelium called _____.

19. The muscularis externa is composed of two opposing layers of smooth muscle: inner _____
    and outer _____.

20. The Intrinsic Enteric Nervous System is subdivided into two Nerve Plexuses: the _____
    Plexus and the _____ Plexus.

21. The Submucosal Plexus stimulates both _____ and
    contractions of the _____ _____.

22. The Myenteric Plexus is located _____ and stimulates
    _____.

23. The oral or _____ cavity is lined by _____ _____
    _____.

24. The lips or _____ are noted as the transition point from the keratinized squamous
    epithelium of the integument to the non-keratinized of the buccal cavity; this transition is called the
    _____ _____.

25. The attachment of the labia to the gum (or _____) is the _____
    _____; that of the tongue to the floor is the _____
    _____.

26. The midline of the hard palate is called the _____. The _____ hangs
    from the soft palate.

27. During swallowing, the uvula moves _____ closing off the _____; the
    opening arch-like to the oropharynx is the _____.

28. How do intrinsic muscles of the tongue differ from extrinsic? _____

_____

29. The three types of lingual papillae are _____, _____, and

_____.

30. The four neurologic tastes associated with Fungiform and Circumvallate papillae are

_____, _____, _____, and _____.

Filiform papillae give the tongue its _____.

31. The anterior two-thirds of the tongue is separated from its posterior third by the _____

_____.

32. The two types of cells that contribute to saliva are _____ and _____ cells;

saliva is _____% water.

33. Unlike the mucus cells, the secretions of serous cells include _____. Intrinsic salivary

glands are also known as _____ glands and are located _____

_____

34. In addition to the numerous buccal glands, saliva is produced by three extrinsic glands: the

_____, _____, and _____ glands.

35. A childhood infection of the parotid glands is known as the _____. Saliva also contains

the digestive enzyme _____ and an anti-microbial secretion, _____.

36. Salivary amylase catabolizes which organic compound? _____ Amylase is produced by

what other accessory digestive organ? _____

37. Starch digestion begins in the _____; salivation is controlled by Cranial Nerves

_____, the _____ nerve, and the _____ nerve.

38. Bad breath is properly termed _____ and may indicate of _____ rather

than poor hygiene.

39. The teeth form _____ joints with the mandible and maxillary bones within their

_____ sockets.

40. The alveolar sockets are lined by the _____ ligament. Chewing is properly termed

_____.

41. Milk or non-permanent teeth are termed _____ indicating that they will fall out. There

are _____ in all.

42. Unlike deciduous teeth, there are _____ permanent teeth. The five types of permanent teeth include

_____, _____, _____, _____, and

_____ _____.

43. The typical tooth is divided into three regions: the _____, which is exposed above the

gum, the _____ within the gum, and the _____, which is embedded

within the alveolar socket.

44. The bulk of the tooth is composed of bone-like _____; only the crown is covered by a layer of _____, the hardest substance in the body.

45. The hollowed-out center of dentin is called the _____ _____. The dentin shaft is connected to the periodontal ligament by _____.

46. The pulp cavity leads into the _____ _____, which is filled with nerves and blood and lymphatic vessels. Caries are more commonly known as _____.

47. The voluntary initiation of swallowing is performed by the _____ _____ muscle.

48. Contraction of the pharyngeal constrictor pushes food into the _____.

49. Food is routed to the esophagus during swallowing by the _____, which prevents it from entering the _____. The esophagus passes through the _____ _____ of the diaphragm to reach the stomach.

50. Food is kept in the stomach by the action of the _____ or _____ _____ Sphincter.

51. The backsplash of gastric contents into the esophagus due to poor function of the cardiac sphincter is called _____; the acidic pH at first creates common indigestion or _____, but if chronic can lead to _____.

52. The concave side of the stomach is called the _____ _____; the convex side is the _____ _____.

53. The _____ sphincter separates the stomach from the _____.

54. Aside from ulcers, refluxed gastric contents can wind up in the trachea, a condition called _____. Displacement of the stomach superiorly through the esophageal hiatus is called a _____ _____.

55. Chewing is properly called mastication; swallowing is called _____.

56. Deglutition is divided into two phases: the _____ and _____ _____ phases.

57. The Buccal Phase involves _____ _____ of swallowing and is mediated by CN _____, the _____ Nerve.

58. The Pharyngeal-Esophageal Phase involves _____ _____ and is innervated by CN _____, the _____ Nerve.

59. Unlike other organs, the muscularis of the stomach has _____, layers: _____, _____, and the outer _____.

60. The gastric mucosa is noted for its folds or _____; the mucosa is lined by _____ _____ _____.

61. Through the columnar epithelium are openings to _____ _____.

62. The gastric pits are lined by four different secretory cells: _____ _____ cells, _____ cells, _____ cells, and _____ cells.

63. Unlike goblet cells of the gastric lining, the pH of the secretion of the mucus neck cells is _____. Parietal cells secrete _____.

64. Chief Cells secrete the inactive enzyme _____. Enteroendocrine cells secrete _____ such as _____, _____, and _____.

65. What is the functional relationship between Parietal Cells and Chief Cells? _____ _____

66. What organic compound does pepsin catabolize? _____ The stomach also secretes the enzyme _____ in young children and _____ _____ for B₁₂ absorption.

67. Without Intrinsic factor, one will eventually develop _____ _____.

68. Define Gastritis: _____.
    Define Ulcer: _____.

69. Although gastric reflux is responsible for most esophageal ulcers, what are 90% of gastric ulcers caused by? _____

70. Gastric secretion is regulated by three regional mechanisms: the _____, _____, and _____ Phases.

71. The Cephalic Phase is noted for collective _____ affecting different sensory regions; the result is gastric stimulation by the _____ nervous system.

72. The Gastric Phase begins by the simple filling of the stomach or _____.

73. Distention of the gastric wall stimulates mechanoreceptors of the _____ plexus; the result is the parasympathetic release of the neurotransmitter _____.

74. Vagal release of ACh stimulates gastric secretion of the hormone _____.

75. Gastrin is secreted _____ cells in response to _____ _____ and rising/lowering pH.

76. Gastrin functions by targeting _____ to produce more _____. Gastrin release is inhibited when pH drops below _____.

77. Gastrin, Ach, and _____ combined stimulate the most _____ secretion.

78. The Intestinal Phase is divided into _____ and _____ stages.

79. The Excitatory stage is initiated by the presence of _____ _____ in the _____.

80. The low pH of chyme stimulates the duodenum to secrete _____ _____, which results in _____.

81. As the duodenum fills and distends it triggers the _____ reflex, which begins the Inhibitory stage.

82. The Enterogastric Reflex inhibits the _____ Nerve while stimulating sympathetic nuclei to close the _____ sphincter.

83. The small intestine is noted for three segments: the proximal _____, the _____, and the distal _____.

84. The duodenum is the shortest segment measuring _____; the jejunum is longer at _____, and the ileum longest at _____.

85. Measuring 10 inches long, the duodenum is noted for the entry of the hepato-pancreatic ampulla at the _____ _____ _____.

86. The Major Duodenal Papilla allows for the entry of _____ and digestive _____ via the _____ _____ _____.

87. The entry of bile from the _____ _____ and enzymes from the _____ through the Common Bile Duct is controlled by the _____ of _____.

88. The duodenum also differs from the other segments by the exclusive presence of _____ Glands. The mucosa and submucosa of the small intestine present three surface modifications to increase surface area: _____ _____ or _____ _____, _____, and _____.

89. Plicae circulares and villi are considered to be permanent/exfoliative modifications. Villi are noted for their central lymphatic _____, which is associated with a slip of _____ _____ to facilitate "milking."

90. Microvilli are considered to be permanent/exfoliative surface modifications; in addition to absorption, they secrete _____ _____ _____.

91. Brush Border Enzymes complete _____, _____, and _____ _____ digestion.

92. In between villi are invaginations called the _____ of _____.

93. Intestinal Crypts of Lieberkuhn secrete _____ _____; they are also noted for _____ cells, which secrete lysozyme.

94. As one progresses from duodenum to ileum villi, crypts increase/decrease in numbers. Lymphatic Follicles called _____ _____ within the intestinal wall increase/decrease as one approaches the ileum.

95. The ileum leads into the _____, but its contents are controlled by the _____-_____ Valve/Sphincter.

96. The caecum connects the ileum to the colon; also connected to the caecum is the _____, which is filled with _____.

97. The colon or large intestine is divided into five segments: _____ colon, _____ colon, _____ colon, _____, and _____.

98. The smooth muscle layers of the colon are known as _____ _____; they form pocket-like sacs called _____.

99. The ascending colon bends at the right upper quadrant forming the _____ flexure; the transverse colon bends at the left upper quadrant forming the _____ flexure.

100. The colon is most noted for _____ _____. This occurs in invaginations of the mucosa called _____.

101. Crypts for water resorption can become impacted with feces causing _____. The naturally occurring bacteria of the colon are collectively referred to as _____.

102. Most bacterial flora are symbiotic/parasitic and complete certain stages of catabolism; they in turn release Vitamin _____ to produce clotting factors and _____ Complex.

103. The rectum possesses _____ _____, which prevent passing feces with air; the anal sphincter is composed of _____ and _____ muscle.

104. Distinguish between Haustral and Mass movements: _____
_____.

105. How does the Gastrocolic Reflex differ from the Defecation Reflex? _____
_____

106. The liver is divided into four lobes: the largest, the _____, and the _____, and _____, and _____.

107. The large right lobe is attached to left by the _____ Ligament. The _____ Ligament is the remnant of the umbilical vein.

108. Bile exits the liver via the _____ _____ _____; it merges with the _____ Duct of the gallbladder to form the _____ _____ Duct.

109. The Porta Hepatis is noted for the entry of the _____ Artery and the _____ _____ Vein.

110. Lobes are subdivided into hexagonal functional units called _____. The functional cells of the liver are called _____; the macrophage of the liver is known as the _____ cell.

111. Hepatocytes are arranged in plates around leaky capillaries or _____ _____. _____ _____ are located at each corner of the lobule.

112. Portal Triads consist of _____ _____, _____ _____, and a _____ _____.

113. Blood from the Portal arteries and veins flows through the sinusoids to the _____ _____. Bile flows from the hepatocytes through bile _____ to drain into the _____ _____.

114. Other functions of hepatocytes besides bile synthesis include storage of _____ and _____-_____ _____, production of _____ _____, and _____.

115. What are the principal causes of Hepatitis? _____

116. Describe the overall affects of Cirrhosis on liver tissue: _____

117. What are the complications of Portal Hypertension? _____

118. The principal constituents of bile include _____ _____, the pigment _____ from RBCs, and _____. Bile functions by _____ fats rather than catabolizing them.

119. Describe emulsification: _____

120. Bile is released by the gallbladder in response to the intestinal hormone _____, which is secreted in response to the presence of _____ _____ in the duodenum.

121. Bile can dehydrate and form _____ _____; inflammation of the gallbladder is called _____.

122. Biliary calculi can cause obstruction of bile flow from the liver; this may cause discoloration of the skin and sclera called _____. Obstruction causing backsplash into the pancreas may result in _____.

123. The exocrine cells of the pancreas are known as _____ cells, which are noted for their _____ granules.

124. The zymogen granules are responsible for producing the inactive enzymes _____, _____, and _____.

125. Trypsinogen is activated into Trypsin by the Brush Border enzyme _____. Trypsin then activates Carboxypeptidase and Chymotrypsin, which complete _____ digestion.

126. The acini cells also produce _____, _____, and _____ in active forms, which don't require enterokinase.

127. The release of pancreatic juice is stimulated by the intestinal hormone _____ as well as by sympathetic/parasympathetic.

128. The chemical process of breaking down complex compounds is _____ or
_____.

129. The four organic compounds are _____, _____, _____,
and _____ _____.

130. The three groups of carbohydrates are: _____, _____, and
_____.

131. Starch digestion begins with _____ _____ in the _____.

132. Salivary Amylase catalyzes starch into small chain _____; amylase is also produced by the
_____.

133. Oligosaccharides are reduced to monosaccharides by the enzymes _____ and
_____.

134. Dextrimase and Glucoamylase are produced by the _____ _____ and are
known as _____ _____ enzymes.

135. Describe the effects of Lactose Intolerance: _____
_____.

136. Protein catabolism begins in the _____ with the enzyme _____.

137. Pepsin reduces proteins to _____ by breaking _____-
_____ bonds.

138. Polypeptides are broken into smaller chains in the _____ by the enzymes
_____ and _____.

139. Individual amino acids are released by the action of _____ and _____.

140. Neutral fats are prepared for catabolism by _____ by _____
_____.

141. Emulsification produces small droplets called _____; bile salts also _____
the droplets.

142. Polarized micelles can now have fatty acids cleaved by _____, leaving absorbable
_____ and _____.

143. DNA and RNA are broken down into _____ by _____
_____.

144. Nucleotides are further reduced to _____, _____,
and _____ by the _____ _____ enzymes
_____ and _____.

145. The movement of nutrients through the intestinal mucosa is called _____
_____.

146. Transepithelial transport of monosaccharides, amino acids, and pentoses requires _____ _____, and is properly called _____ Transport.

147. Unlike other compounds, micelles, fatty acids and cholesterol enter the epithelium by _____ _____; once inside, these components recombine to form water soluble _____.

148. Chylomicrons then diffuse into the _____, enter the _____, and then drain into the _____ system.

149. Once in the venous blood, chylomicrons are hydrolyzed by _____ _____ into _____ _____ and _____.

150. Describe Adult Celiac Disease: _____
_____.

151. How does Crohn's Disease differ from Ulcerative Colitis? _____
_____

152. How does Bulimia differ from Anorexia? _____
_____

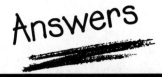

Unit XIII: Digestive System

1. Introduction of food into the digestive system
2. Movement of food through the alimentary tract via peristalsis
3. Segmentation: localized constrictions to mix food and enzymes
4. Catabolic process of enzyme activity yielding monomers
5. The process by which nutrients pass through the intestinal lining
6. Distention; pH, Solute Concentration, Lumen
7. Intrinsic, Extrinsic
8. Enteric Plexus; CNS, ANS
9. Peritoneum, Visceral, Parietal
10. Surface of organs, abdominal wall; Peritoneal Cavity
11. Infection of the peritoneum vs. accumulation of fluid within the peritoneal cavity
12. Double layer of peritoneum which anchors organs in place; do not possess, Retroperitoneal
13. Mucosa, Submucosa, Muscularis Externa, Serosa
14. Adventitia
15. Mucus Membrane, Epithelial
16. Goblet; Lamina Propria
17. Muscularis Mucosae
18. Muscularis Externa; Mesothelium
19. Circular, Longitudinal
20. Submucosal, Myenteric
21. Glandular secretion, Muscularis Mucosae
22. Between layers of Muscularis Externa, Peristalsis
23. Buccal, Stratified Squamous Epithelium
24. Labia; Red Margin
25. (Gingiva) Oral Frenulum; Lingual Frenulum
26. Raphe. Uvula
27. Upward, Nasopharynx. Fauces
28. Intrinsic within tongue for movement; extrinsic outside for anchoring
29. Filiform, Fungiform, Circumvallate
30. Sweet, Salt, Bitter, Sour. Rough
31. Sulcus Terminalis
32. Serous, Mucus; 97–99.5%
33. Enzymes; Buccal, through mucosa
34. Parotid, Submandibular, Sublingual
35. Mumps. Amylase, Defensins
36. Starch; Pancreas
37. Mouth; VII Facial, IX Glossopharyngeal
38. Halitosis, infection
39. Gomphosis, Alveolar
40. Periodontal. Mastication
41. Deciduous; 20
42. 32; 4 Incisors, 2 Canines, 4 Premolars, 4 Molars, 2 Wisdom Teeth (×2)
43. Crown, Neck, Root
44. Dentin; Enamel
45. Pulp Cavity; Cemetin
46. Root Canal; Cavities
47. Pharyngeal Contrictor
48. Oropharynx
49. Epiglottis, Trachea. Esophageal Hiatus
50. Cardiac, Gastro-Esophageal
51. GERD/Reflux; Heartburn, Ulcers
52. Lesser Curvature; Greater Curvature
53. Pyloric, Duodenum
54. Aspiration; Hiatial Hernia
55. Deglutition
56. Buccal, Pharyngeal-Esophageal
57. Voluntary initiation, IX, Glossopharyngeal
58. Involuntary Peristalsis, X, Vagus
59. 3; Oblique, Circular, Longitudinal
60. Ruggae; Simple Columnar Epithelium
61. Gastric Pits
62. Mucus Neck, Parietal, Chief, Enteroendocrine
63. Acidic; HCl
64. Pepsinogen; Hormones, Gastrin, Cholecystokinin, Serotonin
65. Parietal Cells secrete the HCl required to lower the pH to activate Pepsinogen into Pepsin
66. Proteins; Rennin, Intrinsic Factor
67. Pernicious Anemia
68. Inflammation of stomach wall; Break in continuity of wall with erosion
69. Bacteria: Heliobactor pylori
70. Cephalic, Gastric, Intestinal
71. Cues; Parasympathetic
72. Distention
73. Myenteric; ACh
74. Gastrin
75. G, Caffeine, Proteins, Rising

76. Parietal, HCl. 2
77. Histamine, HCl
78. Excitatory and Inhibitory
79. Acidic Chyme, Duodenum
80. Intestinal Gastrin, gastric HCl surge
81. Enterogastric
82. Vagus, Pyloric
83. Duodenum, Jejunum, Ileum
84. 10 inches, 8 feet, 12 feet
85. Major Duodenal Papilla
86. Bile, Enzymes, Common Bile Duct
87. Gallbladder, Pancreas, Sphincter of Oddi
88. Brunner's, Plicae Circularis—Circulat Folds, Villi, Microvilli
89. Permanent, Lacteal, Smooth Muscle
90. Exfoliative; Brush Border Enzymes
91. Protein, Carbohydrate, Nuclei Acid
92. Crypts of Lieberkuhn
93. Intestinal Juice, Paneth
94. Decrease; Peyer's Patches
95. Caecum; Ileocaecal Valve
96. Appendix, Lymphocytes
97. Ascending, Transverse, Descending, Sigmoid, Rectum
98. Taenia Coli; Haustra
99. Hepatic, Splenic
100. Water Resorption. Crypts
101. Diverticulosis. Flora
102. K, B
103. Rectal Valves; Smooth, Skeletal
104. Haustral: move feces from pocket to pocket mixing with water; Mass: move feces towards rectum
105. Gastrocolic: distention of stomach stimulates Haustral movement; Defecation: distention of rectum stimulates Mass movement
106. Right, Left, Caudate, Quadrate
107. Falciform; Round
108. Common Hepatic Duct; Cystic, Common Bile
109. Hepatic, Hepatic Portal
110. Lobules; Hepatocytes; Kuppfer
111. Liver Sinusoids; Portal Triads
112. Portal Arteriole, Portal Venule, Bile Duct
113. Central Vein; Canaliculi, Bile Duct
114. Glycogen, Fat-Soluble Vitamins, Plasma Proteins, Detoxification

115. Viral Infection, Drug and Alcohol Toxicity
116. Scarring and shrinking of liver obstructing blood flow
117. Esophageal Varices and Ascites
118. Bile Salts, Bilirubin, Cholesterol. Emulsifying
119. breaks up fat globules increasing surface area
120. Cholecystokinin, Fatty Chyme
121. Biliary Calculi; Choleystitis
122. Jaundice; Panceatitis
123. Acini, Zymogen
124. Trypsinogen, Carboxypeptidase, Chymotrypsin
125. Enterokinase; Protein
126. Amylase, Lipases, and Nucleases
127. Secretin; Parasympathetic
128. Hydrolysis, Catabolism
129. Carbohydrates, Lipids, Proteins, Nucleic Acids
130. Monosaccharides, Disaccharides, Polysaccharides
131. Salivary Amylase, Mouth
132. Oligosaccharides; Pancreas
133. Dextrimase, Glucoamylase
134. Small Intestine, Brush Border
135. Lactose fermented in colon by bacteria producing gas and symptoms
136. Stomach, Pepsin
137. Polypeptides, Tyrosine-Phenylalanine
138. Duodenum, Trypsin, Chymotrypsin
139. Carboxypeptidase, Aminpeptidase
140. Emulsification, Bile Salts
141. Micelles; Polarize
142. Lipase, Glycerol, Monoglycerides
143. Nucleotides, Pancreatic Nuclease
144. Pentose, Bases, Phosphate, Brush Border, Nucleosidase, Phosphatase
145. Transepithelial Transport
146. Protein Carriers, Facilitated
147. Passive Diffusion; Chylomicrons
148. Lacteal, Lymph, Venous
149. Lipoprotein Lipase, Fatty Acids, Glycerol
150. Gluten Enteropathy, gradual atrophy of intestinal villi, malabsorption
151. Crohn's: regional ileitis; Colitis: hypermotility of colon
152. Bulimia: Ox Hunger, consume 50k calories/day and purges; Anorexia: self imposed starvation

Unit XIII: Take a Test!

1. Chewing is properly called:
   - a) Propulsion
   - b) Segmentation
   - c) Mastication
   - d) Deglutition
   - e) Elimination

2. Which describes the localized contractions of intestinal wall to mix contents:
   - a) Propulsion
   - b) Segmentation
   - c) Mastication
   - d) Deglutition
   - e) Elimination

3. Swallowing is properly called:
   - a) Propulsion
   - b) Segmentation
   - c) Mastication
   - d) Deglutition
   - e) Elimination

4. Peristalsis is mediated by:
   - a) CN V
   - b) CN IX
   - c) CN X
   - d) CN VII
   - e) a and b

5. Mastication is controlled by:
   - a) Trigeminal
   - b) Glossopharyngeal
   - c) Vagus
   - d) Hypoglossal
   - e) a and b

6. Salivation is controlled by:
   - a) Facial
   - b) Glossopharyngeal
   - c) Vagus
   - d) a and b
   - e) a, b and c

7. Deglutition is controlled/initiated by:
   - a) CN V
   - b) CN IX
   - c) CN X
   - d) CN VII
   - e) a and b

8. Amino Acids will depolarize which type of taste receptor:
   - a) Salt
   - b) Sweet
   - c) Sour
   - d) Bitter

9. Overstimulation of which taste bud can initiate the "Gag" Reflex:
   - a) Salt
   - b) Sweet
   - c) Sour
   - d) Bitter

10. Which gland is classified as "intrinsic":
    - a) Buccal
    - b) Parotid
    - c) Sublingual
    - d) Submandibular
    - e) Lacrimal

11. Which of the following enzymes are constituents of saliva:
     a) amylase   b) inactive lipase
     c) pepsin   d) a and b   e) a, b and c

12. The bone-like material of a tooth is called :
     a) enamel   b) cementin
     c) dentin   d) pulp   e) gingiva

13. Which portion of the Alimentary Canal possesses an Adventitia rather than a Serosa:
     a) esophagus   b) stomach
     c) duodenum   d) ileum   e) sigmoid colon

14. The Visceral Peritoneum is also known as the:
     a) Mucosa   b) Submucosa
     c) Serosa   d) Adventitia   e) Muscularis mucosae

15. Fluid accumulation within the peritoneal cavity is known as:
     a) Edema   b) Effusion
     c) Peritonitis   d) Diverticulitis   e) ascites

16. Which is responsible for the formation of Rugae in a relaxed/empty stomach:
     a) Muscularis Mucosae   b) Serosa
     c) Muscularis Externae   d) Submucosa   e) Taenia Coli

17. Which is responsible for of the mass movements of elimination:
     a) Muscularis Mucosae   b) Serosa
     c) Muscularis Externae   d) Submucosa   e) Taenia Coli

18. The Enteric Nervous System includes:
     a) Submucosal Plexus   b) Myenteric Plexus
     c) Celiac Plexus   d) a and b   e) a, b and c

19. The reflux of gastric contents is due to poor tone of the:
     a) Pharyngeal Constrictor   b) Ileocaecal Valve
     c) Pyloric Valve   d) Cardiac Valve   e) Sphincter of Oddi

20. Which of the following is only secreted by nursing infants:
     a) Gastrin   b) Pepsin
     c) Intrinsic Factor   d) Pepsinogen   e) Rennin

21. Intrinsic factor is needed for:
     a) beginning milk digestion   b) activating pepsinogen
     c) B12 absorption in the small intestine   d) lowering pH

22. Which is not associated with Gastric pits:
     a) Mucus Neck Cells   b) Parietal Cells
     c) Chief Cells   d) Enterendocrine Cells   e) Paneth Cells

23. HCl is secreted by:
    a) Mucus Neck Cells
    b) Parietal Cells
    c) Chief Cells
    d) Enterendocrine Cells
    e) Paneth Cells

24. Pepsinogen is secreted by:
    a) Mucus Neck Cells
    b) Parietal Cells
    c) Chief Cells
    d) Enterendocrine Cells
    e) Paneth Cells

25. Gastrin and Cholecystokinin are secreted by:
    a) Mucus Neck Cells
    b) Parietal Cells
    c) Chief Cells
    d) Enterendocrine Cells
    e) Paneth Cells

26. Gastrin secretion is stimulated by:
    a) Gastric Distention
    b) Peptides in the stomach
    c) ACh
    d) CN X
    e) all of these

27. HCl functions by:
    a) breaking peptide bonds
    b) activating pepsinogen into pepsin
    c) activating amylase
    d) activating Trypsinogen into Trypsin
    e) forming micelles

28. Which closes in response to acid chyme entering the duodenum:
    a) Pharyngeal Constrictor
    b) Ileocaecal Valve
    c) Pyloric Valve
    d) Cardiac Valve
    e) Sphincter of Oddi

29. Which structures increase in numbers/concentration approaching the cecum:
    a) Crypts of Lieberkuhn
    b) Intestinal Villi
    c) Microvilli
    d) Peyer's Patches
    e) Plicae Circularis

30. The Crypts of Lieberkuhn are noted for:
    a) producing pancreatic enzymes
    b) secreting intestinal juice
    c) resorption of water
    d) producing CCK and Secretin

31. Brush Border Enzymes are secreted by:
    a) Crypts of Lieberkuhn
    b) Intestinal Villi
    c) Microvilli
    d) Peyer's Patches
    e) Brunner's Glands

32. The exocrine cells of the pancreas are known as:
    a) Paneth Cells
    b) Acini Cells
    c) Crypt Cells
    d) Islet Cells
    e) Duct Cells

33. Pancreatin contains which of the following:
    a) Nuclease
    b) Amylase
    c) Lipase
    d) a and b
    e) a, b and c

34. The entry of bile and pancreatic juice into the duodenum is controlled by the:
    a) Pharyngeal Constrictor
    b) Ileocaecal Valve
    c) Pyloric Valve
    d) Cardiac Valve
    e) Sphincter of Oddi

35. Functions of the Large Intestine include:
    a) water resorption
    b) disaccharide catabolism
    c) emulsification
    d) gas production
    e) all of these

36. Which delivers nutrient rich blood from the spleen and small intestine to the Liver for processing:
    a) Hepatic Arteries
    b) Hepatic Portal Veins
    c) Hepatic Veins
    d) a and b
    e) a, b and c

37. Which of the following is the remnant of the umbilical vein:
    a) Hepatic Artery
    b) Hepatic Portal Vein
    c) Hepatic Vein
    d) Round Ligament
    e) Falciform Ligament

38. Which describe the functions of Bile:
    a) polarize lipids
    b) increase surface area
    c) cleave Fatty Acids
    d) a and b
    e) a, b and c

39. Bile exits the Gallbladder via the:
    a) Common Hepatic Duct
    b) Common Bile Duct
    c) Pancreatic Duct
    d) Cystic Duct
    e) Porta Hepatis

40. Obstruction of the Common Hepatic Duct by Biliary Calculi can lead to:
    a) Cirrhosis
    b) Cholecystitis
    c) Jaundice
    d) Hepatitis
    e) Diverticulosis

41. Which of the following can result from Cirrhosis:
    a) Jaundice
    b) Portal Hypertension
    c) Ascites
    d) Poor Clotting
    e) all of these

42. Cholecystokinin is released in response to:
    a) peptides in the stomach
    b) fatty chyme in the duodenum
    c) peptides in the duodenum
    d) Gastrin in the duodenum

43. Trypsinogen is activated into Trypsin by:
    a) Gastrin
    b) HCl
    c) Enterokinase
    d) Cholecystokinin
    e) Secretin

44. Secretin is released in response to:
    a) distention of the stomach
    b) acid chyme in the duodenum
    c) CCK
    d) Gastrin in the duodenum

45. Amylase functions by:
    a) catalyzing starch into monosaccharides
    b) catalyzing starch into disaccharides
    c) catalyzing starch into oligosaccharides
    d) catalyzing oligosaccharides into monosaccharides
    e) catalyzing monosaccharides

46. Amino acids are released for absorption by:
    a) HCl
    b) Carboxypeptidase
    c) Pepsin
    d) Gastrin
    e) Trypsin

47. Which of the following does not require a protein carrier for absorption:
    a) simple sugars
    b) amino acids
    c) nucleic acids
    d) glycerol and fatty acids
    e) all require a carrier

48. Which enter the lacteals before entering the vascular system:
    a) amino acids
    b) simple sugars
    c) chylomicrons
    d) nitrogen bases
    e) phosphorus

49. Carbohydrate metabolism begins in the:
    a) Mouth
    b) Stomach
    c) Small Intestine
    d) Colon
    e) Gall Bladder

50. Which of the following is characterized by the atrophy of villi due to chronic gluten allergy:
    a) Crohn's Disease
    b) Ulcerative Colitis
    c) Celiac Disease
    d) Halitosis
    e) Pancreatitis

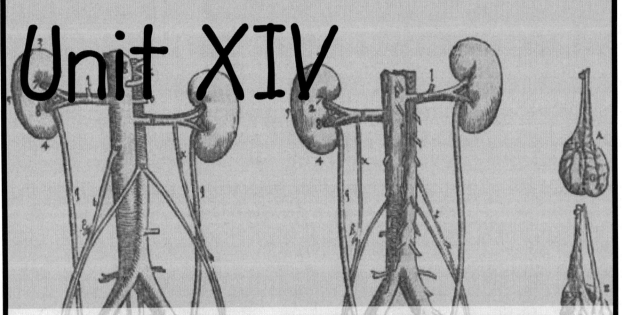

Unit XIV

URINARY SYSTEM AND ELECTROLYTE BALANCE

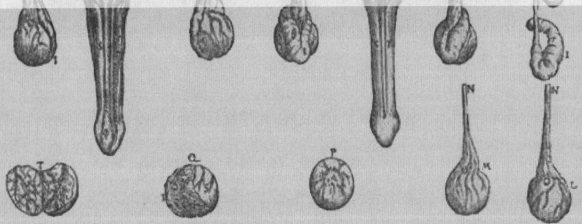

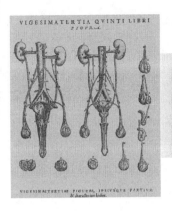

Urinary System and Electrolyte Balance

1. The Urinary System is composed of four main structures: the _____, _____, _____, and the _____.

2. In addition to filtering of blood, the kidney also functions as an _____ gland, metabolizes Vitamin _____, and stimulates _____.

3. The endocrine secretions of the kidney include _____ and _____.

4. Renin functions by _____.

5. After being catalyzed from Angiotensinogen, Angiotensin I is catalyzed into Angiotensin II by _____ _____ _____. Angiotensin II acts by stimulating _____.

6. Erythropoietin functions by _____.

7. The kidney's location is described as _____; it is noted for its concave cleft or _____ _____.

8. The renal hilus opens into the _____ _____ and serves as the entry/exit for _____, _____ _____, and _____ _____.

9. The kidney is surrounded by three protective layers: the inner, fibrous _____ _____, the middle _____ _____, and the outermost fibrous _____ _____.

10. The Renal Capsule overlies the outer region of the kidney, the renal _____; the inner portion of the kidney is called the renal _____. Displacement of the kidney within its adipose capsule and renal fascia is called _____.

11. The Renal Cortex is composed mostly of _____; the medulla is noted for its _____.

12. The medullary pyramids are separated by extensions of cortical tissue, the _____ _____; the apexes of the pyramids are known as _____.

13. A renal pyramid, its two outlining columns, and its overlying cortex and capsule are called a _____. Papillae conduct urine into the _____ _____.

14. The Minor Calyxes conduct urine into the _____ _____, which then deliver it into the _____ _____.

15. The Major Calyxes and the Renal Pelvis are located within the _____ _____. The Renal Pelvis conducts urine into the _____.

16. How does Pyelitis differ from Pyelonephritis? _____

17. After exiting at a right angle from the aorta, the Renal Artery branches into several _____ arteries before entering the Hilus.

18. Segmental Arteries then branch into _____ and then _____ arteries, which run between the lobes to the cortex.

19. The Interlobar Arteries then branch into _____ arteries. These arteries arch over the cortex and form _____ arteries, which will serve the cortical tissue.

20. The Interlobular arteries direct blood to the nephron via the _____ _____.

21. Blood flows from the Afferent Arteriole through the _____ and then into the _____ _____.

22. The blood that passes through the glomerulus to the Efferent Arteriole is joined by blood from the _____ _____.

23. Blood from the Peritubular Capillaries and Efferent Arteriole flow into the _____ _____, the _____ vein, the _____ _____, and then directly into the _____ vein.

24. The Renal Plexus receives parasympathetic innervation from the _____ plexus and sympathetic innervation from Thoracic and Lumbar _____ nerves.

25. The structural and functional unit of the kidney is the _____.

26. Nephrons consist of main principal portions: the _____ _____ and the _____ _____.

27. The Renal Corpuscle consists of the _____ and the surrounding _____ _____. The Renal Tubule is subdivided into three regions: the _____ _____ _____, _____ _____, and _____ _____ _____.

28. The Glomerulus is composed of _____ capillaries, which are best described as "_____." Bowman's (Glomerular) Capsule is composed of two layers, the outer _____ and inner _____.

29. Fenestrated capillaries allow for _____. The inner parietal layer of Bowman's capsule is composed of branching epithelial cells called _____.

30. Podocytes cling to the _____ _____ of the glomerulus and form _____, or _____, pores to allow filtrate to pass through.

31. The _____ epithelium of the Proximal Convoluted Tubule has _____ to increase surface area for enhanced _____.

32. The Loop of Henle is divided into the _____ or _____ segment and _____ or _____ segment, which conveys filtrate into the Distal Convoluted Tubule and on to the _____ _____.

33. Nephrons are subdivided into two groups: _____ nephrons (_____%) and _____ nephrons (_____%).

34. Cortical nephrons are so named because _____
_____.

35. Juxtamedullary nephrons are so named because _____
_____.

Unlike cortical nephrons, juxtamedullary nephrons also possess a _____ _____.

36. The vasa recta and _____ capillaries resorb _____% of the filtrate.

37. Filtrate entering the peritubular capillaries is then directed to the _____ _____ and on to the venous system.

38. The region where the DCT is in direct contact with the Afferent Arteriole is called the
_____ _____.

39. The Juxtaglomerular Apparatus is known for two cell types: _____, or _____, Cells and _____ _____ Cells.

40. Juxtaglomerular (JG) Cells are _____ _____ cells that secrete
_____.

41. The smooth muscle JG cells respond to _____ and act as _____. Macula Densa Cells respond to _____ and act as _____.

42. The Filtration Membrane consists of three layers:
the _____,
the _____ _____, and
the _____.

43. How does filtrate differ from blood? _____

44. How does urine differ from filtrate? _____
_____

45. Of the 1200 ml of blood/minute that pass through the glomerulus, what portion is plasma? _____ ml. How much enters the tubule as filtrate per minute? _____ ml.

46. The BP in the Afferent Arteriole is normally _____ mm Hg and is referred to as the _____ _____ Pressure.

47. Glomerular Hydrostatic Pressure (55 mm Hg) must exceed two opposing pressure gradients: the blood _____ _____ pressure (_____ mm Hg) and the _____ _____ Pressure (_____ mm Hg).

48. The difference from the GHP and the colloid osmotic and capsular hydrostatic pressures determine the _____ _____ _____ Pressure.

49. The Net Filtration Pressure helps to determine the _____ _____ Rate.

50. The Glomerular Filtration Rate increases/decreases with high blood volume to form diluted/concentrated urine. The Glomerular Filtration Rate increases/decreases with dehydration to form diluted/concentrated urine.

51. The GFR is regulated by three mechanisms: _____ or _____ Renal, _____ innervation, and the _____-_____ mechanism.

52. Autoregulation, or Intrinsic renal, uses the _____ Mechanism and _____ Feedback.

53. The Myogenic Mechanism responds to increased BP by causing vasodilation/constriction of the _____ Arteriole, increasing/decreasing GFR. It responds to decreased BP by causing vasodilation/constriction of the _____ Arteriole, increasing/decreasing GFR.

54. The Tubuloglomerular Feedback Mechanism involves the _____ _____ and _____ Cells.

55. In response to low osmolality, the _____ _____ cells release chemicals that cause dilation/constriction of the _____ Arteriole.

56. In response to high osmolality, the macula densa cells release chemicals that stimulate dilation/constriction of the _____ Arteriole. These responses are known as _____ Feedback.

57. Renin's activation of Angiotensin II causes _____. Renin's release by the _____ cells can be triggered by BP below _____ mm Hg, by the _____ _____ cells, by _____ during stress, and by _____ itself.

58. Angiotensin II causes pronounced vasoconstriction everywhere except in the _____ _____. Angiotensin II also stimulates the adrenal cortex to secrete _____ and the hypothalamus to release _____ from the _____ _____.

59. Aldosterone increases _____ and _____ reabsorption; ADH increases _____ reabsorption and stimulates _____.

60. Tubular Reabsorption involves three layers between filtrate and blood: the _____ and _____ membranes of the _____ cells, and the endothelium of _____ capillary.

61. Tubule cells are joined by _____ _____; this prevents substances from squeezing between them. This is also called the _____ pathway.

62. Sodium reabsorption is by _____ _____ _____.

63. Sodium is pumped out of the tubule through the _____ membrane; this creates an ICF gradient allowing for passive diffusion of sodium through the _____ membrane.

64. When substances such as glucose and amino acids are "pushed" through the _____ membrane with sodium along its gradient, it is called _____ _____ Transport.

65. Secondary Active Transport is assisted by protein carriers or _____.

66. Substances reabsorbed through the Luminal Membrane by passive diffusion include _____, _____, and all _____ soluble substances.

67. What is meant by Obligatory Water Reabsorption? _____
_____

68. What is meant by Transport Maximum (T_M)? _____
_____
_____

69. How is T_M involved in Diabetes Mellitus? _____
_____
_____

70. Substances are not absorbed if they don't have _____, are not _____ _____, are _____ _____, or are classified as _____ wastes.

71. Nitrogenous wastes are the by-products of _____ and _____ _____ metabolism and include _____, _____, and _____ _____.

72. Any plasma proteins entering the PCT are removed from filtrate by _____.

73. The PCT is also the site where cotransporters facilitate the reabsorption of large molecules such as _____ and _____ _____. All _____ _____ will also be reabsorbed but will be secreted out later.

74. In addition to glucose, amino acids, and uric acid/urea, _____% of sodium and _____% water is reabsorbed. What percent of Cl^- and K^+ are reabsorbed? _____; Bicarbonate: _____%.

75. The descending segment of Henle's Loop is noted for _____% reabsorption of _____ only. The ascending segment is noted for _____ % of sodium and _____% of Cl⁻ and K⁺.

76. Sodium and water reabsorption in the DCT and Collecting Duct is controlled by _____ and _____.

77. Define Tubular Secretion: _____
_____
_____.

78. What substances are secreted by the tubule cells into the filtrate: _____, _____, _____ _____, and _____.

79. Tubular secretion of H⁺ assists in the maintenance of _____.

80. Define Osmolality: _____.
How is a solution's osmolality expressed? _____

81. The greater a solution's osmolality, the greater its ability to _____ _____.
The solute concentration of filtrate entering the tubule is _____ mOsm.

82. The osmolality of the interstitial fluid increases from 300 mOsm in the cortex to _____ mOsm in the medulla; this results in the reabsorption of _____ from the filtrate in the _____ segment of Henle's Loop.

83. As water is resorbed, the osmolality of the filtrate increases/decreases to _____ mOsm.

84. As the concentrated filtrate passes through the ascending segment, the osmolality of the interstitial fluid increases/decreases to _____ mOsm; this results in the reabsorption of _____.

85. The reabsorption of NaCl reduces the osmolality of the filtrate to _____ mOsm as it enters the DCT. What is the effect of the active transport of NaCl into the interstitial fluid surrounding Henle's Loop?
_____
_____

86. The Collecting Duct is noted for its permeability to _____; the Vasa Recta is permeable to _____ and _____.

87. Filtrate is diluted/concentrated as it flows through the ascending segment. Urine is concentrated by the action of _____.

88. ADH signals secondary messengers in the _____ _____ to facilitate _____ transport.

89. Increased water transport by ADH increases filtrate osmolality to _____ mOsm, resorbing _____% of the water that entered the PCT. This is known as _____ Water Resorption.

90. Define Diuretic: _____
_____.

91. How does alcohol act as a diuretic? _____

92. Define Renal Clearance: _____
    _____.

    What substance is used to test renal clearance? _____

93. Why is Inulin used to test the rate of kidney filtration? _____

94. What substance gives urine is characteristic yellow color? _____ What substance is this a
    metabolite of? _____

95. What causes standing urine to acquire an odor of ammonia? _____
    _____

96. Normal pH of urine: _____
    Normal specific gravity: _____-_____
    Water content: _____%

97. Urine is conducted from the renal pelvis into the _____.

98. Kidney stones or _____ _____ can lodge in the ureter causing a pain
    syndrome known as _____ _____.

99. The opening of the two ureters and the urethra in the wall of the urinary bladder is called the
    _____. The muscular wall of the bladder is called the _____ muscle.

100. A thickened region of the Detrusor Muscle surrounding the urethra forms the _____
    _____ _____; this sphincter is involuntary/voluntary.

101. Unlike the Internal Urethral Sphincter, the External is composed of _____ muscle and is
    involuntary/voluntary.

102. How does Diuresis differ from Micturition? _____
    _____

103. How does Cystitis differ from Urethritis? _____
    _____

104. How does Urgency differ from Incontinence? _____
    _____

105. Define Dysuria: _____.

106. After filling with _____ ml of urine, the stretching of the bladder wall stimulates
    _____, which initiates the _____ Reflex.

107. This partial filling of the bladder signals the micturition center of the _____, which in
    turn stimulates the _____ nervous system.

108. Parasympathetic innervation contracts/relaxes the detrusor muscle and contracts/relaxes the urethral
    sphincters allowing one to _____ the bladder.

109. The Micturition Reflex can be inhibited by _____

_____.

110. The total capacity urinary bladder is _____ ml.

111. Body fluid is divided into two compartments: _____ _____ Fluid and

_____ _____ Fluid.

112. The ICF accounts for _____ % of the total body fluid volume (_____ L). The ECF is subdivided

into two regions: _____ and the _____ Fluid.

113. Adipose tissue is more/less hydrated than muscle; females have higher/lower water: tissue ratio than

males.

114. Define Electrolyte: _____

_____.

115. Define Non-Electrolyte: _____

_____.

Non-electrolytes include _____, _____, and _____.

116. What is the principal cation of the ECF? _____ Of the ICF? _____

What is the principal anion of the ECF? _____ Of the ICF? _____

117. Fluids are driven from the capillaries to the interstitial spaces by _____ pressure; fluids

are drawn from the interstitial spaces into the capillaries by _____ _____

pressure.

118. The average daily water intake is _____ ml of which _____% is ingested as fluids and

_____ % from "solid" foods.

119. The balance of the body's daily water intake (_____%) is derived from chemical processes and is

referred to as _____ _____ of _____.

120. The daily water output is _____ ml of which _____% is urine, _____% feces, and

_____% perspiration.

121. The balance of the daily output of water (_____%) is via vaporization through the

_____ and _____, and is referred to as _____ water loss.

122. Thirst is regulated by the _____.

123. The hypothalamus possesses water-solute receptors called _____.

124. Osmoreceptors respond to _____.

125. Increased osmolality of the ECF triggers the hypothalamus to secrete _____.

126. ADH functions by _____

_____.

127. What is meant by "Obligatory water loss"? _____

_____

128. In addition to insensible water loss and feces, the kidney must excrete _____ ml of fluid to eliminate the _____ mOsm of solute that is produced regardless of water intake.

129. Define Dehydration: _____

_____.

Symptoms include: _____, _____, and _____.

130. How does Hypotonic Hydration (Water Intoxication) differ from Edema? _____

_____

_____

131. How is Hypoproteinemia related to Edema? _____

_____

_____

132. What compound is used to treat Hypotonic Hydration? _____

133. What hormone principally regulates sodium concentration? _____ What gland secretes it? _____

134. Aldosterone functions by _____ ;
its release is inhibited by high/low osmolality and high/low BP.

135. In response to increased BP, _____ within the arterial wall will stimulate dilation/constriction of the afferent arteriole, resulting in increased/decreased filtration.

136. Atrial Natriuretic Peptide functions by _____

_____.

137. How is estrogen similar to aldosterone? _____

138. How is aldosterone related to potassium balance? _____

_____

139. Calcium concentration is controlled by the hormones _____ and _____.

140. PTH controls calcium levels in three areas: _____, _____

_____, and the _____.

141. PTH stimulates the kidneys to convert Vitamin _____ to its usable form, _____. It also stimulates the kidney to increase/decrease calcium resorption.

142. The pH of blood is _____, of Interstitial Fluid _____, and of the ICF, _____.

143. What is meant by "Physiologic Acidosis" (pH = _____)? _____

_____

144. Metabolic sources of acidic pH include: _____ acid, _____ acid, _____ acids, and _____ ions.

145. Define Buffer: _____.

146. What is an acid? _____

147. What is a base? _____

148. Combining a strong base with a weak acid produces a _____ _____
     and _____; combining a strong acid with a weak base produces a _____
     _____ and a _____.

149. The three chemical buffers include _____, _____, and
     _____.

150. Define "Amphoteric": _____
     _____.

151. What portion of the protein acts as a weak acid? _____. Which acts a weak base?
     _____

152. How do the two sodium salts of the phosphate buffer differ? _____
     _____

153. What is Hypercapnia? _____

154. How do increased CO_2 levels affect pH? _____

155. What is meant by "Respiratory Acidosis"? _____
     _____

156. The kidneys control pH by two mechanisms: the elimination of _____
     _____ and by the resorption of _____.

157. What is meant by "Metabolic Acidosis"? _____
     _____

158. What is the normal range for pH? _____-_____

159. What are the consequences of a pH below 7.0 (acidosis/alkalosis)? _____
     _____

160. What are the consequences of a pH above 7.8 (acidosis/alkalosis)? _____
     _____

1. Ureter, Bladder, Kidney, Urethra
2. Endocrine, D, Gluconeogenesis, Erythropoiesis
3. Renin, Erythropoietin
4. Catalyzing Angiotensinogen into Angiotensin I
5. Angiotensin Catalyzing Enzyme, Vasoconstriction
6. Stimulating erythropoiesis
7. Retroperitoneal; Renal Hilus
8. Renal Sinus, Ureter, Blood Vessels, Nerves, Lymph
9. Renal Capsule, Adipose Capsule, Renal Fascia
10. Cortex; Medulla; Ptosis
11. Glomeruli; Pyramids
12. Renal Columns; Papilla
13. Lobe; Minoe Calyxes
14. Major Calyx, Renal Pelvis
15. Renal Sinus; Ureters
16. Inflammation/infection of renal pelvis and calyxes vs. entire kidney
17. Segmental
18. Lobar, Interlobar
19. Arcuate, Interlobular
20. Afferent Arteriole
21. Glomerulus, Efferent Arteriole
22. Peritubular Capillaries
23. Interlobular Vein, Arcuate Vein, Interlobar Vein, Renal Vein
24. Celiac, Splanchnic
25. Nephron
26. Renal Corpuscle, Renal Tubule
27. Glomerulus, Bowman's Capsule; Proximal Convoluted Tubule, Henle's Loop, Distal Convoluted Tubule
28. Fenestrated, Leaky; Parietal, Visceral
29. Filtration; Podocytes
30. Basal Lamina, Slits, Filtration
31. Cuboidal, Microvilli, Absorption
32. Thin/Descending, Thick/Ascending; Collecting Duct
33. Cortical 85%, Juxtamedullary 15%
34. The bulk of the tubule is in the cortex
35. Their tubules extend into the Medulla; Vasa Recta
36. Peritubular, 99%
37. Efferent Arteriole
38. Juxtaglomerular Apparatus
39. Juxtaglomerular/JG, Macula Densa
40. Smooth Muscle, Renin
41. Stretch, Mechanoreceptors. Osmolality, Chemoreceptors
42. Fenestrated epithelium of glomerulus, Basal Lamina, Visceral Membrane of Capsule and Podocytes
43. No cells or Proteins
44. Water and Nitrogenous wastes
45. 625 ml, 125 ml
46. 55 mm Hg, Glomerular Hydrostatic
47. Colloidal Osmotic (30 mm Hg), Capsular Hydrostatic (15 mm Hg)
48. Net Filtration Rate
49. Glomerular Filtration
50. Increases, Diluted; Decreases, Concentrated
51. Autoregulation or Intrinsic, Sympathetic, Renin-Angiotensin
52. Myogenic, Tubuloglomerular
53. Constriction, Afferent, Decreasing; Vasodilation, Afferent, Increasing
54. Macula Densa, JG
55. Macula Densa, Dilation, Afferent
56. Constriction, Afferent
57. Vasoconstriction. JG: 80 mm Hg, Macula Densa, Sympathetic, Angiotensin II
58. Afferent Arteriole. Aldosterone, ADH, Posterior Pituitary
59. Na$^+$, Water; Water, Thirst
60. Luminal, Basoluminal, Peritubular
61. Tight Junctions; Paracellular
62. Primary Active Transport
63. Basoluminal; Luminal
64. Luminal; Secondary Active
65. Cotransporters
66. Water, Urea, Lipid
67. Water always follows Na$^+$
68. Specific substances have a finite number of cotransporters available per unit of time
69. When glucose tops 400 mg/100 ml /min, it exceeds its Tm of 375 mg/100 ml/min and "spills" into urine
70. Cotransporters, Lipid Soluble, too large, nitrogenous wastes

71. Protein, Amino Acids, Urea, Creatinine, Uric Acid
72. Endocytosis
73. Glucose, Amino Acids, Uric Acid
74. 65%, 65%; 55%; 90%
75. 10%, water; 25%, 35%
76. Aldosterone, ADH
77. Substances are secreted back into the filtrate through the peritubular capillaries and/or tubule cells
78. H^+, K^+, Uric Acid, Creatinine
79. pH
80. Concentration of dissolved particles per liter of water; Milliosmols (mOsm)
81. Attract water; 300 mOsm
82. 1200 mOsm; water, Descending
83. Increases, 1200 mOsm
84. Decreases, 300 mOsm; NaCl
85. 100 mOsm; Creates a Countercurrent Multiplier, the NaCl from the ascending segment creates the gradient for water in the descending
86. Urea; Water, NaCl
87. Diluted; ADH
88. Collecting Duct, Water
89. 1400 mOsm, 99%. Facultative
90. Any substance that increases urinary output
91. Inhibits ADH
92. Rate at which a substance is filtered from the blood; Insulin
93. Not resorbed
94. Urochrome; Bilirubin
95. Bacterial action on Urea
96. 6.0; 1.001–1.035; 95%
97. Ureter
98. Renal Calculi; Renal Colic
99. Trigone; Detrussor
100. Internal Urethral Sphincter; Involuntary
101. Skeletal Muscle; Voluntary
102. Urine formation vs. voiding the bladder
103. Inflammation/infection of bladder vs. Urethra
104. Sudden need to void vs. inability to control urinary sphincter
105. Pain during urination
106. 300 ml, Mechanoreceptors, Micturition
107. Pons, Parasympathetic
108. Contracts, Relaxes, Void
109. Voluntary contraction of external urinary sphincter
110. 500 ml
111. Internal Cellular Fluid and External Cellular Fluid
112. 66% (25 ml); Plasma, Interstitial

113. Less; Lower
114. Substances that disassociate in water to bear a net charge +/−
115. Any substance that does not disassociate and bear a net charge; Glucose, Urea, Lipids
116. Na^+; K^+. Cl^-, HPO_4^- (phosphate)
117. Hydrostatic; Colloidal Osmotic
118. 2500 ml, 60%, 30%
119. 10% Water of Oxidation
120. 2500 ml, 60%, 4%, 8%
121. 28%, Lungs and Skin, Insensitive
122. Hypothalamus
123. Osmoreceptors
124. Increased osmolality
125. ADH
126. Increases water resorption in the collecting duct and stimulates thirst
127. Loss via Insensible, feces and to enough urine to pass solute
128. 500 ml, 1200 mOsm
129. Fluid output exceeds input creating negative fluid balance
130. Excess water intake creates Acute Hyponatremia causing cells to swell with water vs. increased water retention in interstitial spaces
131. Reduced plasma proteins reduce Colloidal Osmotic Pressure gradient leaving excess water in interstitial spaces
132. Mannitol
133. Aldosterone, Adrenals
134. Increasing Na^+ and water resorption; High, High
135. Baroreceptors, Dilation, Increased
136. Inhibits vasoconstriction and water and Na^+ retention
137. enhances NaCl Resorption
138. Enhances K^+ secretion
139. Calcitonin, PTH
140. Bones, Small Intestine, Kidneys
141. D, D_3, Increase
142. 7.4, 7.35, 7.0
143. pH = 7.0: pH reduced due to metabolic factors
144. Phosphoric, Lactic, Fatty, H^+
145. Substances that resist changes in pH
146. Proton donors, free H^+
147. Proton acceptors, free OH^-
148. Weak base and water; Weak acid and a salt
149. Phosphate, Protein, Bicarbonate
150. Proteins can act as either weak acid or weak base

151. Carboxyl; Amino

152. $NaHPO_4$ weak base; Na_2HPO_4 weak acid

153. Increased CO_2

154. Release H^+ reducing pH

155. Acidic pH due to respiratory induced increased CO_2

156. Metabolic acids, Bicarbonate

157. Acidic pH due to factors other than CO_2

158. 7.0–7.8

159. Acidosis: depressed NS, Coma

160. Alkalosis: Tetany, Convulsions, Respiratory arrest

1. Which is not a function of the kidney:
   a) Erythropöeisis
   b) Activate Vitamin D_3 into Calcitriol
   c) BP regulation
   d) pH balance
   e) All are functions

2. The kidney regulates pH balance by:
   a) excreting uric acid
   b) resorbing H_2CO_3
   c) secreting Renin
   d) a and b
   e) a, b and c

3. Which is considered the functional unit of the kidney:
   a) Lobe
   b) Pyramid
   c) Nephron
   d) Column
   e) Pelvis

4. Which does not exit/enter at the hilus:
   a) urethra
   b) renal Vein
   c) renal artery
   d) ureter
   e) all enter

5. Which is not part of a renal lobe:
   a) pyramid
   b) column
   c) papilla
   d) ureter
   e) all are part

6. The filtration membrane is composed of all of the following except:
   a) Podocytes
   b) Basal Lamina
   c) Macula Densa
   d) Fenestrated Epithelium

7. Which of the following acts as a chemoreceptor:
   a) JG Cells
   b) Vasa Recta
   c) Macula Densa
   d) Peritubular Capillaries
   e) Bowman's Capsule

8. Which contains smooth muscle-like cells which act as mechanoreceptors:
   a) JG Cells
   b) Vasa Recta
   c) Macula Densa
   d) Peritubular Capillaries
   e) Bowman's Capsule

9. Which is the correct order:
   a) interlobar a., arcuate a., interlobular a., efferent arteriole glomerulus, afferent arteriole, interlobular v.
   b) interlobular a., interlobar a., arcuate a., afferent arteriole, glomerulus, efferent arteriole, interlobular v.
   c) arcuate a., interlobar a., interlobular a., efferent arteriole interlobular a., glomerulus, interlobular v.
   d) interlobar a., arcuate a., interlobular a., afferent arteriole, glomerulus, efferent arteriole, interlobular v.

10. Which is the correct order of structures:
    a) papillary duct, collecting duct, major calyx, minor calyx, renal pelvis
    b) collecting duct, papillary duct, minor calyx, major calyx, renal pelvis
    c) major calyx, minor calyx, renal pelvis, papillary duct, collecting duct
    d) collecting duct, minor calyx, major calyx, papillary duct, renal pelvis

11. Renin is secreted by:
    a) JG Cells   b) Macula Densa Cells
    c) Podocytes   d) Glomerular Cells

12. Renin functions by:
    a) Increasing Na^+ reabsorption in the DCT
    b) Increasing water reabsorption in the DCT
    c) Catalyzing Angiotensinogen into Angiotensin I
    d) Stimulate dilation of the afferent arteriole
    e) Inhibit Na^+ reabsorption

13. Which occurs in response to slow flow rate and low osmolality:
    a) JG cells release Renin causing peripheral vasoconstriction
    b) JG cells release Renin causing constriction of the afferent arteriole
    c) Macula Densa cells release Renin causing constriction of the afferent arteriole
    d) Macula Densa cells stimulate dilation of the afferent arteriole
    e) Macula Densa cells stimulate JG cells to constrict afferent arteriole

14. Which occurs in response to the BP dropping below 80mm Hg:
    a) JG cells release Renin causing peripheral vasoconstriction
    b) JG cells release Renin causing constriction of the afferent arteriole
    c) Macula Densa cells release Renin causing constriction of the afferent arteriole
    d) Macula Densa cells stimulate dilation of the afferent arteriole
    e) Macula Densa cells stimulate JG cells to constrict afferent arteriole

15. Which of the following help create the Net Filtration Pressure:
    a) the BP in the Afferent Arteriole
    b) the Parietal Layer of Bowman's Capsule
    c) the osmotic gradient created by Albumin in blood
    d) a and b
    e) a, b and c

16. Which of the following is resorbed by Primary Active Transport:
    a) Na^+ b) water
    c) K^+ d) Glucose   e) plasma proteins

17. Which is resorbed by Secondary Active Transport using cotransporters:
    a) Na^+ b) water
    c) K^+ d) Glucose   e) plasma proteins

18. Which is secreted into the filtrate by the distal collecting tubule:
a) Na^+ b) water
c) K^+ d) Glucose   e) plasma proteins

19. Which is removed from filtrate in the PCT by endocytosis:
a) Na^+ b) water
c) K^+ d) Glucose   e) plasma proteins

20. Juxtamedullary nephrons differ from Cortical nephrons in that they possess:
a) Juxtaglomerular Cells   b) Vasa Recta
c) Macula Densa   d) Peritubular Capillaries   e) Bowman's Capsule

21. The Descending segment of Henle's Loop is:
a) permeable to Na^+ b) permeable to water
c) permeable to urea   d) impermeable to water

22. The Collecting Duct is noted for being:
a) permeable to Na^+ b) permeable to water
c) permeable to urea   d) impermeable to water

23. What is meant by Obligatory Water Resorption:
a) the minimum volume of water to excrete nitrogenous wastes
b) the maximum percentage water of water resorbed from filtrate
c) the water which accompanies resorbed Na^+
d) the volume of water needed to balance osmolality

24. Aldosterone functions principally by:
a) Increasing Na^+ resorption in the DCT
b) Increasing water resorption in the DCT
c) Catalyzing Angiotensinogen into Angiotensin I
d) Stimulate dilation of the afferent arteriole
e) Increasing Na^+ excretion

25. Atrial Natriuretic Peptide functions principally by:
a) Increasing Na^+ resorption in the DCT
b) Increasing water resorption in the DCT
c) Catalyzing Angiotensinogen into Angiotensin I
d) Stimulate dilation of the afferent arteriole
e) Increasing Na^+ excretion

26. How is Diabetes Mellitus related to Glycosuria:
a) reduced insulin causes glomerular dysfunction
b) reduced insulin increases normal glucose excretion
c) increased glucose exceeds transport maximum
d) increased glucose inhibits ADH
e) increased glucose inhibits Aldosterone

27. ADH functions principally by:
    a) Increasing Na$^+$ resorption in the DCT
    b) Increasing water resorption in the DCT
    c) Catalyzing Angiotensinogen into Angiotensin I
    d) Stimulate dilation of the afferent arteriole
    e) Increasing Na$^+$ excretion

28. Estrogen:
    a) Increases Na$^+$ resorption in the DCT
    b) Increases water resorption in the DCT
    c) Catalyzes Angiotensinogen into Angiotensin I
    d) Stimulates dilation of the afferent arteriole
    e) Increases Na$^+$ excretion

29. Which tem best describes the production of urine:
    a) Diuresis   b) Dysuria
    c) Polyuria   d) Cystitis   e) Incontinence

30. The Micturation Reflex results in:
    a) Voiding of the bladder   b) Formation of filtrate
    b) Concentration of urine   d) Diluting of urine
    e) none of the above

31. The External Urethral Sphincter is formed from:
    a) smooth muscle   b) skeletal muscle
    c) thickened portion of the Detrusor   d) Rugae

32. Which tissue is the least hydrated:
    a) Muscle   b) Areolar
    c) Adipose   d) Lymphatic

33. Which is a non-electrolyte:
    a) Na+   b) Glucose
    c) Acids   d) Bases   e) all are electrolytes

34. Which is the principal cation of the ECF:
    a) Na$^+$ b) K$^+$ c) Cl$^-$ d) HPO$_4^-$

35. Which is the principal cation of the ICF:
    a) Na$^+$ b) K$^+$ c) Cl$^-$ d) HPO$_4^-$

36. Fluid moves from the ECF into the capillaries by:
    a) Colloid osmotic pressure   b) Hydrostatic pressure
    c) Active Transport   d) Secretion   e) Electrochemical gradient

37. What percentage of water intake is due to metabolic oxidation:
    a) 4%   b) 8%
    c) 10%   d) 28%   e) 30%

38. What percentage of water output is considered insensible:
    a) 4%   b) 8%
    c) 10%   d) 28%   e) 30%

39. Insensible water loss refers to water output via:
    a) feces   b) vaporization through the lungs
    c) bedwetting   d) active perspiration   e) micturation

40. Osmoreceptors of the hypothalamus respond to:
    a) increased osmolality of the ECF   b) decreased osmolality of the ECF
    c) decrease in plasma volume   d) a and c   e) b and c

41. Which of the following will most likely cause edema:
    a) Hyponatremia   b) Hypoproteinemia
    c) Reduced Na^+ d) Dehydration

42. How is liver disease related to edema:
    a) reduced plasma protein production   b) reduced Aldosterone production
    c) increased plasma protein production   d) increased Aldosterone production
    e) increased portal hypertension

43. Hypotonic Hydration will result in:
    a) hypocapnia   b) hyponatremia
    c) hypokalemia   d) hypernatremia   e) hypercapnia

44. Combining a strong base with a weak acid results in the formation of:
    a) Weak acid and a salt   b) Weak acid and water
    c) Weak base and a salt   d) Weak base and water
    e) Salt and water

45. The body is in a state of "physiologic acidosis" when the blood pH measures:
    a) 7.45   b) 7.4   c) 7.35   d) 7.30

46. Which of the following does not contribute to "metabolic acidosis":
    a) Phosphoric acid   b) Lactic acid
    c) CO_2 d) Ketones
    e) Fixed acids

47. Which compound is described as "Amphoteric":
    a) Bicarbonate   b) Phosphate
    c) Protein   d) Inulin   e) Mannitol

48. A state of "physiologic alkalosis" can result from:
    a) hypocapnia   b) hyponatremia
    c) hypokalemia   d) hypernatremia   e) hypercapnia

49. Inability to control the External Urinary Sphincter is properly called:
a) Hesitancy b) Urgency
c) Enuresis d) Cystitis e) Incontinence

50. Which will not contribute to metabolic acidosis:
a) uric acid b) CO_2
c) ketones d) lactic acid e) all do

1: e, 2: d, 3: c, 4: a, 5: d, 6: c, 7: c, 8: a, 9: d, 10: b, 11: a, 12: c, 13: d, 14: a, 15: e, 16: a, 17: d, 18: c, 19: e, 20: b, 21: b, 22: c, 23: c, 24: a, 25: e, 26: c, 27: b, 28: a, 29: a, 30: a, 31: b, 32: c, 33: b, 34: a, 35: b, 36: a, 37: c, 38: b, 39: b, 40: d, 41: b, 42: a, 43: b, 44: d, 45: d, 46: c, 47: c, 48: a, 49: e, 50: b

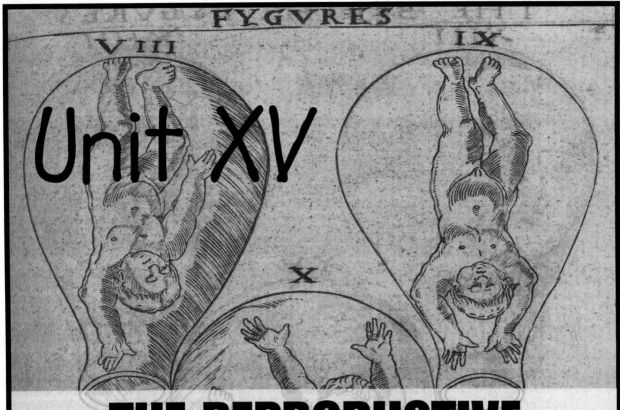

Unit XV

THE REPRODUCTIVE SYSTEM

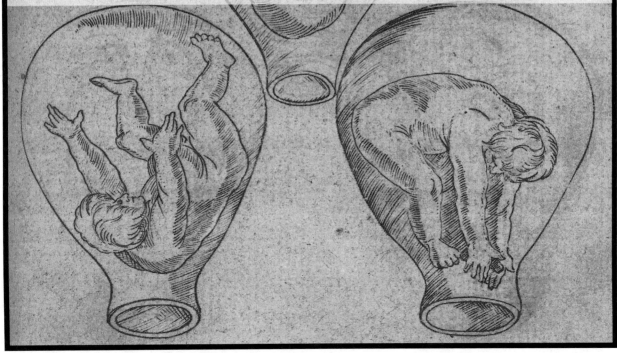

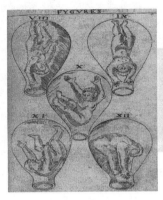

Part 1: Genetics and Embryology

1. Mitosis is defined as the reduction/duplication of genetic material yielding the _____ count; Meiosis is defined as the reduction/duplication of genetic material yielding the _____ count.

2. Mitosis is also referred to as _____ _____ in single-celled organisms; it is also descriptively referred to as _____.

3. The period of time that a cell spends preparing for mitotic division is known as _____; the time spent in preparation and dividing is collectively referred to as the _____ _____.

4. Interphase is subdivided into three periods: _____, _____, and _____.

5. The principal events include:
   Growth 1: _____,
   Synthesis: _____, and
   Growth 2: _____.

6. The typical human body cell possesses _____ chromosomes in _____ _____ pairs. This is known as the _____ count and is represented by the symbol _____.

7. At the start of mitosis there are _____ chromosomes, or more properly, _____ paired _____ _____ in the nucleus.

8. The 46 pairs of sister chromatids are joined at the _____; this will be the point of attachment for the _____ _____.

9. The spindle apparatus is formed by the _____, which was duplicated during _____.

10. Mitosis is divided into four phases: _____, _____, _____, and _____.

11. The four principal events of Prophase are:

_____,

_____,

_____, and

_____.

12. The principal event of Metaphase is: _____

_____.

13. The principal event of Anaphase is: _____

_____.

14. The four principal events of Telophase are:

_____,

_____,

_____, followed by

_____, which yields two identical daughter cells.

15. Meiosis is also referred to as _____ _____ in higher order organisms; during Meiosis _____ cells undergo _____ modified mitotic divisions to produce _____, also known as sperm and ova.

16. Gametes possess the _____ chromosome count, which is represented by the symbol _____.

17. At the beginning of Meiosis there are a total of _____ chromosomes in _____ groups or _____.

18. Tetrads consist of duplicated _____ _____; each tetrad consists of _____ chromosomes: _____ maternal and _____ paternal.

19. In addition to reducing the chromosomal count to (N), Meiosis also produces _____ _____ by exchanging regions of homologous maternal and paternal chromosomes. This is known as _____ _____ or _____.

20. Crossing over/Synapsis of tetrads occurs during _____; Telophase I ends by producing _____ cells, each containing _____ chromosomes.

21. Meiosis II begins with _____ cells, each containing _____ chromosomes; Telophase II ends by producing a total of _____ cells, each containing _____ chromosomes, the _____ count; each cell is genetically _____.

22. Homologous pairs 1–22 are referred to as _____; pair #23 is referred to as the _____ _____. The nomenclature for the female genotype is _____ and for the male genotype _____.

23. "Maleness" is carried by the _____ chromosome; this gene is known as _____ or _____ _____.

24. Phenotypic sex is determined at _____; however, during the first six weeks of gestation the embryo appears _____, each sex possessing identical primitive structures and duct systems.

25. Internally, both possess the _____ _____, the _____ or _____ duct, and the _____ or _____ duct.

26. Externally both possess the _____ _____, _____ _____, the _____ _____, and the _____ _____.

27. During the sixth week, TDF causes the XY embryo to produce _____, which changes the androgynous embryo into a phenotypic _____.

28. Due to testosterone, the Gonadal Ridges differentiate into the _____ and the Mesonephric/Wolfian duct into the internal _____ reproductive structures; the Paramesonephric/Mullerian duct _____.

29. Also due to TDF, the Genital Tubercle differentiates into the _____ _____, the Urethral Groove fuses/remains open forming the _____, the Urethral Folds fuse/remain open forming the _____, and the Labioscrotal Folds fuse/remain open forming the _____.

30. Without testosterone, the XX individual becomes a phenotypic _____, the Gonadal Ridges differentiate into the _____, the Paramesonephric/Mullerian duct into the internal _____ reproduction structures, and the Mesonephric/Wolfian duct _____.

31. Also without TDF/Testosterone, the Genital Tubercle differentiates into the _____, the urethral groove fuse/remain open forming the _____, the urethral folds fuse/remain open forming the _____ _____, and the labioscrotal folds fuse/remain open forming the _____ _____.

32. An XY individual with a non-functional TDF will ultimately develop as a phenotypic _____; a dysfunctional TDF producing insufficient testosterone will result in an _____ individual.

33. Similarly, an XX individual whose mother's endocrine system has a testosterone surge can produce an Intersex phenotype, known as the _____ _____ Syndrome.

34. The nucleus of all female body cells possesses a _____ _____, which is an _____ ____ chromosome.

35. Primary sex characteristics are the _____ _____; secondary sex characteristics are associated with _____ and develop in response to _____ changes.

36. Secondary sex characteristics in females include _____
_____
_____.

37. Secondary sex characteristics in males include _____
_____
_____.

38. Failure of chromosomes to separate during Meiosis is known as _____, the result of which is known as a _____ _____.

39. An XO individual's primary sex characteristics are _____, secondary _____, and is fertile/sterile. This is referred to as _____ Syndrome.

40. An XXY individual's primary sex characteristics are _____, secondary _____, and is fertile/sterile. This is referred to as _____ Syndrome.

41. An XYY individual's primary sex characteristics are _____, secondary _____, and is fertile/sterile. This individual is noted for _____.

42. An XXX individual's primary sex characteristics are _____, secondary _____, and is fertile/sterile. This individual is noted for _____.

43. During the seventh month of gestation, the _____ _____ of the male fetus descends, dragging the _____ and _____ with it into the _____.

44. As the testes and duct system descend they are surrounded by layers of _____, which form the _____ _____ and _____ _____.

45. Failure of the testes to descend is called _____; if not corrected secondary sex characteristics will/will not develop.

46. During early fetal development stem cells from the _____ _____ migrate to the _____ _____, the future ovaries and testes. These cells will become the _____ _____ in males and _____ _____ in females.

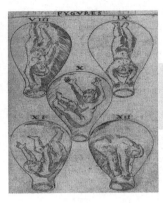

Part 2: Male

47. The outer fibrous capsule of the teste, the _____ _____, is surrounded by the two-layered _____ _____, which is formed from the _____ Process and _____ as the testes descended.

48. The seminiferous tubules are grouped in _____, which direct spermatids into the _____ _____, the _____ _____, and then the _____ _____ to exit the teste.

49. After exiting through the efferent ductules, spermatids enter the _____, which measures _____. Immotile spermatids are conveyed via _____ until they develop _____ and are properly referred to as _____.

50. Spermatozoas are conveyed into the pelvic cavity via the _____ or _____ _____, which continues behind and over the _____ as the _____. These in turn merge with the _____ ducts of the _____ _____.

51. The Vas/Ductus Deferens enters the pelvic cavity along with nerves and blood and lymphatic vessels within the _____ _____; the testes are lifted by the _____ muscle.

52. The merged Ampulla and Ejaculatory Duct then merge with the _____ within the _____. The 3 joined ducts exit as the _____ _____.

53. The Prostatic Urethra becomes the _____ _____ within the lower pelvic cavity, joins with the ducts of the 2 _____ Glands, and then becomes the _____ _____ within the shaft of the penis.

54. The Spongy Urethra is surrounded by the _____ _____; the erectile tissue of the penis is known as the _____ _____.

55. Within the surrounding CT in between the Seminiferous Tubules are the _____ Cells of _____ are the _____ cells of the testes; these produce the hormone _____.

56. The _____, or _____, cells support the developing spermatids.

57. The accessory glands of the male reproductive system include the paired _____ _____, the _____, and the paired _____ Glands. Their collective secretions and spermatozoa are referred to as _____.

58. The seminal vesicles supply _____ % of the semen volume. Semen has an _____ pH and contains _____, _____ Acid, and the hormone _____.

59. Prostaglandins function by _____.

60. The prostate supplies _____ % of the semen volume and is noted for the enzyme _____ _____.

61. Elevated Acid Phosphatase in combination with elevated Alkaline Phosphatase is indicative of _____ _____ with _____.

62. The Bulbourethral Glands supply _____ % of the semen volume; they release their secretions _____ in order to _____ _____.

63. Premature puberty is inhibited by the _____ gland. Secondary male sex characteristics develop in response to the hormone _____.

64. Testosterone is secreted by the testes in response to the hormone _____, which is secreted by the _____ _____. Testosterone is also secreted by the _____ _____.

65. In addition to ICSH, the Anterior Pituitary secretes _____, which stimulates the _____ _____ to begin spermatogenesis. it commences with _____.

66. The stem cells lining the Seminiferous Tubules are _____. These cells undergo mitosis yielding two cell types:
A, which _____ and
B, which _____, and
are properly called _____ _____.

67. Primary Spermatocytes entering Meiosis I possess _____ chromosomes; Secondary Spermatocytes entering Meiosis II possess _____ chromosomes. Meiosis II ends by yielding ____ immotile _____ possessing the _____ count.

68. Spermatids mature within the _____ becoming motile _____.

69. Spermatozoa are comprised of three regions: the _____ head , the _____ midsection, and the _____ tail or _____.

70. The genetic region or head of the spermatozoa is covered by the _____ _____, which secretes _____ to allow for chromosomes to enter the ova. The middle/metabolic region is composed of _____.

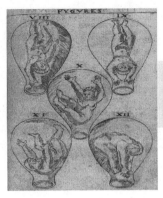

Part 3: Female

71. The ovary differentiates from the _____ _____; the Fallopian Tube and uterus differentiate from the _____ or _____ Duct.

72. During the _____ month of gestation stem cells that migrated from the _____ _____ to the Gonadal Ridges become _____ _____.

73. Primordial follicles formed during the seventh month each contain a single _____ _____, which begins _____.

74. All primary oöcytes are "frozen" in _____ of _____; at this time there are approximately _____ primordial follicles located within the _____ of each ovary. By birth this number is reduced to a total of _____ and by puberty to _____.

75. Starting with puberty the hormones _____ and _____, which is secreted by the _____ _____, stimulates approximately _____ primary oöcytes to complete Meiosis. These Primordial Follicles are now called _____ Follicles.

76. Of the 20 primary follicles only one will develop supportive _____ Cells. The follicle is now called a _____ follicle.

77. As the Secondary Follicle expands it forms a fluid-filled cavity, the _____; the oöcyte is surrounded by the _____ _____ and the follicle is now called a _____ or _____ Follicle.

78. The Primary oöcyte within the Vesicular/Graafian Follicle completes Meiosis I with the formation of a viable _____ _____ and non-viable _____ _____.

79. The Polar Body _____ whereas the Secondary Oöcyte begins Meiosis II but halts in _____. During this time the follicle migrates from the ovary's _____ to the _____ .

80. The secondary oöcyte will progress from Metaphase II only following _____ _____; Meiosis II then ends by yielding a viable _____ containing the _____ count, and another polar body.

81. In response to a surge in _____ levels, the ovum with its surrounding Corona Radiata is ejected from the Vesicular Follicle onto the external surface, rupturing the fibrous _____ _____, which is covered by the _____ _____. This process is called _____. The characteristic pain associated with it is called _____.

82. The germinal layer is noted for its specialized _____ _____, which will convey the ovum to the uterine tube. The Graafian/Vesicular Follicle now differentiates into a _____ _____, which will secrete _____ and _____.

83. The Corpus Luteum will secrete Estrogen and Progesterone over the next _____ days, stimulating the _____ _____ of the endometrium to give rise to the _____ _____. It will also stimulate development of the _____ _____ of the breast.

84. The ovary is anchored to the uterus by the _____ Ligament and to the pelvic wall by the _____ Ligament. The uterus is anchored to the pelvic wall by the _____ Ligament. ; it and other structures are covered by a fold of peritoneum called the _____ Ligament.

85. Ova are swept into the Fallopian Tube by the _____ at its opening; the three segments of the tube are the _____, the middle _____, and the _____, which leads into the _____ of the uterus.

86. Unlike the Fimbriae, the tube is composed of three layers: the inner _____ lined by _____ _____, the middle _____, which produces peristaltic contractions, and the outer _____.

87. Fertilization generally occurs in the _____ producing a _____, which secretes _____, the hormone tested for in pregnancy.

88. A zygote that implants in the ampulla is referred to as an _____ _____.

89. HCG directly stimulates the _____ to stimulate the _____ _____ to secrete _____.

90. LH stimulates and maintains the Estrogen and Progesterone secretions of the _____ _____ for the next _____ until the _____ fully develops and takes over.

91. The placenta fully develops after 2–3 months after which it takes over the CL's secretion of Estrogen as well as secreting _____ which relaxes /softens the _____ _____ and _____ ligaments.

92. After 14 days without HCG/pregnancy, the corpus luteum will _____ becoming a _____ _____, which appears as a whitish scar on the surface of the ovary.

93. Without HCG after 14 days the corpus luteum's secretion of _____ and _____ ceases, resulting in the degeneration of the _____ _____, which is shed as the _____ _____.

94. The three main regions of the uterus are the _____, the _____, and the _____.

95. The wall of the Body is composed of three layers: the outer _____, the middle _____, and the inner _____. The opening to the cervix is called the _____.

96. The Endometrium is composed of two layers: the permanent _____ _____, which gives rise to the _____ _____, which exfoliates as the _____ Flow.

97. The Uterine Cycle begins with _____; the Stratum Functionalis begins developing after Day _____ in response to estrogen. This developmental stage is referred to as the _____ phase and ends with _____ on Day _____.

98. After Ovulation on Day 14, the endometrium begins the _____ phase in response to rising _____ levels; this phase is noted by the development of _____ _____.

99. The Secretory Phase ends on Day _____ due to _____. The absence of menstruation is called _____; pain during menstruation is called _____.

100. The vagina is composed of three layers: the outer _____, the middle _____, and the inner _____.

101. The Mucosa is further lubricated by secretions of the _____ Glands. The Muscularis produces _____ _____, which inhibits _____ _____ _____.

Unit XV: The Reproductive System

Part 1: Genetics and Embryology

1. Duplication, Diploid; Reduction, Haploid
2. Asexual Reproduction; Division
3. Interphase; Cell Cycle
4. Growth 1, Synthesis, Growth 2
5. Synthesis of Organic Compounds; Replication of DNA; Formation of Organelles
6. 46, 23 Homologous. Diploid, (2N)
7. 92, 46 Sister Chromatids
8. Centromere; Mitotic Spindle
9. Centriole, Interphase
10. Prophase, Metaphase, Anaphase, Telophase
11. Chromatin condenses, Nuclear membrane disappears, Centrioles migrate to the poles, Spindle begins to form
12. Sister chromatids line up on the Equator
13. Sister chromatids split; Chromosomes migrate to the poles
14. Cell Plate forms, Nuclear Membrane reforms, Chromosomes unravel into chromatin, Cytokinesis
15. Sexual Reproduction; Stem, 2, Gametes
16. Haploid, (N)
17. 92, 23, Tetrads
18. Homologous Chromosomes; 4, 2, 2
19. Genetic Variation. Crossing Over, Synapsis
20. Prophase I; 2, 46
21. 2, 46; 4, 23, Haploid; Different
22. Autosomes; Sex Chromosomes. XX, XY
23. Y; TDF, Testes Determining Factor
24. Fertilization; Androgynous
25. Gonadal Ridges, Wolfian/Mesenephric, Mullerian/ Paramesenephric
26. Genital Tubercle, Urethral Groove, Urethral Fold, Labioscrotal Fold
27. Testosterone, Male
28. Testes, Male; Degenerates
29. Glans Penis, Fuses--Urethra, Fuses--Shaft of Penis, Fuses--Scrotum
30. Female, Ovaries, Female, Degenerates
31. Clitoris, Remains open--Vestibule, Remain open-- Labia Minora, Remain open--Labia Majora
32. Female; Intersex
33. Maternal Adrenal
34. Barr Body, Inactive X
35. External genitalia; Puberty, Hormonal
36. Onset of Ovulation and Menstruation, Breast Development, Changes in bone structure and adipose distribution, Body hair
37. Onset of Spermatogenesis, Changes in bone structure, Enlargement of external genitalia, Deepening of Voice, Body hair
38. Non-Disjunction, Chromosomal Aberrancy
39. Female, Fail to develop, Sterile. Turner's
40. Male, Fail to develop, Sterile. Kleinfelter's
41. Male, Develop normally, Fertile. Aggressive and violent behavior
42. Female, Develop normally, Fertile. Profoundly mentally handicapped
43. Vaginal Process, Testes, Epididymis, Scrotum
44. Peritoneum, Tunica Vaginalis, Spermatic Cord
45. Cryptorchidism; Will Not Develop
46. Yolk Sac, Gonadal Ridges. Seminiferous Tubules, Primary Oöcytes

Part 2: Male

47. Tunica Albuginea, Tunica Vaginalis, Vaginal, Peritoneum
48. Lobules, Tubulus Rectus, Rete Testes, Efferent Ductule
49. Epididymis, 22 ft. Peristalsis, Flagella, Spermatozoa
50. Vas/Ductus Deferens, Bladder, Ampulla; Ejaculatory Ducts, Seminal Vesicles
51. Spermatic Cord; Cremasteric
52. Urethra, Prostate; Prostatic Urethra
53. Membranous Urethra, Bulbourethral, Spongy Urethra
54. Corpus Spongiosum; Corpus Cavernosa
55. Interstitial, Leydig; Endocrine, Testosterone
56. Sertoli, Sustentacular
57. Seminal Vesicles, Prostate, Bulbourethral. Semen
58. 60%; Alkaline, Fructose, Ascorbic, Prostaglandin
59. Reversed Uterine Contractions
60. 30%, Acid Phosphatase.
61. Prostate Cancer, Metastasis to Bone

62. 10%; prior to ejaculation, Clear the urethra of acidic urine
63. Pineal. Testosterone
64. ICSH, Anterior Pituitary. Adrenal Cortex
65. FSH, Seminiferous Tubules, Puberty
66. Spermatogonia; Remain at the baseline to continue dividing; Migrate toward lumen, Primary Spermatocytes
67. 92; 46. 4, Spermatids, Haploid
68. Epididymis, Spermatozoa
69. Genetic, Metabolic, Locomotor, Flagella
70. Acrosomal Cap, Enzymes. Mitochondria

Part 3: Female

71. Gonadal Ridge; Paramesenephric, Mullerian
72. 7th, Yolk Sac, Primordial Follicles
73. Primary Oöcyte, Meiosis
74. Prophase I, Meiosis I; 7 million, medulla. 2 Million, 400,000
75. FSH, LH, Anterior Pituitary, 20. Primary
76. Granulosa; Secondary
77. Antrum, Corona Radiata, Vesicular/Graafian
78. Secondary oöcyte, Polar Body
79. Degenerates, Metaphase II. Medulla, Cortex
80. Sperm Penetration; Ovum, Haploid
81. LH, Tunica Albuginea, Germinal Layer. Ovulation; Mittelshmertz

82. Ciliated Epithelium. Corpus Luteum, Estrogen, Progesterone
83. 14, Statum Basalis, Startum Functionalis. Lactiferous Glands
84. Ovarian, Suspensory. Round, Broad
85. Fimbria; Infundibulum, Ampulla, Isthmus, Fundus
86. Mucosa, Ciliated Epithelium, Muscularis, Serosa
87. Ampulla, Zygote. HCG
88. Ectopic Pregnancy
89. Hypothalamus, Anterior Pituitary, LH
90. Corpus Luteum, 2–3 months, Placenta
91. Relaxin, Pubic Symphysis, Pelvic
92. Degenerate, Corpus Albicans
93. Estrogen, Progesterone, Stratum Functionalis, Menstrual Flow
94. Fundus, Body, Cervix
95. Perimetrium, Myometrium, Endometrium. Os
96. Stratum Basalis, Stratum Functionalis, Menstrual
97. Menstruation; 6. Proliferative, Ovulation, 14.
98. Secretory, Progesterone; uterine glands and spiral arteries
99. 28, reduced progesterone. Amenorrhea, dysmenorrhea
100. Adventitia, Muscularis, Mucosa
101. Bartholin's. Lactic Acid, Bacterial, and Fungal Growth

Time allowed: 30 minutes

1. A human body cell contains:
   a) 46 chromosomes
   b) 23 pairs of chromosomes
   c) 23 chromosomes
   d) a and b

2. A human gamete contains:
   a) 46 chromosomes
   b) 23 pairs of chromosomes
   c) 23 chromosomes
   d) a and b

3. Meiosis I ends with:
   a) 2 genetically identical diploid daughter cells
   b) 2 genetically different diploid daughter cells
   c) 4 genetically identical haploid daughter cells
   d) 4 genetically different haploid daughter cells

4. Meiosis II ends with:
   a) 2 genetically identical diploid daughter cells
   b) 2 genetically different dipolid daughter cells
   c) 4 genetically identical haploid daughter cells
   d) 4 genetically different haploid daughter cells

5. Crossing over occurs during:
   a) prophase
   b) prophase I
   c) prophase II
   d) metaphase I
   e) metaphase II

6. Sex is determined at:
   a) puberty
   b) birth
   c) month seven of gestation
   d) week six of gestation
   e) fertilization

7. Primary sex characteristics develop at:
   a) fertilization
   b) 6-7th week of gestation
   c) 7th month of gestation
   d) birth
   e) puberty

8. Secondary sex characteristic begin developing:
   a) puberty
   b) birth
   c) month seven of gestation
   d) week six of gestation
   e) fertilization

9. Which will differentiate into the Fallopian Tubes and Uterus:
   a) genital tubercle
   b) Urethral folds
   c) Mullerian Ducts
   d) Gonadal ridges
   e) Wolfian Ducts

10. Which of the following will differentiate into the testes under the influence of TDF:
    a) genital tubercle
    b) urethral folds
    c) yolk sac
    d) gonadal ridges
    e) urethral folds

11. Which fuses in males to form the Corpus Cavernosum:
    a) Genital Tubercle
    b) Urethral Groove
    c) Yolk Sac
    d) Gonadal Ridges
    e) Urethral Folds

12. Which remains open in females as the vestibule:
    a) Genital Tubercle
    b) Urethral Groove
    c) Yolk Sac
    d) Gonadal Ridges
    e) Urethral Folds

13. Which will differentiate into the Labia Minora:
    a) Genital Tubercle
    b) Urethral Folds
    c) Mullerian Ducts
    d) Gonadal Ridges
    e) Wolfian Ducts

14. Which will differentiate into the Clitoris:
    a) Genital Tubercle
    b) Urethral Folds
    c) Mullerian Ducts
    d) Gonadal Ridges
    e) Wolfian Ducts

15. The Cremasteric muscle develops from the:
    a) Labioscrotal Folds
    b) Wolfian Ducts
    c) Urethral Folds
    d) Genital Tubercle

16. Which of the following can result in a genotypic male with mixed primary sex characteristics:
    a) dysfunctional "Y" chromosome
    b) maternal adrenal/testosterone syndrome
    c) "XXY" genotype
    d) Trisomy 21
    e) all of these

17. "Klinefelter's", a phenotypic male that fails to develop secondary sex characteristics has which genotype:
    a) XX
    b) XXX
    c) XXY
    d) XO
    e) YO

18. Which of the following can result in a genotypic female with mixed primary sex characteristics:
    a) dysfunctional "Y" chromosome
    b) maternal adrenal/testosterone syndrome
    c) "XXY" genotype
    d) Trisomy 21
    e) all of these

19. Stem cells of the seminiferous tubules and primordial follicles originate from the:
    a) genital tubercle
    b) urethral folds
    c) yolk sac
    d) gonadal ridges
    e) urethral folds

20. "Turner's", a phenotypic female that fails to develop secondary sex characteristics has which genotype:
    a) XX
    b) XXX
    c) XXY
    d) XO
    e) YO

21. Secretions of which gland will signal the onset of puberty:
    a) Anterior Pituitary
    b) Posterior Pituitary
    c) Hypothalamus
    d) Pineal
    e) Adrenal Medulla

22. The testes descend through the inguinal canal during:
    a) puberty   b) birth
    c) month seven of gestation   d) week six of gestation   e) fertilization

23. Failure of the testes to descend is called:
    a) Intersex   b) Cryptorchidism
    c) Testosterone Insufficiency   d) Pseudohermaphrodism

24. Spermatogenesis occurs in the:
    a) seminal vesicles   b) seminiferous tubules
    c) interstitial cells   d) serotoli cells   e) bulbourethral

25. Which of the following is the endocrine portion of the male reproductive system:
    a) seminal vesicles   b) seminiferous tubules
    c) interstitial cells   d) serotoli cells   e) bulbourethral

26. Which is the longest portion of the male reproductive duct system::
    a) epididymis   b) ductus deferens
    c) ampulla   d) membranous urethra

27. Which carries sperm from the scrotum into the pelvic cavity:
    a) epididymus   b) ductus deferens
    c) ampulla   d) membranous urethra

28. Immature sperm travel through the duct system via:
    a) flagella   b) cilia
    c) peristalsis   d) fluid medium

29. Acid Phosphatase is produced by which accessory gland:
    a) Prostate   b) Seminal Vesicles
    c) Bulbourethral   d) Cowper's

30. Prostaglandins are produced by which accessory gland:
    a) Prostate   b) Seminal Vesicles
    c) Bulbourethral   d) Cowper's

31. The portion of the uterine tube closest to the fundus is the:
    a) fimbria   b) infundibulum
    c) ampulla   d) isthmus

32. Which is the correct order of structures:
    a) ampulla, fimbria, isthmus, infundibulum, fundus
    b) fimbria, ampulla, infundibulum, isthmus, fundus
    c) fimbria, infundibulum, ampulla, isthmus, fundus
    d) fundus, infundibulum, isthmus, ampulla, fimbria

33. Secretion of which hormone will lead to the development of the breasts during puberty:
    a) GH   b) estrogen
    c) oxytocin   d) prolactin   e) FSH

34. Which hormone will signal the start of the monthly ovarian cycle:
    a) GH   b) estrogen
    c) oxytocin   d) prolactin   e) FSH

35. Oogenesis' begins:
    a) puberty   b) birth
    c) month seven of gestation   d) week six of gestation   e) fertilization

36. Ovulation is in response to secretions by:
    a) anterior pituitary   b) posterior pituitary
    c) Graafian follicle   d) corpus luteum   e) corpus albicans

37. Ovulation is directly stimulated by which hormone:
    a) FSH   b) LH
    c) Estrogen   d) Progesterone   e) GH

38. Ovulation produces:
    a) primordial follicle   b) primary follicle
    c) primary oocyte   d) secondary oocyte   e) ovum

39. Rising levels of which hormone signals the hypothalamus to signal the release of LH:
    a) FSH   b) estrogen
    c) prolactin   d) oxytocin   e) TSH

40. LH will lead to the development of the :
    a) primary follicle   b) secondary follicle
    c) vesicular follicle   d) corpus luteum   e) corpus albicans

41. Estrogen and progesterone are secreted by:
    a) anterior pituitary   b) posterior pituitary
    c) Graafian follicle   d) corpus luteum   e) corpus albicans

42. Rising levels of estrogen and progesterone bring about which layer during the uterine cycle:
    a) stratum functionalis   b) stratum basalis
    c) myometrium   d) perimetrium

43. In which segment does fertilization usually occur;
    a) fimbria   b) infundibulum
    c) ampulla   d) isthmus   e) uterus

44. Pregnancy is determined by checking levels of:
    a) FSH   b) LH
    c) Prolactin   d) Progesterone   e) HCG

45. If fertilization does not occur the corpus luteum will:
   a) continue to grow until fertilization does occur
   b) become enlarged over the next three months
   c) degenerate within the next 14 days
   d) release another ova during the next cycle

46. Which represents the greatest number of ova which could be fertilized in a woman's lifetime:
   a) 10   b) 60   c) 400   d) 800

47. Ectopic pregnancies are those that implant within the:
   a) endometrium   b) fundus
   c) fallopian tube   d) ovary   e) vagina

48. The outer most layer of the uterine wall is known as the:
   a) stratum functionalis   b) stratum basalis
   c) myometrium   d) perimetrium   e) endometrium

49. Which of the following layers exfoliates as the menstrual flow:
   a) stratum functionalis   b) stratum basalis
   c) myometrium   d) perimetrium

50. Which appears as a whitish scar on the surface of a normal ovary:
   a) corpus luteum   b) corpus albicans
   c) endometriosis   d) ectopic pregnancy

1. d, 2. c, 3. b, 4. d, 5. b, 6. e, 7. d, 8. a, 9. c, 10. d, 11. e, 12. b, 13. b, 14. a, 15. a, 16. a, 17. c, 18. b, 19. c, 20. d, 21. d, 22. c, 23. b, 24. b, 25. c, 26. a, 27. b, 28. c, 29. a, 30. b, 31. d, 32. d, 33. d, 34. d, 35. c, 36. a, 37. b, 38. b, 39. b, 40. d, 41. d, 42. a, 43. c, 44. e, 45. c, 46. c, 47. c, 48. d, 49. d, 50. a